Bilharziasis

International Academy of Pathology · Special Monograph

Edited by

F. K. Mostofi

With 160 Figures

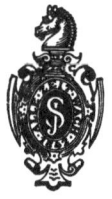

Springer-Verlag Berlin Heidelberg New York 1967

F. K. MOSTOFI, *M. D., Chief, Division of Special and General Pathology, Armed Forces Institute of Pathology and Veterans Administration Central Laboratory for Anatomic Pathology and Research, Washington, D. C., Clinical Professor of Pathology, Georgetown Medical School, Washington, D. C., Assistant Professor of Pathology, Johns Hopkins University, Baltimore, Maryland, and Secretary-Treasurer, International Academy of Pathology, Washington, D. C., U. S. A.*

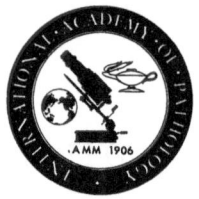

ISBN 978-3-642-49492-5   ISBN 978-3-642-49777-3 (eBook)
DOI 10.1007/978-3-642-49777-3

Softcover reprint of the hardcover 1st edition   1967

Foreword

During the past decade there has been an increasing awareness of the need for a different approach to the problem of bilharziasis. We do know that 180—200 million people are infected and that the infection is increasing but we have not as yet been able to answer the question: Are they suffering from a disease.

Study of vital statistics or hospital records, mass biochemical or immunological tests and community surveys have not yet provided the full answer. Gradually and perhaps begrudgingly, we have come to realize that we must study the man — initially by means of well controlled clinical observations to obtain evidence for the altered physiology, if any, due to bilharzial infection; secondly and equally important through pathological studies on individual patients to determine the structural changes, if any, as a result of infection with this parasite; and by post mortem studies.

Experimental studies of bilharzial infection in animals, valuable as they may be for the elucidation of the pathogenesis of the lesions in the laboratory animal and in man cannot serve as a substitute for the precise information on the nature of the possible lesions induced by bilharziasis in man. Basically, the significance of any clinical observation can be evaluated only through reliable pathological confirmation.

Dr. MOSTOFI, who has been a pioneer in efforts to focus attention on the need for pathological studies in bilharziasis, has succeeded admirably to bring together in this monograph much of the known information on the pathology of this disease. Such information is valuable for those who are working in the field but essential as a basis for future clinical, pathological and experimental research.

To Dr. MOSTOFI and the outstanding team of contributors, my best wishes for continued success.

Geneva, Switzerland   N. ANSARI M. D.

Preface

This monograph represents, in part, the proceedings of a symposium on bilharziasis organized by the editor at the invitation of the International Academy of Pathology for the Fifth International Congress held at the Royal College of Surgeons, London, England, in June 1964. Although the publication of the proceedings had not been seriously contemplated at the time, the large number of requests received for the material presented at the symposium and the expression of disappointment by many who had been unable to attend led to publication.

A number of scientists who had not been able to participate in the symposium have contributed, and the material presented in 1964 has been brought up to date, resulting in a comprehensive and broad coverage of bilharziasis unequalled in any publication to date.

Dr. N. Ansari, Chief, Parasitic Diseases, World Health Organiziation, Geneva; Dr. Chapman Binford, Medical Director, Leonard Wood Memorial Foundation, Washington, D. C., and Dr. Gustave Dammin, Friedman Professor of Pathology, Harvard Medical School, Boston, provided invaluable guidance and advice. Dr. Damaris Russell (Mrs. Brian N. Purser) assisted materially in the extensive editorial revision of many of the manuscripts and in proof reading all. Dr. David Byar accomplished the indexing of the monograph. The wholehearted support of General Joe M. Blumberg, the Director of the Armed Forces Institute of Pathology, made it possible to fully utilize the secretarial, library and other facilities of the AFIP.

All the authors relinquished their royalties. This and the generous financial assistance from F. Hoffmann-La Roche & Co. (Switzerland), Burroughs Wellcome & Co., Inc. (USA), and the U. S. Army Medical Research and Development Command made it possible not only to have the color plates but to affect a substantial reduction in the price of the book.

It is the hope of the Editor and the authors that this monograph will be valuable in the fight against bilharziasis.

Washington, D. C.   F. K. Mostofi, M. D.

Table of Contents

Contributing Authors

ANDRADE, Z. A., M.D., Head, Department of Pathology, Hospital Prof. Edgard Santos, University of Bahia School of Medicine, Bahia, Brazil.

ANSARI, N., M.D., Chief, Parasitic Diseases, World Health Organization, Geneva, Switzerland.

ATTA, A. H. A., M.D., M.R.C.P., Professor of Endemic Medicine, Faculty of Medicine, Cairo University, Cairo, Egypt.

BARBOSA, J., Fo., M.D., Head, Heart Laboratory, Department of Cardiology, Guanabara State University Hospital, Rio de Janeiro, Brazil.

BHAGWANDEEN, S. B., M.D., Senior Lecturer, Department of Pathology, University of Natal, Durban, South Africa.

BOGLIOLO, L., M.D., Chairman, Department of Pathology, Faculty of Medicine, University of Minas Gerais, Belo Horizonte, Brazil.

BRADLEY, D. J., M.A., M.B., B.Chir., M.I.Biol., Senior Lecturer, Department of Preventive Medicine, Makerere College Medical School, Kampala, Uganda.

CAMAIN, R., M.D., Chief, Laboratory of Histopathology, Institut Pasteur, and Professor of Histology and Embryology, Faculty of Medicine and Pharmacology, Dakar, Senegal.

CHEEVER, A. W., M.D., Pathologist, Laboratory of Parasitic Diseases, National Institutes of Health, Bethesda, Maryland. Formerly Eleanor Roosevelt Cancer Research Fellow, Department of Pathology, Hospital Prof. Edgard Santos, University of Bahia School of Medicine, Bahia, Brazil.

COUTINHO, S. G., M.D., Assistant, Department of Tropical Medicine, University of Brazil, Rio de Janeiro, Brazil.

DE PAOLA, D., M.D., Professor and Head, Department of Pathology, Service of Tropical Medicine and Infectious Diseases, University of Brazil, Rio de Janeiro, Brazil.

EDINGTON, G. M., M.B.E., M.D., F.C.Path., M.R.C.P., D.C.P., D.T.M. & H., Professor and Head, Department of Pathology, University of Ibadan, Nigeria.

ELSDON-DEW, R., M.D., F.R.S., S.Af. Director, Amoebiasis Research Unit, Institute for Parasitology, Durban, South Africa.

ELWI, A. M., M.D., Chairman and Professor, Department of Pathology, Cairo University Faculty of Medicine, Cairo, Egypt.

FODA, M., M.D., Clinical Demonstrator, Department of Chest Diseases, Alexandria University, Alexandria, Egypt.

FORSYTH, D. M., F.R.C.P.E., D.T.M. & H., Biharzia Research Unit, The Ross Institute of Tropical Hygiene, London, England. Formerly B.R.U., Ross Institute of Tropical Hygiene, Zanzibar, Tanzania.

EL-GAREM, A. A., M.D., D.M., D.T.M. & H., Lecturer of Endemic Medicine, Faculty of Medicine, Cairo University, Cairo, Egypt.

GAZAYERLI, M., M.D., Ph.D., F.R.C.P. (Edin.), Professor and Head, Department of Pathology, Alexandria University, Alexandria, Egypt.

GEAR, J. H. S., B.Sc., M.B., B.Ch., D.P.H., D.T.M. & H. Dipl.Bact., Director, South African Institute for Medical Research, Johannesburg, South Africa.

GELFAND, M., C.B.E., M.D., F.R.C.P., Professor of Medicine, University College of Rhodesia and Nyasaland, Salisbury, Rhodesia.

EL-HENEIDY, A. R., M.D., Assistant Professor of Chest Diseases, Alexandria University, Alexandria, Egypt.

ISHAK, K. G., M.B., Ch.B., Ph.D., Chief, Hepatic Pathology Branch, Armed Forces Institute of Pathology, Washington, D. C., USA.

JORDAN, P., M.D., D.T.M. & H., (Lond. + Eng.), Director, Research and Control Department, Castries, St. Lucia, West Indies. Formerly Director, East African Institute for Medical Research, Mwanza, Tanzania.

KHALIL, M., M.B., Ch.B., M.D., Demonstrator, Chest Diseases, Alexandria University, Alexandria, Egypt.

KORAITUM, M., M.Ch., Demonstrator, Department of Urology, Faculty of Medicine, Alexandria University, Alexandria, Egypt.

LE GOLVAN, P. C., M.D., Assistant Director, Pathology and Allied Sciences Service, Veterans Administration Central Office, Washington, D. C., USA.

MAKAR, N., M.B., Ch.B., F.R.C.S., Emeritus Professor of Urology, Cairo University, and Senior Urologist, The Coptic Hospital, Cairo, Egypt.

MENEZES, H., M.D., Associate Professor of Pathology, University of Sao Paulo, Faculty of Medicine, Ribeirao Preto, Brazil.

MIDDLEMISS, J. H., M.D., M.R.C.P., D.M.R.D., F.F.R., Director of Radiology, United Bristol Hospitals, and Professor of Radiology, University of Bristol, Bristol, England.

MIYAKE, M., M.D., Professor and Head, Department of Pathology, Faculty of Medicine, The University of Tokyo, Hongo, Tokyo, Japan.

MOORE, D. V., Ph.D., Department of Microbiology, University of Texas, Southwestern Medical School, Dallas, Texas, USA.

MOSTOFI, F. K., M.D., Chief, Division of Special and General Pathology, Armed Forces Institute of Pathology and Veterans Administration Central Laboratory for Anatomic Pathology and Research, Washington, D. C., Clinical Professor of Pathology, Georgetown Medical School, Washington, D. C., and Assistant Professor of Pathology, Johns Hopkins University, Baltimore, Maryland, USA.

MOUSA, A. H., M.D., M.R.C.P., D.T.M. & H., Professor and Head, Endemic Medical Unit, Kasr el Ainy Medical Faculty, Cairo University, Cairo, Egypt.

OLIVIER, L., Ph.D., Regional Advisor in Parasitic Diseases, Pan American Health Organization, Washington, D. C. Formerly Consultant, Parasitic Diseases, World Health Organization, Geneva, Switzerland.

PAYET, M., M.D., Dean, Faculty of Medicine and Pharmacology, Director, Institute of Applied Tropical Medicine, and Professor of Clinical Medicine, University of Dakar, Dakar, Senegal.

EL-RAZIKY, S. H., M.D., D.M., D.T.M. & H., Lecturer of Endemic Medicine, Faculty of Medicine, Cairo University, Cairo, Egypt.

RODRIGUES DA SILVA, J., M.D., Professor and Head, Clinic of Parasitic and Infectious Diseases, University of Brazil, and Director, Institute of Rural Endemic Diseases, Ministry of Health, Rio de Janeiro, Brazil.

EL-ROOBY, A. S., M.D., D.M., D.T.M. & H., Assistant Professor of Endemic Medicine, Faculty of Medicine, Cairo University, Cairo, Egypt.

SAAD, E. A., M.D., Assistant, Departments of Tropical Medicine and Cardiology, University of Brazil and Guanabara State University Hospital, Rio de Janeiro, Brazil.

SADUN, E. H., Sc.D., B.S., Bi.M., M.A., Chief, Department of Medical Zoology, Walter Reed Army Institute of Research, Washington, D. C., USA.

EL-SEBAI, I., M. B., Ch.B., M.Ch., Surgeon, Kasr el Ainy and Manial University Hospitals, and Professor of Surgery, Cancer Institute University of Cairo, Cairo, Egypt.

TARABEIH, A. A., M.B., Ch. B., M. D., Department of Chest Diseases, Alexandria University, Alexandria, Egypt.

VON LICHTENBERG, F., M.D., Assistant Professor, Department of Pathology, Harvard Medical School, Peter Bent Brigham Hospital, Boston, Massachusetts, USA.

WAHAB, M. F. ABDEL, M.D., D.M., D.T.M. & H., Lecturer of Endemic Medicine, Faculty of Medicine, Cairo University, Egypt.

WINSLOW, D. J., M.D., Chief, Infectious Disease Branch, Armed Forces Institute of Pathology, Washington, D. C., USA.

WRIGHT, C. A., Ph.D., D.I.C., Head, Experimental Taxonomy Unit, Department of Zoology, British Museum (Natural History), London, England.

ZAKY, H. A., T.D.D., M.R.C.P., Professor and Head, Department of Chest Diseases, Alexandria University, Alexandria, Egypt.

The Aim of the Symposium

F. K. MOSTOFI*

Despite the extensive literature on bilharziasis — the life cycle, the host, the diagnosis, the treatment, the immunological response, the pathology, and the prevalence of infection in various communities — many questions remain un-answered. Among these the most significant are: Is bilharziasis really a disabling disease and does it have any socio-economic effects?

A disease can be a public health problem in its acute or in its chronic phase and in either event, the evaluation of its significance is dfficult. As the reports of WHO Scientific Advisory Groups have emphasized [1, 2], the problem is magnified in bilharziasis because it is not characterized by acute, easily recognizable episodes of disability as seen in malaria or meninigitis, in which the exposure date and the interval between exposure and the appearance of the symptoms can be readily determined, since the pathophysiology and the pathology of these diseases are well recognized. In bilharziasis such information is available only under special conditions. The Australian experience in Egypt during World War I, and the American and the British experiences in the Far East and West Africa, respectively, during the second war demonstrated that there is a significantly high casualty rate from the acute phase of bilharziasis when a large body of men previously unexposed to the parasite is suddenly brought into an endemic area. Such information, however, is not readily available on those living in endemic areas.

The evaluation of public health importance of certain chronic diseases — heart diseases, tuberculosis, and cancer — has been accomplished in more advanced countries. In each of these, the condition is clinically easily recognizable, its pathophysiology and pathology well defined. Moreover, medical, hospital, and laboratory facilities are readily available for the comprehensive study of the disease.

Such an assessment of bilharziasis in its late stages is greatly complicated because the disease usually occurs in communities where hygiene is inadequate, where poverty prevails, where malnutrition and infection with other parasites are all too common, and where the medical, hospital, and laboratory facilites are often limited.

Yet the long standing need for information on the socio-economic impact of the disease has become imperative when it appears that 180 to 200 million people may be infected, that there is a substantial increase in cases in developing coun-tries, and that the infection is spreading with new irrigation projects.

The public health importance of any disease must be measured in terms of the community and the individual, but basically it is the effect of the condition

* Armed Forces Institute of Pathology, Washington, D. C. U.S.A.

on the individual that must be measured. Recognizing that this can be done only through field investigation, the WHO Scientific Advisory Group recommended [1] and the Ross Institute of Tropical Hygiene initiated certain cross sectional studies in Tanganyika (now Tanzania), using parasitological, clinical, radiological, and laboratory technics. Forsyth and his associates [3] have described important lesions in children. These were serious enough to suggest a high mortality but the clinical course, the pathogenesis, the pathology, and the exact outcome could not be determined by such cross sectional studies. Obviously, there is a great need for a comprehensive longitudinal study. Before such studies can be effectively organized, however, we must know what has transpired.

Bilharziasis, in all its manifestations, is of such magnitude as to be beyond the scope of any single group or a single monograph. But while certain aspects of bilharziasis have been emphasized in the past, the clinical and pathological manifestations, observed only through longitudinal studies, have been relatively ignored. These are the areas which this symposium wishes to emphasize, for they offer an important line of inquiry into the areas of public health.

The purpose of the symposium then is to focus attention on the functional and structural changes found in patients infected with the schistosome, to determine the role of the parasite in producing these changes, and to provide a scientific basis for evaluating the socio-economic importance of bilharziasis.

References

[1] *World Health Organization*. Scientific Group on Research in Bilharziasis. (Assessment of medical and public health importance) Geneva, 18—22 July 1960.
[2] *World Health Organization*. Scientific Group on Research in Bilharziasis (Mesaurement of public health importance) Geneva, 9—14 August 1965.
[3] Forsyth, this monograph.

The Schistosome Life-Cycle

C. A. WRIGHT*

The parasitic worms which cause bilharziasis in man and domestic animals belong to the genus *Schistosoma*, a somewhat unusual group of digenetic trematodes or flukes. All of the Digenea have complex life-cycles involving one or more intermediate hosts in addition to the definitive host in which they attain sexual maturity; a universal character of these parasites is that at least one of the intermediate hosts must be a mollusc, usually either a snail or a bivalve, and in this molluscan host there is always a phase of asexual larval multiplication.

The schistosomes differ from most other flukes in two important respects. The first is that, apart from a small and rather obscure group parasitic in the gill-cavities of some Pacific marine fishes, they are the only trematodes in which the sexes are separate in the adult worms. The males are shorter and more fleshy than the narrowly elongate females and, when mature, the females are carried by the males in a ventral groove of the body known as the gynaecophoric canal. The other unusual character of the schistosomes is their adoption of the blood system of the definitive host as their adult habitat. They are not unique in this respect because there are blood-flukes of fish, turtles and birds but it is an unusual environment for the Digenea as a whole and it presents special problems both in initial access and in the dispersal of eggs. It is particularly this character that makes the schistosomes of greater pathological importance than the other trematode parasites of man.

There are three species of schistosome commonly parasitic in man. *Schistosoma japonicum* occurs in parts of China, Japan, Taiwan and the Phillipine islands with sparse foci reported from Thailand and the Celebes. This species shows little host-specificity in its adult stages and it infects a range of domestic animals including water buffalo and dogs as well as man. The adult worms live in the blood vessels draining the intestine and the snail intermediate hosts of *S. japonicum* are species of the amphibious prosobranch genus *Oncomelania*. *Schistosoma mansoni* is also parasitic in the veins of the intestinal wall but it is much more restricted in its host-distribution than *S. japonicum* and is almost confined to man. In parts of its range this host-specificity appears to be a little less strict and infections in wild rodents and some other animals occasionally occur. *S. mansoni* is widespread in Africa, Arabia, Eastern and Northern South America and some of the Caribbean islands. The snail intermediate hosts of *S. mansoni* are aquatic planorbids belonging to the genera *Biomphalaria* (in Africa) and *Australorbis* and *Tropicorbis* (in the New World). This is not the place to elaborate on problems of nomenclature but it must be pointed out that these three genera should be united because there is no adequate distinction between them. The matter is at present before the International Commission on Nomenclature and until a decision has been given the

---

* British Museum (Natural History), London, England.

commonly-used names are still applied. The causative organism of urinary schistosomiasis is called *Schistosoma haematobium* but there is increasing evidence that this is a composite species of two morphologically similar forms, *S. haematobium* sensu stricto and *S. capense*. Both species are parasitic in the veins of the bladder-wall, both are markedly host-specific to man and both use snails of the planorbid genus *Bulinus* for intermediate hosts. However *S. haematobium* develops only in snails of the *Bulinus truncatus* and *Bulinus forskali* species groups while *S. capense* undergoes larval development in members of the *Bulinus africanus* complex. *S. haematobium* occurs in North Africa and the Middle East, parts of West Africa and on Mauritius and Madagascar while *S. capense* occurs generally in Africa south of the Sahara. In West Africa there is a mosaic distribution of both species.

Several other species have been reported in human infections but only two are of much interest here. One is *Schistosoma intercalatum* a parasite of the intestinal blood vessels of man but resembling the urinary parasites in the terminal position of the egg-spine and in its development in bulinid snails. *S. intercalatum* is so far known only from a few foci in the Congo basin and West Africa. The other species of some medical interest is *S. mattheei* normally parasitic in the mesenteric veins of cattle and sheep in South Africa. This species also belongs to the group of schistosomes with terminal-spined eggs and it develops in snails of the *Bulinus africanus* complex. Mixed urinary infections of *S. mattheei* and *S. capense* have been found in man in South Africa and there is evidence of hybridisation between the two [3].

The schistosome life-cycle is relatively simple and follows the same general pattern as that of most flukes. Eggs produced by female worms have to pass through the wall of the fine blood vessels in which they are laid and thence through the wall of the bladder or intestine (according to the species of schistosome concerned) until they fall into the lumen of the organ and are eventually voided with either the faeces or urine. Not all of the eggs laid are successful in achieving this passage, some are carried back in the venous blood and become lodged in the liver or other organs while others may be held in the wall of the bladder or intestine and remain there until they die. During their passage through the tissues the embryos within the eggs develop and by the time that they are voided the enclosed larvae are mature and ready to hatch. Hatching will only occur if the eggs fall into fresh water and the process is stimulated by warmth and light. The eggs lack opercula and the cilated larvae or miracidia emerge through rents in the thin capsules brought about by a combination of osmotic effects and active movements of the larvae. Once free the miracidia swim actively; they respond positively to the stimulus of light and they are negatively geotropic, thus they reach the surface layers of the water in which most of their potential snail hosts live. A single case of *Schistosoma haematobium* infection from an area in Iraq where the intermediate hosts tend to live on the bottom of the irrigation canals yielded miracidia which did not rise to the surface. These miracidia were used to infect snails which in due course produced normal cercariae and the infection was passaged into hamsters. Miracidia derived from both the first and second passages in experimental animals still retained the behaviour of the original specimens. This suggests that in certain areas the usual cycle has become modified to suit local conditions [9].

Once within the intermediate host environment the miracidia undergo a phase of random movement, usually in long sweeping lines, but if they pass close to a potential host the behaviour pattern changes and they follow an irregular path, turning frequently, until contact with the snail is achieved [10]. The free-swimming life of a miracidium is short and if a suitable host is not encountered within a few hours of hatching the larva dies. Recently CHERNIN and DUNAVAN [1] have suggested that under laboratory conditions there is a relationship between the chances of a miracidium locating its snail host and the perimeter of the vessel in which the "search" takes place. Under field conditions this re-lationship may apply in a few closely defined habitats but it is unlikely to be of much singificance in the majority of circumstances. The fecundity of schistosomes is great and there is undoubtedly a considerable wastage of miracidia. It seems likely that in any given transmission site there will be a time/concen-tration factor affecting miracidial density. Ova of the species infecting the bladder hatch rapidly on reaching water and there will be high concentrations of miracidia for relatively short periods of time. Ova of the intestinal parasites will hatch as the faeces in which they are passed disintegrate and there will therefore be a more prolonged output of these miracidia at a lower density. Once contact with the snail has been established the miracidium attaches itself to the surface of the body by a sticky secretion from gland cells at its anterior end and entry through the skin of the snail is achieved with the aid of enzymes secreted from the so-called "miracidial gut" [7]. If the larva has succeeded in entering the correct species of snail development proceeds but if the snail is not a suitable host the mira-cidium is destroyed by phagocytic attack. This host-parasite relationship be-tween larval schistosomes and their snail hosts is extremely delicate and, in many cases, is strain-specific so that development of the next larval stages will not occur even in an unusual strain of the normal host-species.

Within the snail the miracidium remains not far from the point of penetration and develops into a mother sporocyst, a small, sac-like structure within which balls of cells are budded off from the epithelial lining. These germ-balls develop into young daughter sporocysts which leave the mother and migrate to other parts of the snail's body, usually the digestive gland, where they grow and in turn produce germ-balls which develop into the final larval stage or cercaria. Thus, from a single miracidium the processes of asexual multiplication within both mother and daughter sporocysts will result in the production of many cercariae, one estimate puts the number as high as 100,000 [6].

Determination of sex is genetically controlled in the schistosomes and, although no morphological differences have been detected between male and female larvae, all cercariae arising from a single miracidium will mature into adults of one sex only. The cercaria is in effect a juvenile schistosome in which the rudiments of the adult organs already exist in addition to the characteristic larval structures of a large, forked tail for swimming and a battery of gland cells whose secretions assist in penetrating the skin of the definitive host. Entry through the skin is rapid, successful penetrations following ten seconds exposure have been recorded for *Schistosoma japonicum* in experimental animals but in these cases it is probable that entry was effected via hair follicles. The exact route by which the schistoso-mulae (as the young flukes are now called) reach their final destination in the defi-nitive host is not known but, in mice, after traversing the dermis they have been observed to enter lymphatic vessels and thus eventually gain access to the cir-culatory system [5]. In due course they reach the liver where they mature and

mate before migrating through the portal system into the mesenteric or vesicle
veins to commence egg-laying.

This, then, is the broad outline of the life-cycle of schistosomes parasitizing
man. There are two aspects of the cycle which, because of their probable influence
on pathology of the infection in the final host, deserve a little more attention here.
I have already mentioned the extremely close host-parasite relationship between
larval schistosomes and their snail hosts. One effect of this very specific association
is that a population of schistosomes is usually better adapted to its local race of
snail than it is to other races of the same species. This leads to segregation of
populations of the parasite with reduced genetic interchange between one group
and another and, as a result of this close parallel evolution of worm and snail host,
local races of parasite may become differentiated. Differences between such races
need not necessarily be morphological and there may be no way of distinguishing
between them by visual comparison but small alterations in the physiology of the
parasites may have considerable influence on their relationship with their definitive
hosts. This has been clearly shown by Hsu and Hsu [2] for the four main geographical races of *Schistosoma japonicum*. The Taiwan race of this species does not
develop to maturity in man or certain monkeys and in this respect it differs from
the Chinese, Japanese and Phillipine forms. In experimental infections in mice
the parasite eggs are deposited in various organs and the percentage distribution
of the eggs differs between the strains. Thus the Chinese form shows the highest
percentage of eggs deposited in the lungs and large intestine, the Japanese strain
has the highest deposition in the small intestine, the Taiwan strain shows the
highest rates in liver, spleen and stomach and the Phillipine strain has moderately
high percentages in the large and small intestine. The mean prepatent periods
in mice for the Japanese and Phillipine strains are 35—36 days and 41—42 days
for the Taiwan and Chinese strains. The relative virulence of the Chinese, Taiwan
and Japanese strains in mice has been estimated by the longevity of animals with
a standard infection of cercariae after the appearance of eggs in the faeces. The
period for the Chinese and Taiwan strains is about 7—8 days but only 4.5 days
for the Japanese strain indicating that this last is considerably more virulent than
the other two. Additional morphological evidence of distinctions between the
races of *S. japonicum* has been obtained; there are statistically significant differences in size of the adult worms, number and position of the testes, occurrence
of hermaphrodite males and egg dimensions. The situation in *S. mansoni* and
S. haematobium is less clear-cut but snail-infection experiments have given conclusive evidence of the existence of different races within these species [9], and
current work shows that some races of *S. haematobium* differ in the lesions
which they cause in experimental animals [10].

The second aspect of the life-cycle which may be important in its pathological
consequences is the periodicity of the transmission cycle. This is, of course,
merely another aspect of the evolution of local intermediate host-parasite associations and is dependent upon the ecological requirements of the snails. Some
species of snail hosts occur exclusively in temporary water-bodies which are
completely dry for long periods of the year while others live in permanent habitats
and may have their breeding cycles influenced by factors such as floods and temperature. Thus there are places where snail population densities are at their
maxima during the rains, others where the greatest numbers are found during

the dry season and still others where snails may be breeding throughout the year but with fluctuations in total density. Such differences in transmission cycle may occur within a restricted geographical area. SMITHERS [4] has shown that in the Gambia there are at least two distinct transmission cycles of urinary schistosomiasis, one by *Bulinus senegalensis* during the wet season in temporary pools on the laterite plateau and another by *Bulinus jousseaumei* during the dry season in small tributary streams to the main river. WEBBE [8] has also demonstrated wet and dry season transmission in different areas of Tanganyika and there are undoubtedly many other regions where there is pronounced local variation in transmission. As a result of these variations there are some areas in which transmission is brief and intense while in others it is prolonged and less concentrated. The effects of these differing types of exposure on antibody responses of the final hosts have not been studied in sufficient detail but there can be little doubt that they have an influence on the pathology of the disease.

This is an aspect of schistosomiasis research requiring a great deal of investigation. Even in experimental animals our present knowledge of immune responses to schistosome infections is meagre, in man such information is almost entirely lacking. When adequate critera for assessing the pathogenic effects of schistosome infection have been established it will be of great interest to carry out comparative studies in carefully selected areas. The areas should be chosen well in advance so that thorough knowledge of the pattern of transmission is available, also information about peculiarities of the local strain of schistosome and its behaviour in experimental animals.

In conclusion I would ask that should there be any apparent conflict between the observations of different workers presented during the course of this symposium let us first be sure that they are dealing with the same parasite under similar circumstances before we search further for explanations of the disparity of their views.

References

[1] CHERNIN, E., and C. A. DUNAVAN: The influence of host parasite dispersion upon the capacity of *Schistosoma mansoni* miracidia to infect *Australorbis glabratus*. Amer. J. Trop. Med. Hyg. 11, 455—471 (1962).

[2] HSU, H. F., and S. Y. L. HSU: Characteristics of geographic strains of *Schistosoma japonicum* in the final hosts. Proc. VI Int. Cong. Trop. Med. Mal. Lisbon 2, 58—66 (1959).

[3] PITCHFORD, R. J.: Obervations on a possible hybrid between the schistosomes, *S. haematobium* and *S. mattheei*. Trans. Roy. Soc. Trop. Med. Hyg. 55, 44—51 (1961).

[4] SMITHERS, S. R.: On the ecology of schistosome vectors in the Gambia, with evidence of their role in transmission. Trans. Roy. Soc. Trop. Med. Hyg. 50, 354—365 (1956).

[5] STANDEN, O. D.: The penetration of the cercariae of *Schistosoma mansoni* into the skin and lymphatics of the mouse. Trans. Roy. Soc. Trop. Med. Hyg. 47, 292—298 (1953).

[6] — The transmission of Schistosomiasis. In: Biological aspects of the transmission of disease. Horton-Smith, C., (Ed.) London: Oliver & Boyd 1957.

[7] WAJDI, N. A. K.: Studies on the larval development of schistosomes. Ph. D. thesis. University of London 1963.

[8] WEBBE, G.: Population studies of intermediate hosts in relation to transmission of bilharziasis in East Africa. In: Ciba Foundation Symposium, Bilharziasis, WOLSTENHOLME, G. E. W., and M. O'CONNOR (Eds.) pp. 7—22. London: Churchill 1962.

[9] WRIGHT, C. A.: The significance of infra-specific taxonomy in bilharziasis. In: Ciba Foundation Symposium, Bilharziasis. WOLSTENHOLME, G. E. W., and M. O'CONNOR (Eds.) pp. 103—120. London: Churchill 1962.

[10] — Miracidial responses to molluscan stimuli. Proc. 1st Int. Cong. Parasit. Rome. (1965).

The Epidemiology of Bilharziasis

Louis Olivier*[1] and Nasser Ansari*

There are three species of schistosomes which commonly infect man. *Schistosoma haematobium* occurs in various parts of Africa and the Middle East and in Madagascar and Mauritius. A small focus is found in Southern Portugal and a similar one in Maharashtra State in India. *Schistosoma mansoni* is distributed in many areas in Africa, in some countries of the Middle East, in some of the Caribbean Islands and in Venezuela, Surinam and Brazil. *Schistosoma japonicum* is endemic in Japan, China, the Philippines, Celebes and Thailand. The parasite occurs in lower animals in Formosa but human infections have not been reported.

S. mansoni and *S. japonicum* inhabit the mesenteric veins, and the eggs are found mainly in the liver and the wall of the intestinal tract. They are discharged in the faeces. *S. haematobium* invades the veins of the pelvic plexus and the eggs usually pass in the urine. Besides these common locations, eggs of all species may reach other organs. Potentially, *S. japonicum* is of greater pathological importance because of the greater egg output on the part of the female worm. Second in this respect is *S. mansoni*, while egg production in *S. haematobium* is lowest of the three species.

As a brief orientation, it may be well to review the basic facts of the life cycle. Viable schistosome eggs passing out with the excreta hatch on reaching water and a free-swimming miracidium emerges to seek a suitable molluscan host. If penetration is effected, the organism undergoes asexual reproduction within the snail, usually requiring four weeks or more, depending on temperature and other conditions. Finally, free swimming cercariae emerge from the infected snail. On coming in contact with the human skin, the cercariae penetrate through the action of proteolytic enzymes. Those which succeed in reaching the venous capillaries are carried to the right heart, thence across the capillary bed of the lungs to enter the general circulation. In the intrahepatic portal venous system, the larvae continue to develop. On approaching maturity, the worms, in the case of *S. japonicum* and *S. mansoni*, migrate to the mesenteric vessels while those of *S. haematobium* find their way to the veins of the vesical and pelvic plexus. The prepatent period for *S. japonicum* averages 5 to 6 weeks, that for *S. mansoni* 7 to 8 weeks, and that for *S. haematobium* 10 to 12 weeks.

The epidemiology of bilharziasis involves three main components, viz: the environment, the molluscan intermediate host and the human host. Because each of these components is subject to considerable variability, the epidemiology of the disease presents perplexing aspects not encountered in many other infectious diseases. The factors responsible for the varying transmission dynamics will be

* Parasitic Diseases, Division of Communicable Diseases, World Health Organization, Geneva, Switzerland.
*[1] Presently: Pan American Health Orgauzalien, Washington, D. C., U.S.A.

discussed in some detail, because nearly all of them have some bearing, directly or indirectly, on the pathology of resultant human infections.

The environment

The environment has an influence on both the intermediate and definitive hosts. Temperature and rainfall are important elements. Bilharziasis occurs over areas with isotherms of 20—35° C, but it flourishes best in areas in which consistently warm temperatures prevail. In Japan, the molluscan intermediate host hibernates during the winter, thus halting transmission. Winter closure of irrigation canals in Egypt also tends to decrease transmission. In many endemic areas seasonal drying of snail habitats interrupts transmission. The type of geological formation probably has some influence, ill-defined at present, on the distribution of the disease. Certainly at least, vector snails require calcium for shell formation.

The disease seems to thrive best in areas with rich alluvial deposits, which are most advantageous for agricultural exploitation. Irrigation offers favourable conditions for intensive crop production but at the same time offers favourable habitats for the molluscan hosts and opportunities for disease transmission. However, these factors are not prime criteria for the establishment of bilharziasis, since it is present in many kinds of environment. The various environmental patterns may well be illustrated by certain samples, many of which have little in common and some of which are distinctly disparate.

There are, for instance, in Northeastern Mindanao extensive forested areas in which *Oncomelania quadrasi*, the snail host of *S. japonicum*, is found. In these areas, there is little or no transmission of infection until the forests are cleared and the areas opened to settlers. When infected individuals move into the area to cultivate the land, intensive transmission follows.

The classic man-made transmission environment is represented in Egypt and some other countries of Africa, where irrigation systems promote the spread of infection. The same situation has evolved in Iraq and in the Far East in China and Japan.

In contrast to man-promoted transmission closely related to agriculture, there are areas, such as Northern Brazil, where transmission is not closely linked with agriculture. The host snails live in natural water courses and transmission occurs primarily through casual contact with infested water or through household activities. In St. Lucia, also, infection is contracted from small streams and pools through recreational and domestic activities.

Bilharziasis occurs in isolated, restricted foci in oases where intensive transmission can result because all the population must frequent a small source of water. In some oases where the water supply is adequate to permit its use for irrigation, the endemicity may be enhanced. This has occurred in Mauritania and in areas in North Africa.

Finally, there may be cited the casual pattern of transmission which takes place from reservoirs or lakes, such as in Salvador, Bahia, Brazil and along the shores of Lake Victoria. The same type of transmission probably also occurs in the small farm reservoirs in Rhodesia and at Lake Lindöe in Celebes. An even more bizarre type of exposure is that in the ablution pools in the mosques of Yemen.

The molluscan intermediate host

The snail is an essential link in the bilharzia transmission chain. However, there are marked differences in efficiency of the snails as intermediate hosts. The ability of a snail to serve as an effective transmitter of infection depends on a number of factors, chief among which appear to be its genetic and physiologic constitution and the strain of parasite. There exists a peculiar affinity on the part of snail hosts for the local strain of parasite and such snails may be partially or completely refractory to infection with exotic strains. Certain species of snails have been shown to be susceptible to infection even though bilharziasis does not exist within their known areas of distribution.

The density of the snail population and their reproductive capacity are important factors in transmission. Population density varies greatly from time to time and from place to place, depending on local biotic and climatic factors. In many localities snail population density has a strong seasonal rhythm. Drastic changes in population density, especially sudden declines in snail populations, may occur for no apparent reason, — an indication that we lack sufficient knowledge of the factors regulating snail populations.

The status of bilharzial infection in the snail will have an effect epidemiologically since the prevalence of infection in the snail host and the number of cercariae being shed govern, to some extent, opportunities for exposure of the human population. However, our knowledge of cercarial production, the shedding of cercariae and their ultimate behaviour and fate in the immediate environment is exceedingly meager. Search for infected snails in what seemingly are ideal habitats will frequently provide disappointing results. The percentage of infected snails can sometimes be surprisingly low. Difficulties have been encountered in securing infections in animal exposed in areas where numerous infected snails occur and facile transmission might be expected. Heavy infections produce some mortality in the snail and infected snails are less able to withstand unfavourable environmental influences.

Predators, parasites and diseases probably serve in nature to limit the snail population but little is known concerning these deleterious influences. In only one instance has such an organism been shown in the field to be useful in control of intermediate hosts of bilharziasis: The snail, *Marisa cornuarietis*, has controlled the snail host in Puerto Rico under certain conditions.

The environment and the intermediate host

The snail host cannot escape changes in its aquatic or semi-aquatic environment since its voluntary movements within such habitats are considerably restricted. Although we know much about factors favourable and unfavourable for the snails we are not able to define with any precision the ecological limits within which the intermediate hosts can live nor can we predict with any precision where snails can become established.

Static or slow-flowing water is usually preferred to fast-flowing water. Mild organic pollution is apparently favourable to the snails but heavy pollution is inimical.

Water plants are a desirable adjunct to the environment but are not essential. When plants are present the snails tend to live among them, a fact which indicates the advantages of a molluscicide-herbicide combination in snail control. Certain algae appear to be an important food source of the snails.

It is rather surprising that observations to date have failed to indicate clear relationships between the chemistry of the water and its suitability for the snails. There is a large tolerable range of hydrogen ion concentration, although very acid water is unsuitable. A high salt content is generally not well tolerated. The snails can colonize water with a wide range of hardness, expressed as $CaCO_3$. Probably, oxygen tension seldom plays a significant role. The copper content, and perhaps that of other metals, may be a limiting factor in waters low in dissolved solids.

Water velocity, which is governed in general by stream gradient, is an important factor of snail ecology. For aquatic species, it would seem that the maximum tolerable velocity lies between 30 and 35 cm per second. Beyond this range, the snails are unable to maintain their position within the stream, or can only do so with difficulty.

With this brief review of snail ecology, it will be seen that many factors involving the well-being of the vectors are still obscure. An elucidation, at least of some of these factors, would no doubt constitute a considerable contribution to improvement of snail control methods.

The human host

Humans are the only final host for *S. mansoni* and *S. haematobium* in most endemic foci but, as will be discussed later, reservoir hosts in lower animals may possibly play a small role in maintaining infection in some areas. Reservoir hosts are important in the epidemiology of schistosomiasis japonica.

Sex differences in prevalence are noted in some areas in which the males show a significantly higher infection prevalence than females. However, in most endemic areas the differences are very small and are insignificant, since they depend on a multiplicity of factors which differ from one community to another.

Infection prevalence usually reaches its peak in children in the decade between 10 and 19.

Migratory propensities on the part of the human host have played a role in the extension of the disease into virgin territories. In Brazil, for instance, the extensive migration from the arid lands of the Northeast into the South, especially to the State of São Paulo, has led to the establishment of many new foci.

Population density and proximity to water are significant factors. Heavily populated areas adjacent to water containing efficient intermediate hosts usually show high prevalence, especially if the hygienic habits of the people are such as to promote snail infection and subsequent exposure to cercariae. When populations are located at some distance from water sources and take their household water from wells, there is much less opportunity for exposure.

Higher prevalence of infection in teen age and young adult groups is not necessarily a sign that such groups are the major contributors to transmission. The young children, infected for the first time, are probably the main culprits.

In these early age groups, pathological processes have not yet been activated. There is as yet little inflammatory reaction and practically no cellular infiltration in the intestine and bladder to trap eggs, such as consistently occurs in more chronic infections. Furthermore, young children with new-found freedom from maternal vigilance not only tend to play in the water but are totally uninhibited in their excretory habits.

The relation of transmission dynamics to the extent of pathological processes in the individual or population group cannot be gauged quantitatively at this time. There are many unknown factors. We do not usually know, for instance, the exact point where exposure takes place, how frequently it takes place, or its intensity at any one time or in the aggregate over a period of time. Also, we know very little about the concentration of cercariae in the water at any one time or the effect of various factors, such as water velocity and temperature, on their dispersal. We are quite ignorant concerning the influences which either impede or facilitate penetration. It is of some interest, in this connection, that suceptible mice exposed in habitats containing infected snails do not always become infected.

As the prevalence of infection in an area increases the output of eggs per person also increases and very heavy infections tend to occur most frequently in areas of very high prevalence. This can be taken to mean that where prevalence is high the number of worms per person also tends to be high. Although convincing data concerning the prevalence of clinical disease is lacking for most endemic areas, it is reasonable to believe that the prevalence of clinical disease will be relatively greater when the prevalence of infection is very high.

Bilharziasis is a chronic disease and the pathologic process usually evolves slowly, being governed more or less by the frequency and intensity of exposure over a period of time. Nevertheless, we know that a single exposure, if of sufficient magnitude, can produce dire results. As indicated previously, no marked pathological processes can usually be expected in young children. However, as exposure continues one begins to find ureteral deformity, bladder calcification and hydronephrosis in children infected with *S. haematobium*. Severe liver damage and other symptoms of advanced disease may occur in children infected with *S. mansoni* and *S. japonicum*.

There is a suspicion that strains of schistosomes vary in infectivity. If such is the case, differences in this regard might account for varying clinical manifestations and pathological processes. There is, in fact, some evidence that infectivity can be changed by passage through a snail host other than the accustomed one.

The factor of host resistance also has a bearing on prevalence and degree of infection, on the resulting pathology and on transmission potentials. Possibly certain individuals are inherently less susceptible than others. Moreover, studies on lower primates and other animals have demonstrated the acquisition of a certain degree of resistance to superinfection. The tendency for the prevalence curve to fall after its early peak offers indirect evidence for acquisition of resistance to superinfection in man, but at present there is no precise technique for measuring the speed or degree of such a reaction in the human host.

Nutrition may have an influence on the severity of the disease. Symptoms appear to be more severe in populations on restricted diets, especially those low in protein. In a study done in Puerto Rico liver function tests rapidly returned to normal or showed marked improvement after infected individuals were placed on an enriched diet. Animal experiments have provided some interesting results. *S. mansoni* lowers the efficiency of fat and protein utilization in mice. In mice with deficient diets, especially those low in protein, adult worms were stunted and egg production was markedly reduced. Swiss mice on a high protein diet showed severe local reactions to multiple cercarial exposure. Similarly enhanced reactions occurred around eggs in the liver but regeneration of liver tissue followed more rapidly. It is reasonable to assume that dietary factors may be concerned to some extent with bilharzial pathology in man.

A low socio-economic status plays a considerable role in the epidemiology of bilharziasis. Along with such a condition go poor housing, inadequate nutrition, sub-standard hygienic levels, dearth of sanitary facilities, inadequate water supply and concomitant disease conditions and parasitisms which tend to lower the resistance of the individual.

Reservoir hosts

Schistosoma japonicum has been found frequently in rats, dogs, swine and cattle and occasionally in other animal including carabao and goats. It has been shown in Leyte in the Philippines that the reservoir hosts play a role in maintaining the life cycle of the parasite, and that the life cycle could persist there in the absence of reservoir hosts only if a dense population of humans existed with a dense snail population.

Schistosoma mansoni has been found in naturally infected rodents, baboons, insectivores and dogs in Africa. In South America *S. mansoni* has been found in naturally infected rodents, marsupials and cattle. The role of these animals in maintaining the life cycle of *S. mansoni* is unknown but in most endemic foci reservoirs probably have little or no influence on maintenance of the life cycle.

In the case of *Schistosoma haematobium* occasional animals have been found infected but it is believed these were accidental infections and of no consequence epidemiologically.

Conclusion

Effort has been made to analyse the factors involved in the epidemiology of bilharziasis. Examples have been cited of the varying circumstances under which transmission takes place. The three main components have been reviewed. The environment exerts multiple influences both on the molluscan and human hosts. The snail host has little means of escape from unfavourable conditions in the aquatic or semi-aquatic environment. The human host on the other hand has freedom of movement but his habits and customs, which contribute so materially to the spread of the disease, are for the most part fixed and resistant to change. In spite of much knowledge concerning the broad pattern of transmission, many details have escaped observation. Some of these lacunae have been discussed.

With regard to the snail host, more needs to be known concerning its genetic and physiologic constitution in relation to its susceptibility to infection by various strains of schistosomes. Much more remains to be learned about the ecology of the snail hosts and we should know with greater exactitude their chemical and biotic requirements. More precise data are needed on the mechanisms which govern exposure and infection of the human host. These data concern the exact points of exposure, its frequency and intensity at any one time or in the aggregate, the concentration of cercariae, their movements and behaviour, as well as the influences which either impede or facilitate their penetration.

Bilharziasis tends to reach its greatest prevalence and seriousness in areas where water is used intensively and where agriculture depends on irrigation. This occurs because intensive water use and irrigation provide conditions that favour widespread establishment of the snail hosts and tend to place large numbers of people near these snail colonies. Pollution of the water and extensive water contact then assure transmission of infection. However, it does not necessarily follow that most infections are acquired during agricultural pursuits. Rather, infections are usually acquired at an early age through casual water contact and it is the young children who are the prime sources of infection for the snail hosts.

A more precise knowledge is needed concerning the role of lower animals in the perpetuation of the transmission cycle in different areas, as well as the part played by schistosome strain differences in the epidemiology, symptomatology and pathology of the disease.

Clinico Pathological Aspects of Hepatosplenic Bilharziasis

A. H. Mousa, A. A. Ata, A. El Rooby, A. El Garem, M. F. Abdel Wahab
and E. El Raziky*

With 9 figures

The first reference to hepatosplenic bilharziasis in Egypt was made by Symmers [38] followed by Day and Ferguson [7] based on autopsy material.

As early as 1923, the relation between Schistosoma mansoni and this syndrome
was suggested by Elkadi [12] and later by Day [8, 9], mainly on the parallel
incidence of both conditions based on clinical and epidemiological grounds.

Hashem [22, 23, 24] in a series of papers since 1931 has studied the pathology of this syndrome intensively, both in autopsy material and experimentally
and found the histology of the hepatic lesions different from that of other forms
of cirrhosis, being an interstitial hepatic fibrosis mostly concentrated around the
smaller or larger tracts and producing the fine and coarse forms of the disease.

The disease occurs at all ages between 10 and 70 years. The *incidence gradually*
rises after the age of 10 to reach a maximum in the fourth decade after which it
falls gradually. Males predominate in the proportion of 9 to 1.

The disease is commoner in Lower Egypt especially the Northern part of the
Nile Delta where both species of Schistosomes exist, while it is very rare in Upper
Egypt, where haematobium infection predominates. In areas heavily infested
with mansoniasis about 50% of the people show splenic enlargement and a firm
liver. In pure urinary bilharziasis the liver is involved in about 15% of the cases.

The clinical course of this disease may be divided into three stages, corresponding to the pathological stages of infiltration, fibrosis and complications as follows:
1. Hepatosplenomegalic stage. 2. Splenomegalic stage. 3. Ascitic and terminal
stage. However, the course is a slow progressive one, and the disease may be
arrested and become latent with early treatment. Such early arrested cases can
lead a normal active life, but if neglected and exposed to reinfection, the disease
will follow its course until there is well established fibrosis with splenomegaly
and portal hypertension.

The introduction of needle biopsy of the liver [15, 16], the battery of liver
function tests and haemodynamic studies of the liver have thrown new lights on
the etiology and pathogenesis of hepatosplenic affection. In 147 cases with hepatosplenomegaly studied in our Department in the last two years, we were able
to classify them according to histological examination of a biopsy obtained from
the liver by Vim Silvermann needle into the following: bilharzial (90 cases),
mixed bilharzial (13 cases), portal cirrhosis (20 cases), inconclusive findings
(18 cases) and normal histology in 6 cases (Table 1).

The reliability of the liver biopsy technique in establishing the pathological
nature and type of liver affection, has been also tested in 13 cases in our series;

* Endemic Medical Unit, Cairo University, Cairo, Egypt, U.A.R. — This study was supported
by Research Grant PL 480,83 D Contract Funds between U.S.A. N.I.H. and Cairo University.

a wedge biopsy was taken from the liver during surgical interference and the findings were compared to those shown in the needle biopsy specimen (Table 2). The findings were identical in 8 cases, in 2 cases the needle biopsy showed the bilharzial nature of the disease while the wedge specimens were able to show

Table 1. *Analysis of 147 cases of hepatosplenic affection according to liver biopsy findings*

Type	Early	Late	Total
Pure Bilharzial	66	24	90
Mixed Bilharzial	5	8	13
Portal Cirrhosis	9	11	20
Inconclusive	12	6	18
Normal	6	0	6

an additional cirrhotic element rendering the pathological diagnosis a mixed one. In the remaining 2 cases which were inconclusive by the needle biopsy, the wedge specimen revealed their bilharzial nature.

Table 2. *Pathological findings in the liver as compared by the needle and wedge biopsy techniques*

Ser. No.	Needle biopsy findings	Wedge biopsy findings
1.	Early bilharzial periportal fibrosis	Bilharzial periportal fibrosis
2.	Inconclusive	Bilharzial periportal fibrosis
3.	Early bilharzial periportal fibrosis	Bilharzial periportal fibrosis
4.	Inconclusive	Inconclusive
5.	Inconclusive	Bilharzial periportal fibrosis
6.	Bilharzial periportal fibrosis	Bilharzial periportal fibrosis
7.	Bilharzial periportal fibrosis	Bilharzial periportal fibrosis
8.	Bilharzial hepatic fibrosis	Mixed pathology
9.	Normal findings	Inconclusive findings
10.	? Laennec	Laennec
11.	Bilharzial hepatic fibrosis	Mixed pathology
12.	Bilharzial hepatic fibrosis	Bilharzial hepatic fibrosis
13.	Bilharzial hepatic fibrosis	Bilharzial hepatic fibrosis

The main presenting symptoms are general weakness, gradual loss of weight, epigastric discomfort and abdominal distension after meals, discomfort, pain and heaviness in the left hypochondrium, diarrhea, swelling of lower limbs and hematemesis. In its pure form, the bilharzial liver is at first enlarged, firm, and tender, with smooth surface and well defined edge. The spleen is also enlarged; firm and not tender. Enlargement of these two organs, usually starting early in life and progressing over several years in due time leads to widening of the subcostal angle, divarication of the recti and a barrel shaped chest. Later, the liver shrinks until it may become impalpable, becomes firmer with a sharp border and may have a finely granular surface. The presence of bilharzia ova in the liver can be more easily demonstrated by the newly adopted technique of liver print (Fig. 1 and 2). The spleen may reach a huge size, but with the onset of ascites, it usually diminishes. Splenic puncture is also applied particularly to exclude suspected reticulosis.

Ascites appears towards the end, and may be very excessive. The fluid has the characteristics of a transudate with a low specific gravity and low protein content. Oedema of the legs often follows. Dilated abdominal wall veins may

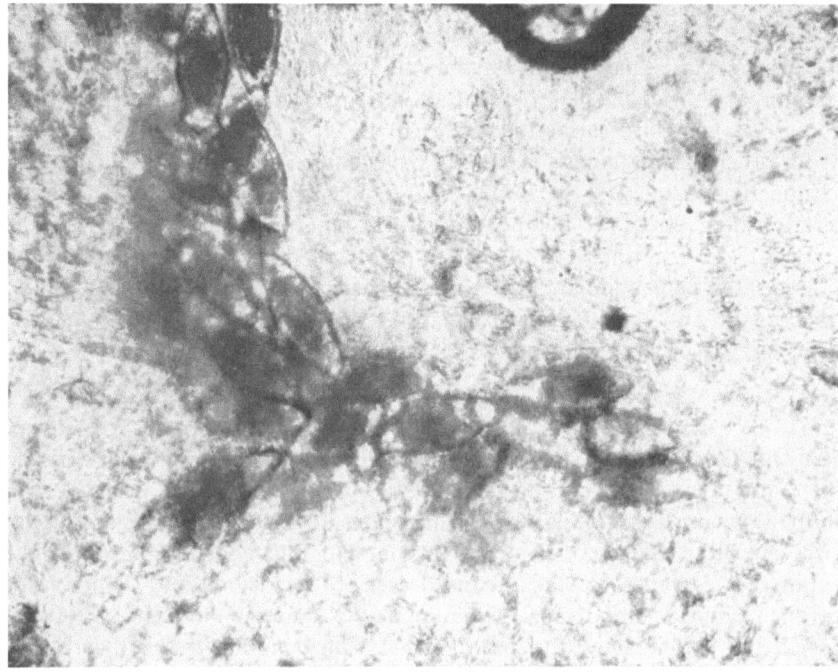

Fig. 1. Liver print showing many bilharzia ova. (Low Power)

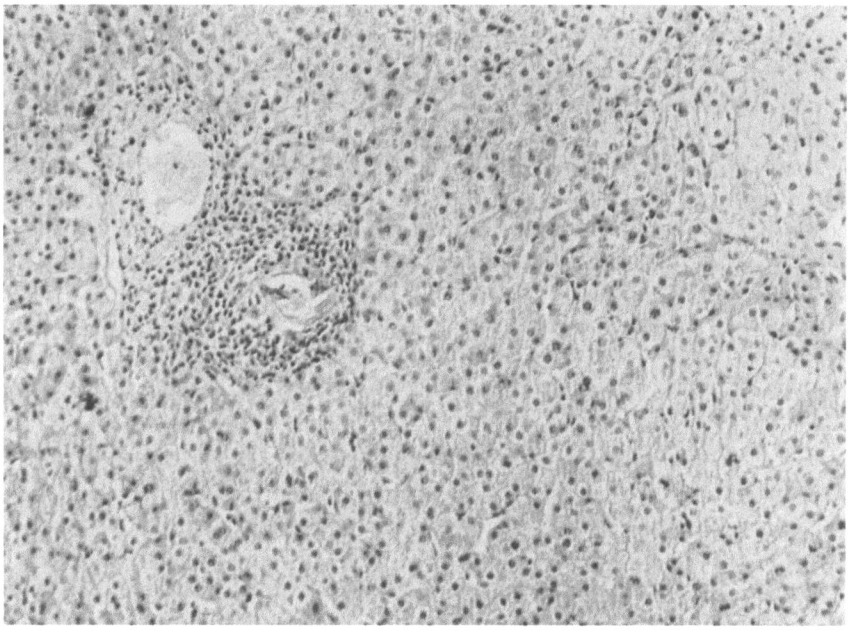

Fig. 2. Stained section from the same specimen of liver biopsy shown in Fig. 1 showing a single bilharzia ovum surrounded by specific cellular infiltration. (Low Power)

2   Bilharziasis

become visible, and there may be a venous thrill and hum over the lower sternum. Clubbing of the fingers is occasionally observed; as is intestinal polyposis. Oeso-phagogastric varices are demonstrable in many cases, and may lead to he-matemesis and melena. Their incidence is variously reported by different workers; but may be generally estimated to be 10 to 20% for hematemesis and twice that for others. Hematemesis is usually recurrent and is rarely fatal at onset.

Endocrine changes in the form of gynecomastia, alopecia, palmar erethyma, arterial spiders, etc., may be encountered in some pure bilharzial cases. MAHDY and BASALY [30] admit that more than half of the cases with endocrine changes had associated parasitism and nutritional deficiencies.

Porta-systemic encephalopathy may occur in patients with extensive col-laterals but are otherwise uncommon in uncomplicated cases.

Haematology

EL DEWI et al. [11] reported two morphological types of anaemia, normocytic in 40% and microcytic hypochromic in 60% but not a single case of macrocytosis. Malnutrition, ancylostomiasis, chronic infections, bleeding from piles or esophageal varices are often associated and may account for this anaemia. Leucopenia was encountered in moderate and advanced cases of hepatic fibrosis, usually due to neutropenia and lymphopenia. Eosinophilia is common and the platelets are reduced, but never below the critical level. The bone marrow is mostly hyper-plastic due to increased normoblasts, with some increase in plasma cells and bone marrow. Eosinophilia is a constant finding even in absence of blood eosinophilia. No maturation arrest is found in any elements. The coagulative mechanism is normal or very slightly affected.

SALAH [36] relates the presence of hypersplenism to the reduction of neu-trophils and platelets, but probably not to that of the red cells as there is no evidence of haemolysis in these cases and splenectomy does not improve their anaemia.

ATA [4, 5], from a study of 300 cases of this syndrome, concluded that the enlarged spleen in this disease does not result in any decrease of functions. The leucopenia and thrombocytopenia are a release phenomena probably due to a humoral effect of the spleen unchecked by a failing liver, or through portasystemic shunts directly affecting the bone marrow.

FARID et al. [18] studied the red cell half life and organ uptake of chromium[51] radioactivity in such patients and found no convincing evidence of haemo-lytic anaemia due to hypersplenism.

Biochemistry

As would be expected in a disease which affects mainly mesenchyme and spares the parenchyme until very late, liver function tests usually reveal little impair-ment of the hepatocellular unit.

ERFAN et al. [17] found that serum albumin is slightly lowered in nonascitic cases, and more so in ascitic ones. The hypo-albuminaemia is generally con-sidered to result not so much from hepatocellular dysfunction as from protein malnutrition, blood loss and haemodilution from salt and water retention. Serum globulins on the other hand, are raised through the gamma fraction, which reflects reticulo-endothelial activity, so that the A/G ratio is markedly reduced and inverted. The dysproteinaemia of bilharzial hepatic fibrosis is responsible for positive seroflocculation tests in a high percentage of cases. Hippuric acid test, prothrombin synthesis and carbohydrate metabolism are usually normal. Occasionally hypoprothrombinaemia occurs, but is easily correctable by vitamin K administration.

SAIF et al. [35] studied both S.G.O.T. and S.G.P.T. in a series of cas es of bilharzial affection of liver, intestine, and bladder. Significant elevation in both enzymes was found in all bilharzial cases, and generally ran parallel to the course of the disease, being more marked in intestinal than in urinary and in ascitic than in non-ascitic cases and antibilharzial treatment resulted in a further rise.

Cholangiolar implication is rare and very late. The icterus index and serum bilirubin are usually normal, but the alkaline phosphatase, sensitive to focal cholangiolar involvement, is moderately raised in 30% of non-ascitic cases. The bromsulphthalein test is normal in over 2/3 of the cases. This test reflects not only hepatocellular function but also hepatic blood flow, so much so that in this disease it may be an indication of portocaval collateral vessels [6].

Finally, most liver function tests show further deterioration with onset of ascites or after a bout of hematemesis. Serum sodium and potassium levels are within normal limits, in non-ascitic cases of the disease, but with the onset of ascites, serum sodium tends to fall.

PRASSAD et al. [34] showed that dwarfism and hypogonadism associated with hepatosplenic bilharziasis conserve zinc by reducing its excretion in the urine, the plasma and red cell levels being nevertheless low.

Biochemical evidence of pancreatic involvement was mostly masked by the presenting symptomatology of associated bilharzial liver.

17-Ketosteroids were reported to be low, and F.S.H. was markedly diminished in cases with endocrine disturbances. They are related either to prolonged malnutrition or to liver insufficiency leading to insufficient inactivation of certain hormones especially the antidiuretic hormone, aldosterone and oestrogens.

Haemodynamics

The total blood volume was estimated in cases of bilharzial hepatic fibrosis and was found to be from 13 to 74.7% higher than the average blood volume of normal controls [29]. This was related to dilated portal tributaries and tendency to water retention. Hypervolemia may be a contributing factor to the congested neck veins and pulmonary hypertension seen in some of these cases. In 49 bilharzial hepatosplenic cases studied in our Department, it was quite evident that the later stages of the disease with shrunken livers were associated with relatively higher values of total blood volume than the early hepatosplenomegalic cases; this increase is mainly due to increase in the plasma volume, rather than to increase in the cellular elements of the blood (Table 3).

The total volume of collateral circulation was calculated [26] by a method using percutaneous intrasplenic injection of isotopes and scintillation probing over the liver and heart and it was found to be contributing to the increase in blood volume in such cases.

Table 3. *Total blood volume and plasma volume in the various stages of hepatosplenic bilharziasis*

Stages	Total blood volume in ml/m²			Plasma volume in ml/m²		
	No. of cases	Range	Average	No. of cases	Range	Average
Early Pure Hepatosplenic Bilharzial cases	32	1159.7 5381.8	3140	30	1062.6 3229.0	1979.9
Late pure Hepatosplenic Bilharzial cases	17	1893.3 5128.4	3570	10	1387.9 2777	2333.6

The intrasplenic pressure was found to be raised and Mousa and Garem [32] found a discrepancy between the elevated intrasplenic pressure and the unchanged occluded hepatic vein pressure in bilharzial cases. This pattern suggested the portal hypertension in these cases to be due to a presinusoidal rather than a peri- or post-sinusoidal lesion, well known in Laennec cirrhosis.

Table 4 demonstrates this finding in the pure bilharzial cases belonging to our recently studied series in contrast to the mixed bilharzial and portal cirrhotic cases.

Table 4. *Intrasplenic pressure (I.S.P.) and occluded hepatic vein pressure (O.H.V.P.) in hypertensive cases of hepatosplenic affection*

Type	Case No.	The I.S.P. in cm/saline	The O.H.V.P. in cm/saline
Pure bilharzial	7	37	15
	11	30	16.5
	12	29	14
	13	27	15
	17	27	17
	19	30	11
Mixed bilharzial	97	20	19
	100	37	24
	101	29	17
	103	32	12
Portal cirrhosis	104	29	27
	105	38	31.5
	110	32	22
	123	27	22

The portal circulation time was found to be prolonged at the start but shortened later with the establishment of collateral circulation. Double responses was noted in some cases.

Hepatic blood flow as measured by the B.S.P. clearance technique or the isotope method was found to be slightly reduced in this syndrome. The degree of reduction was found to vary directly with the size of the liver and its pathological changes and with the extent of collaterals. In our recently studied series, both methods of estimating the effective hepatic blood flow were utilized in the study of some pure hepatosplenic bilharzial cases, the results of which are shown in Table 5.

Table 5. *Effective hepatic blood flow in ml/m/m² in early and late hepatosplenic bilharziasis by the B.S.P. and Radiogold methods*

| Stages | B.S.P. Clearance Technique | | | Radiogold Clearance Technique | | |
	No. of cases	Range	Average	No. of cases	Range	Average
Early hepatosplenic bilharzial cases	14	158.8 1322.8	672	22	225.7 2049.3	724.7
Late hepatosplenic bilharzial cases	11	284 1216.19	840.1	7	484 1923	1069.3
Total	25	158.8 1322.8	752.36	29	225.72 2049.3	796.3

Portal venography by the percutaneous splenic route shows the degree of hepatic fibrosis and the patency of the splenic and portal veins as well as the extent of collaterals.

Barium swallow will show the oesophago-gastric varices if the oesophagoscope is considered risky.

Pathology and pathogenesis

Apart from an early transitory stage of cercarial invasion in which the liver may be involved by isolated discrete or diffuse cellular infiltration, the pathology of hepatic bilharziasis passes through two stages: an early infiltrative or granulomatous and a late advanced fibrotic. In the early phase, ova are impacted in the main, medium or fine portal tracts, usually in or around small portal tributaries and excite a histiocytic and eosinophilic cellular reaction which is gradually replaced by fibroblasts. The fibrocellular infiltration in and around the portal tracts extends toward similar lesions in neighboring portal tracts. There is hypertrophy and hyperplasia of Kupffer's cells and bilharzial pigment is seen engulfed by reticuloendothelial elements. The sinusoids are engorged and contain eosinophils. The parenchymal liver cells show no signs of fatty infiltration, degeneration, necrosis, or regeneration (Fig. 3).

In the advanced fibrotic stage, in addition to the above mentioned changes there is thickening of the portal tracts, with mild cloudy swelling and wasting of liver cells at the periphery of the lobules (Fig. 4).

Thus bilharzial hepatic fibrosis differs from genuine cirrhosis in that the parenchyma is spared and shows neither apparent degeneration or any attempt at regeneration. The lobular pattern is also preserved until very late in the disease when some distortion may occur as a result of excessively contracting fibrous tissue. Whether fine (diffuse) or course (pipe stem) fibrosis results appears to

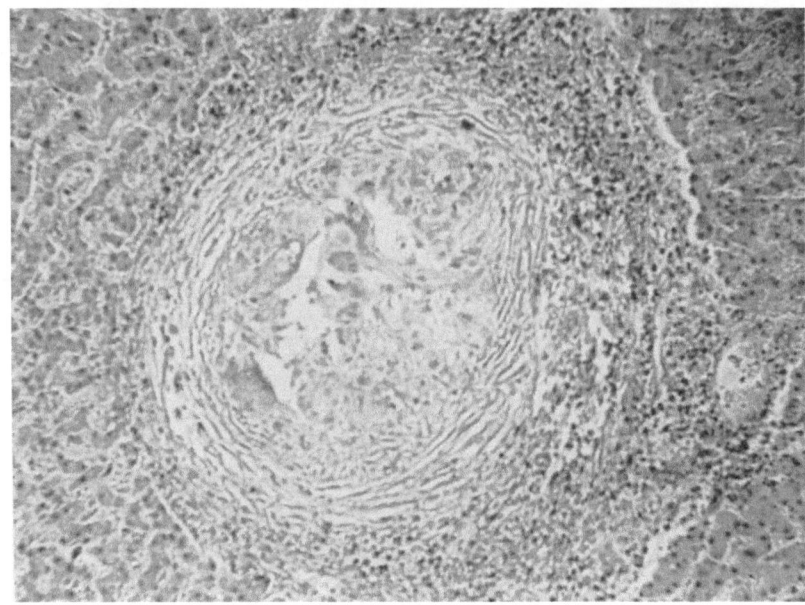

Fig. 3. Liver section of early bilharzial infiltration. (High power)

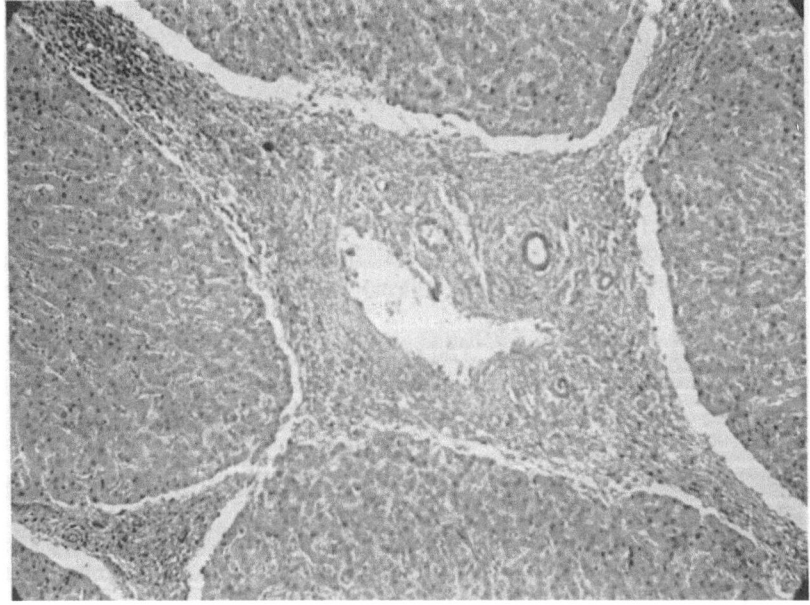

Fig. 4. Liver section of bilharzial periportal fibrosis. (Low Power)

depend on whether the small or large portal tracts are mainly involved and this in turn may be related to the rate and number of ova or worms deposited. Very often they are combined and sometimes one lobe shows periportal and the other diffuse fibrosis.

In the early stage of active bilharziasis there is hyperplasia of the splenic reticular tissue in response to bilharzial toxins, associated with active congestion and leucocytic cellular infiltration rich in eosinophils; very rarely B. ova are found, surrounded by their specific reaction in the pulp of the spleen. With prolongation of the bilharzial infection, further enlargement of the spleen results from progressive hyperplasia of its reticulum, to which is added another element of mild portal congestion consequent to the presence of infiltrative bilharzial lesions in the liver. These two stages of splenic enlargement are usually reversible on specific treatment. In the third stage, the hyperplastic splenic reticular tissue has now given way to diffuse fibrosis associated with marked destruction of the musculoelastic tissue of the trabeculae and capsule. This leads to diminution of the elasticity and excessive distensibility of the spleen under the much increased portal pressure due to the progressive periportal fibrosis of the liver.

As a result of excessive congestion and occasionally thrombosis of the smaller vessels haemorrhages occur which on healing result in the fibrosiderotic nodules. Haemorrhages occurring in the capsule and in the pericapsular tissues on healing result in dense, hyaline, sometimes cartilagenous scar tissue in the capsule and adhesions with surrounding tissues. Congestion of the gastro-intestinal tract, oesophagogastric varices and other portocaval collaterals and ascites are common findings in advanced cases with portal hypertension and need no special comment.

There is pathological evidence of bilharziasis of the pancreas in 50% of cases of bilharzial hepatic fibrosis in the form of bilharzial fibrosis, acinar atrophy or interstitial fibrosis.

HASHEM [23] studied experimentally the effect of schistosomal worm extract injected intraperitoneally into rats and rabbits and through the portal veins of rabbits compared with that of S. haematobium ova suspension injected into the portal vein of dogs. The former produced no significant liver changes, while the latter resulted in pathological lesions exactly similar to those seen in the evolution of the human disease. He carried out studies of the vascular anatomy of the bilharzial liver, by injection of colored gelatin into the portal vein and hepatic artery. He concluded that all the stages of evolution of bilharzial hepatic fibrosis can well be explained by the local effects of ova impacted in the portal venules. Dead ova cause little or no reaction. It is the toxin of living miracidia that excites the specific response. Their diffusion from the affected tracts along the liver divisions of Glisson's capsule explains the common observation in diffuse bilharzial hepatic fibrosis that this fibrosis is usually out of proportion to the number of ova deposited. HASHEM [24, 25] was also able experimentally to produce pure bilharzial hepatic fibrosis in animals on normal diets with ample supply of proteins and vitamines thus excluding malnutrition as the main factor in producing hepatic fibrosis in this syndrome.

DEWITT [10] showed in experimental animals that diets deficient in certain amino acids and vitamins have profound effect on the course of S. mansoni infection. In some cases the worms did not undergo normal development and sexually immature worms did not produce eggs. Since eggs are the major cause of tissue damage, the pathological consequences of the infection were greatly reduced.

Abdine [1], however, suggested an antigen-antibody reaction, possibly the result of death of worms, to explain the marked and diffuse portal thickening where ova are few or absent. In this connection, it should be noted that Andrade et al. [2] were able, by immunocytochemical methods, to demonstrate antigen-antibody complexes in the liver of mice injected with Schistosoma mansoni, which provides support for the immunological nature of the self prepetuating hepatic involvement in schistosomiasis. Andrade and Barka [3] found antigenic material with specific binding affinity to circulating antibodies present in sera of patients with active hepatic schistosomiasis and they demonstrated immunocytochemically the presence of these antibodies in the ova and hepatic granulomata.

It appears that antimony treatment of bilharziasis, introduced in 1919 in Egypt, has increased the incidence of periportal pipe-stem bilharzial fibrosis of the liver [17]. Thus, of cases of liver cirrhosis seen at post mortem in Kasr El-Aini Hospital, bilharzial pipe-stem fibrosis accounted for 1 to 2% in 1909 [7], 22% in 1927 [37], 49% in 1947 [23] and 50% in 1962 [14]. This may be related, among other factors, to the hepatic shift of worms seen in experimental animals infected with bilharziasis when given antimony compounds.

The immediate and late effects of antibilharzial treatment had been demonstrated histologically in experimental animals [13] (Figs. 5, 6, 7 and 8).

Fikry et al., [19] tested the effect of four antimonials used in the treatment of bilharziasis on portal hypertension and found that they induced a sustained rise of portal pressure specially if given intravenously. This has been confirmed by El-Razky et al., [13]. Any parenchymal change including fatty metamorphosis, focal necrosis, swelling of liver cells with loss of granules, cellular regeneration and architectural distortion seen occasionally in liver biopsy material is in our experience due to other etiological factors associated with the disease (Fig. 9). Actually patients with hepatic Schistosomiasis are not immune, if not more susceptible, to hepatic injuries.

Gholmy et al., [21] analysed 54 cases of liver cirrhosis among children; 22 were bilharzial, 14 were due to infantile liver cirrhosis, 8 were post hepatitis, 2 were biliary cirrhosis and 8 were of undetermined etiology. Some of the children surviving their liver affection can get bilharzial infection superadded during adolescence with modification of the previous hepatic pathology.

The pathogenesis of the splenomegaly associated with hepatic bilharziasis has been the subject of much controversy. Day, [8, 9] considered it essentially congestive due to portal venous obstruction. Onsy [33] believed it was due to reaction of the spleen to B. ova deposited in the pulp. The rarity of finding ova in sections from the spleen was explained as due to the phagocytic action of its reticulo-endothelial structures. Khalil [27, 28] regarded the cirrhosis and splenomegaly as a complication of bilharzial infection of the intestine caused by toxins absorbed from the bilharzial intestinal tract. Girgis [20] ascribed the hepatic lesion and splenic enlargement to male Schistosomal infection of the liver and portal veins. Meleney [31], after experimenting with unisexual and bisexual infections, concluded that the fertilized eggs and dead worms produce most of

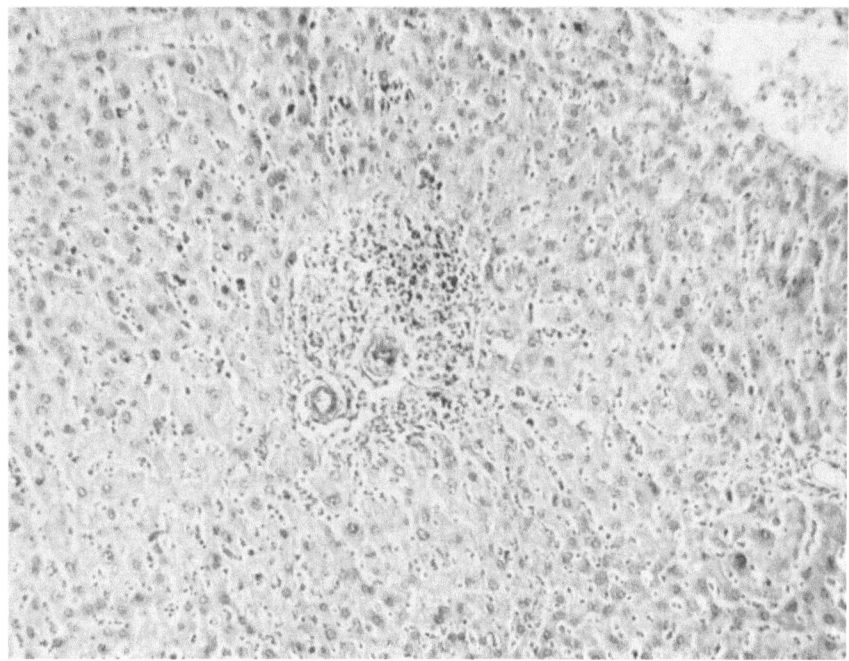

Fig. 5. Liver of hyperinfected mouse 6 weeks after infection

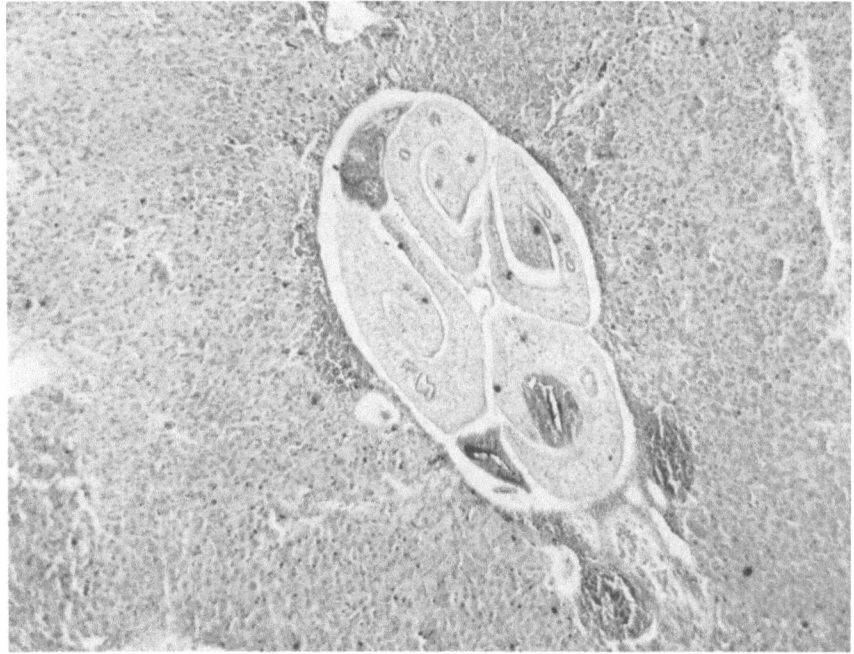

Fig. 6. Liver of hyperinfected mouse with massive hepatic shift of the parasite and rapid portal embolism leading to death of the animal 24 hours after a single full dose of Foadin

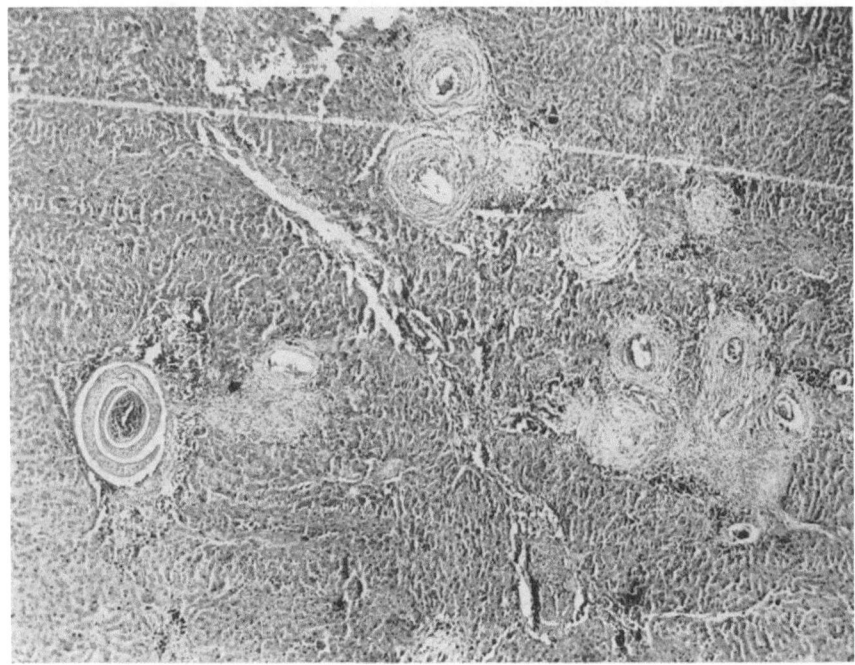

Fig. 7. Liver of untreated hyperinfected mice 6 months after infection, showing a section of male and female bilharzia worms in copulation together with multiple bilharzial granulomata

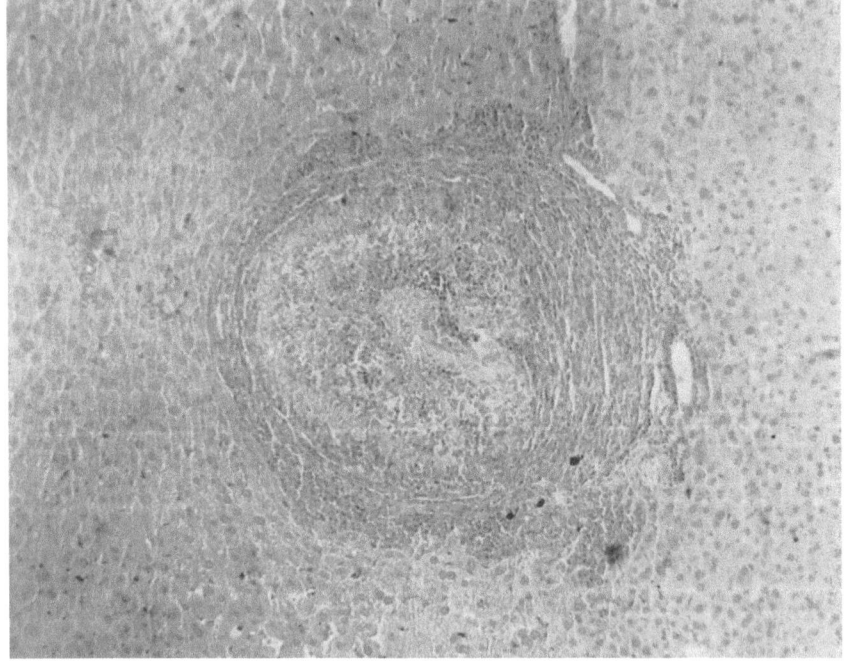

Fig. 8. Liver of hyperinfected mouse sacrificed 6 months after the end of full course of antimony; thrombophlebitis of one of the portal tributaries, liver otherwise is free

the pathological changes in the liver. The development of the full picture of this syndrome has been repeatedly proved in different experimental animals.

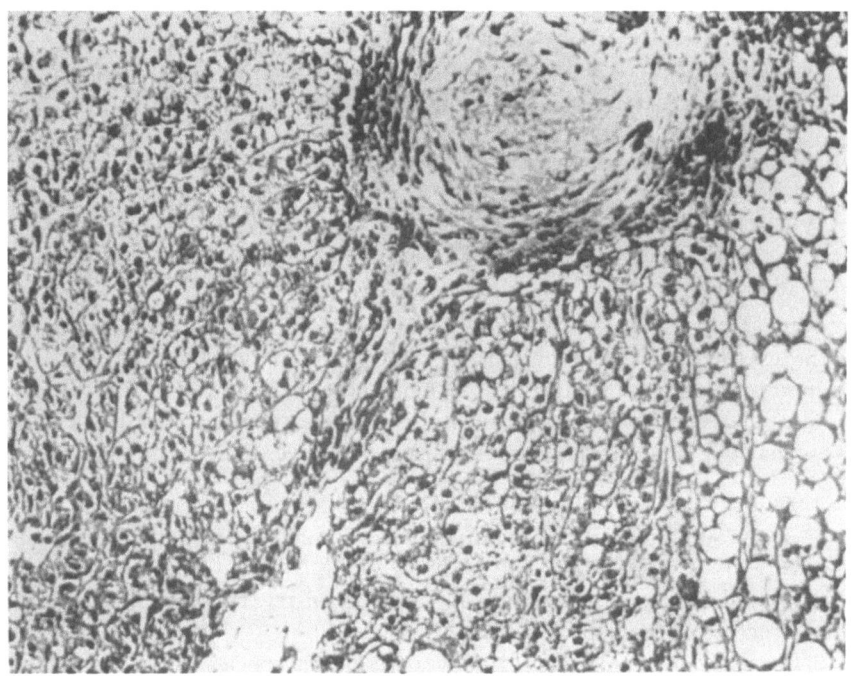

Fig. 9. Liver biopsy of a mixed bilharzial periportal fibrosis

Summary and conclusions

The true nature of the etiological factors in Egyptian or endemic hepatosplenomegaly has long remained a mystery. Even after the discovery of the role of bilharzia in its production, many other factors are still suspect. It has been found that not every case presenting with hepatosplenomegaly in Egypt is bilharzial, and even in the bilharzial cases other etiological factors such as nutritional disorders, viral infections and others may be contributory.

The clinical picture, the biochemical and haemodynamic studies as well as the liver biopsy findings are essential for the differential diagnosis of such disorder. Such differentiation is of great importance for the proper management. The relative sizes of liver and spleen though helpful in the clinical grading of the disease cannot be solely relied upon. Thus a more dynamic and a functional approach must be adopted in classifying this syndrome as follows:

1. Non progressive bilharzial hepatic fibrosis

The reticulo-endothelial evidence of activity and the bilharzial manifestations terminate especially if the patient changes his residence and occupation. These mild forms are of very high incidence among urban inhabitants and they do not need medical or surgical management. Antimonials do not induce eosinophilia or portal hypertension in such cases. The prognosis is different.

2. *Progressive bilharzial fibrosis*

It occurs in two forms

a) The compensated form. This form lasts from the early invasive phase through the phase of gross vascular involvement.

b) The decompensated form. In this form there will be hepatocellular failure, hematemesis or ascites, due either to severe parenchymal and/or vascular involvement.

3. *Complicated bilharzial hepatic fibrosis*

When the disease is associated with extrahepatic splenic or portal vein thrombosis or the condition is mixed with parenchymal liver disorder induced by other associated factors.

The medical and surgical management of these different forms varies according to the extent of portal hypertension, the degree of porto-systemic collaterals, the functional reserve of the liver parenchyme and the availability of modern facilities necessary for thorough diagnosis and treatment. But still, we have to stress that the best treatment of this disease is prevention.

Several frontiers are still unexplored:

1. Does autoimmunity play an important role in the pathogenesis of this disease?

2. Would electron microscopy and cytochemistry throw more light on the ultra structure of the hepatic lesions?

3. Can experimental work utilizing various animal species elucidate the different pathological haemodynamic factors controlling the ultimate clinical picture?

4. Would it be possible by more elaborate study of the vascular pathology utilizing modern isotope techniques and injection corrosive studies to give a better understanding of the disturbed vasculature of this disease?

Such questions are the subject of research projects in the different centers concerned with the study of this disease in Egypt, U. A. R, and it is hoped that some of the anwers will be forthcoming in the near future.

References

[1] Abdin, F. H.: Needle biopsy in cirrhosis of the liver. J. Egypt Med. Ass. **46**, 45—52 (1963).

[2] Andrade, Z. A., F. Paronetto, and H. Popper: Immunocytochemical studies in schistosomiasis. Amer. J. Path. **39**, 589—598 (1961).

[3] —, and T. Barka: Histochemical observations in experimental schistosomiasis of mouse. Amer. J. Trop. Med. Hyg. **11**, 12—24 (1962).

[4] Ata, A. A.: Haematological study in bilharzial hepatolienal fibrosis. J. Egypt Med. Ass. **42**, 285—301 (1959).

[5] — Anaemias in Egypt (UAR). Gaz. Kasr-El-Aini Fac. Med. **27**, 237—250 (1961).

[6] Badawi, H., A. Nomier, and R. Zaher: Evaluation of portal hypertension in hepatic schistosomiasis. Alexandria Med. J. **8**, 208—219 (1962).

[7] Day, H. B., and A. R. Ferguson: An account of a form of splenomegaly with hepatic cirrhosis, endemic in Egypt. Ann. Trop. Med. Parasit. **3**, 379—394 (1909).

[8] — The etiology of Egyptian splenomegaly and hepatic cirrhosis. Trans. Roy. Soc. Trop. Med. Hyg. **18**, 121—130 (1924).

[9] — Bilharzial cirrhosis (Egyptian splenomegaly). J. Trop. Med. Hyg. **36**, 17—23 (1933).

[10] DEWITT, W. B.: Schistosomiasis mansoni in mice with nutritional fatty liver disease. Amer. J. Trop. Med. Hyg. 7, 239—240 (1958).
[11] EL DEWI, S., E. BEBAWI, and A. HABIB: Preliminary report on some of the hematological aspects of hepatosplenic bilharziasis in Egypt. Gaz. Kasr-El-Aini Fac. Med. 23, 52—56 (1957).
[12] EL KADI, A.: Egyptian splenomegaly, the result of intestinal bilharziasis. J. Egypt. Med. Ass. 6, 273—279 (1923).
[13] EL RAZKI, E.: M. D. Thesis, Cairo University 1964.
[14] ELWI, A., and O. M. ATTIA: Pathology of hepato-splenic bilharziasis. Procedings of the Ist International Symposium on Bilharziasis. Cairo 2, 93—114 (1962).
[15] ERFAN, M.: Hepatic bilharziasis. J. Trop. Med. Hyg. 50, 104—109 (1945).
[16] —, and S. TALAT: Demonstration of schistosome ova in the liver by biopsy. J. Egypt. Med. Ass. 30, 663—664 (1947).
[17] —, M. HASHEM, A. EL MOFTY, A. H. MOUSA, and M. KHATTAB: Clinico-pathological study of bilharzial cases with hepatosplenic affection. Gaz. Kasr-El-Aini Fac. Med. 23, 1—13 (1957).
[18] FARIS, Z., A. PRASSAD, A. SCHULERT, H. SANSTEAD, and A. EL ROOBY: Bilharzial splenomegaly. Arch. Intern. Med. 113, 37—41 (1964).
[19] FIKRY, E., M. MONTASER, M. SALEM, and K. DORRY: Egypt. J. Gastro. (in press).
[20] GIRGIS, R.: Pathology of schistosomiasis mansoni. J. Trop. Med. Hyg. 33, 1—7 (1930).
[21] GHOLMY, A., M. NABAWAY, M. GABR, S. AIDROS, and A. OMAR: Hepatic schistosomiasis in children. Gaz. Kasr-El-Aini Fac. Med. 23, 14—25 (1957).
[22] HASHEM, M.: M. D. Thesis, Cairo University, 1931.
[23] — Etiology and pathogenesis of endemic form of hepatosplenomegaly; Egyptian splenomegaly. J. Roy. Egypt. Med. Ass. 30, 48—79 (1947).
[24] — The present status of the so-called Egyptian splenomegaly. J. Egypt. Med. Ass. 40, 860—869 (1957).
[25] — The etiology and pathogenesis of bilharzial bladder cancer. J. Egypt. Med. Ass. 44, 857—966 (1961).
[26] IBRAHIM, M. S., and M. ABDEL WAHAB: Intrasplenic isotopes in study of portal systemic collateral circulation. Brit. Med. J. 2, 623—625 (1961).
[27] KHALIL, M.: The prevention of bilharzia in Egypt. Congres Intern. Med. Trop. Hyg. (Resumé published) Cairo 3, 370 (1928).
[28] — Discussion of paper by Salah. Types of splenomegaly in Egypt and their diagnosis. J. Roy. Egypt. Med. Ass. 18, 264—265 (1935).
[29] KHATTAB, M., V. FANOUS and M. A. ABOUL FADL: Blood volume studies in bilharzial hepatosplenomegaly. J. Egypt. Med. Ass. 43, 280—293 (1960).
[30] MAHDY, A., and M. BASSALY: Endocrinal imbalance in hepatosplenic bilharziasis. Proc. Pharm. Soc. Egypt 37, 53—57 (1955).
[31] MELENEY, H. A., J. H. SANDGROUND, D. V. MOORE, H. MOST, and B. H. CARNEY: The histopathology of experimental schistosomiasis. 2. Bisexual infection with S. mansoni, S. japonicum and S. hematobium. Amer. J. Trop. Med. Hyg. 2, 883—915 (1953).
[32] MOUSA, A. H., and A. GAREM: The haemodynamic study of Egyptian hepatosplenic bilharziasis. J. Egypt. Med. Ass. 42, 444—455 (1959).
[33] ONSY, A. B.: The pathogenesis of endemic (Egyptian) splenomegaly. Trans. Roy. Soc. Trop. Med. Hyg. 30, 597—600 (1937).
[34] PRASSAD, A., H. SANDSTEAD, A. SCHULBERT, and A. EL ROUBY: Urinary excretion of zinc in patients with the syndrome of anaemia, hepatosplenomegaly, dwarfism and hypogonadism. J. Lab. Clin. Med. 62, 591—599 (1963).
[35] SAIF, M., A. ABDALLAH, A. EL ROUBY, M. SHAKIR, J. TAWFIK, and S. SABET: Serum transaminases in bilharziasis and the immediate effect of antibilharzial treatment thereupon. Z. Trop. Med. Paras. 15, 199—207 (1964).
[36] SALAH, M.: The bilharzial liver. Alexandria Med. J. 8, 177—194 (1962).
[37] SOROUR, M. F.: The pathology and morbid histology of bilharzial lesions in various parts of the body. Congres Intern. Med. Trop. Hyg. Cairo 4, 322—377 (1928).
[38] SYMMERS, W. ST. C.: Note on a new form of liver cirrhosis due to the presence of the ova of B. haematobia. J. Path. Bact. 4, 237—239 (1903).

Cardio-Pulmonary Bilharziasis

H. A. ZAKY, A. R. EL HENEIDY, M. FODA, M. KHALIL and A. A. TARABEIH*

With 8 figures

Manifest cardio-pulmonary bilharziasis as seen in Egypt almost always develops in conjunction with hepato-splenomegaly; hence the name of porto-pulmonary bilharziasis is suggested. The disease was first described clinically by AZMY and EFFAT in 1932 [2] under the name of Bilharzial Ayerza. Repeated showers of bilharzia ova are deposited in the peripheral branches of the pulmonary artery and are responsible for the subsequent occlusive angeitis in and around the arterioles along with the formation of angiomatoids [12]. Early in our studies it was noticed that the size of a main pulmonary artery bore little or no relationship to the sustained pressure, that is, the pressure in an aneurysmal pulmonary artery which may even contain large fibrin clots may be distinctly lower than in a correspondingly smaller artery in another patient [14]. In the former group, the oxygen saturation in the pulmonary artery showed a significant increase as the catheter was advanced from proximal to distal [17], the sampling site being kept carefully away from the wedged position. Evidence for the left to right shunt was demonstrated by two procedures [15].

A. Two catheters were introduced in the patient — one in the aorta via the brachial artery and the other through an arm vein to reach a wide branch of the pulmonary artery. Evans blue dye was injected in the aortic catheter opposite the hilum, meanwhile a sample was drawn from the pulmonary artery catheter for a period of five seconds. The amount aspirated was 4 cc and the capacity of the catheter was 2.8 cc. Since the rate of withdrawal was 0.8 cc. per second it follows that 1.2 cc were drawn from the pulmonary artery. This sample represented $1^{1}/_{2}$ seconds and it showed the presence of the dye on the spectrophotometer. Another 2 cc. were withdrawn which represented a further $2^{1}/_{2}$ seconds. In the latter sample the dye could be easily seen by the naked eye.

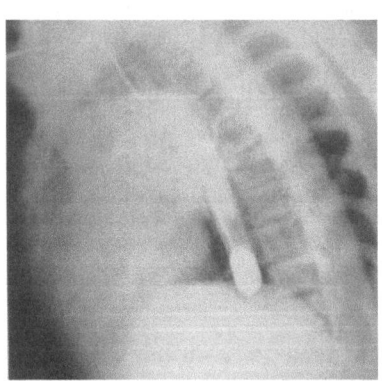

Fig. 1. Aortography with balloon catheter (left oblique view). Contrast materia is seen in both aorta and pulmonary artery [15].

B. A special catheter was made in which a balloon was fitted to the distal end and 2 holes were perforated proximal to it (Fig. 1). The catheter was introduced via the brachial artery into the aorta to a level distal to the hilum and urographin 70% was injected. Radiographs were taken every second. Within 2 seconds the

---

* Department of Chest Diseases, Alexandria University Alexandria, Egypt. U.A.R.

urographin could be seen in the pulmonary artery. The balloon was inflated as long as the injection pressure was applied. It blocked the aorta during the escape of the dye but was deflated by the aortic pressure as soon as the injection was accomplished. The occurrence of such left to right shunt creates an increase in the

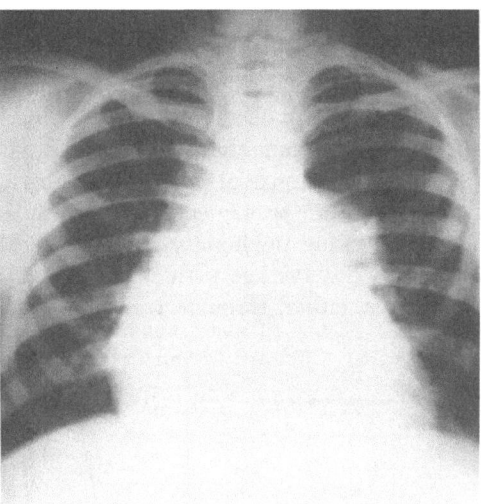

Fig. 2a. Chest radiograph taken before splenectomy

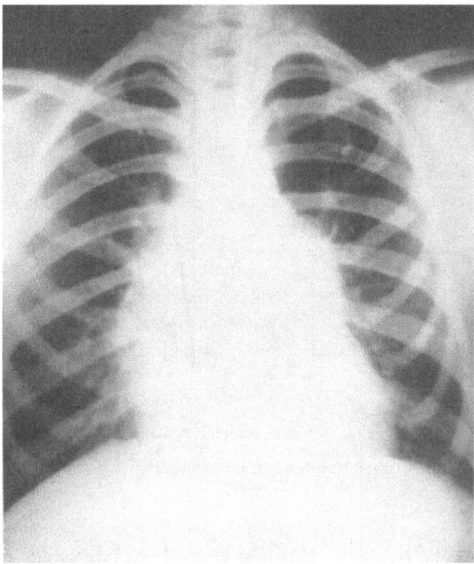

Fig. 2b. Chest radiograph of the same patient taken 18 months after splenectomy, showing reduction in heart size and smaller left pulmonary artery

systolic work of the right ventricle and doubtless contributes to the development of cor pulmonale. The picture of cardio-pulmonary bilharziasis, however, is more complex. In some cases there is an abnormally high oxygen saturation in the inferior or the superior vena cava. In one case the saturation was 14% higher in the inferior vena cava. However, when the spleen was removed and the patient catheterized 18 months later, there was a distinct change [6] (Figs. 2a and b). The pulmonary artery pressure dropped, the size of the heart was smaller and there was a reversal in the pattern of the E.C.G. which previously showed a severe right heart strain. Furthermore, the difference in the oxygen saturation fell to normal or 4% higher in the inferior vena cava.

In other words important vascular shunts exist between the portal circulation and the right heart in a manner that creates diastolic overloading of the right ventricle. The enlarged spleen presumably acts as an exaggerated arterio-venous fistula. The presence of these porto-caval communications was further demonstrated when radioactive Krypton[85] was injected into the spleen [16]. The isotope was recovered from an indwelling pulmonary artery catheter in 7—11 seconds (Fig. 3). In normal subjects the average period was 20—25 seconds. The short circuits join the vena cava either through transabdominal veins or by way

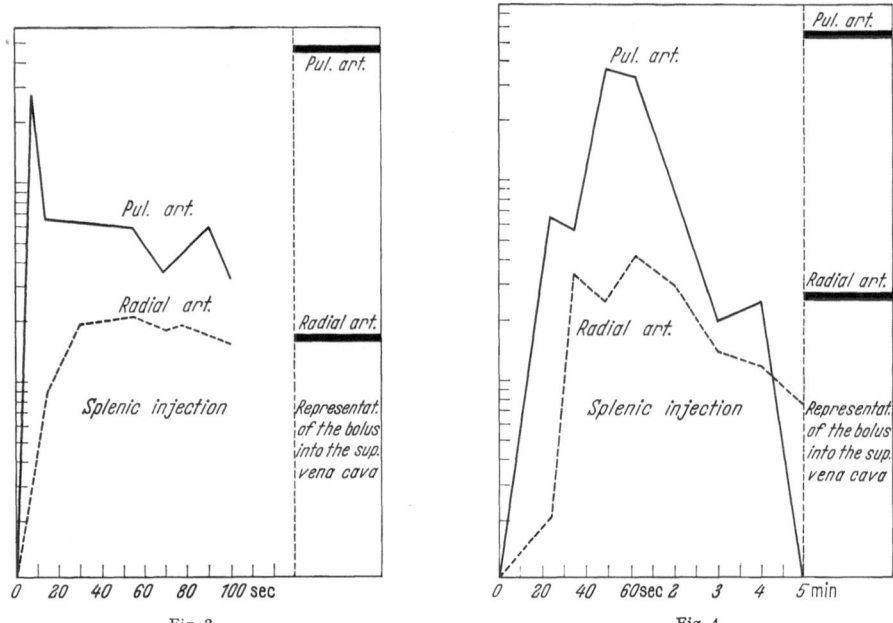

Fig. 3. A graph showing the high peak in the pulmonary artery 7 seconds after Krypton[85] followed by multiple peaks

Fig. 4. A graph showing the continuation of Krypton[85] in the systemic artery and its disappearance in the pulmonary artery

of various channels leading to the azygos veins. There may be an enormous pooling in the portal circulation as shown by the continuous discharge of the isotope for over 5 minutes in the pulmonary artery [16] (Fig. 4). It was also found that there was no relation between the portal pressure as measured from a splenic puncture and the size of the spleen or the liver or the occurrence of hematemesis [10]. It looked as if the pressure in the portal circulation represented the outcome of a race between splenic excessive flow and the shunts that by-pass the blood to the vena cava against the hepatic obstruction. These portacaval shunts doubtless provide an easy route for showers of bilharzia ova to the lungs leading to the ultimate picture of porto-pulmonary bilharziasis.

About 10% of cases of porto-pulmonary bilharziasis show an arterial oxygen saturation of 94% or lower [10] which is not corrected to complete saturation on 100% oxygen inhalation. This finding is rather mysterious, since a Krypton[85]

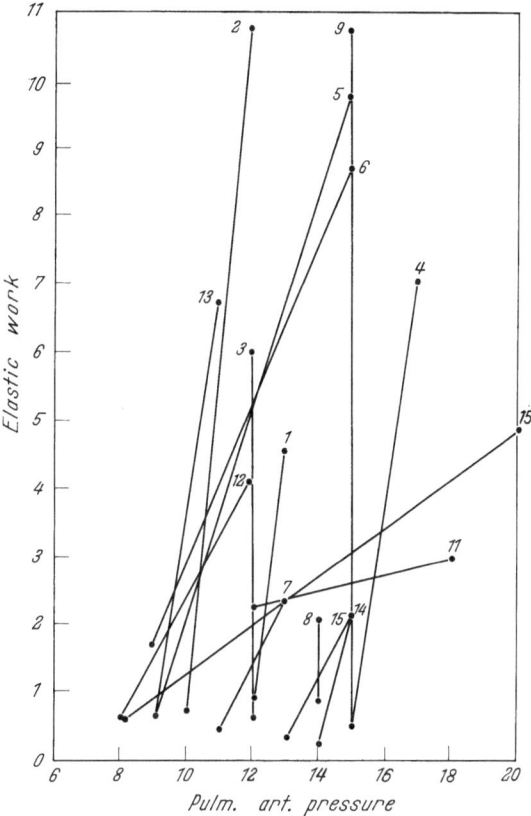

Fig. 5a. Elastic work at rest and during exercise in Bilharzial non cor-pulmonale patients in relation to mean pulmonary artery pressure

cum dye bolus injected in the superior vena cava and recovered within one circulation from the radial artery according to the method of FRITTS and COURNAND [7] showed in only 2 cases out of 15 a pulmonary artery-pulmonary vein shunt of 10% [16]. The others were within the normal range or nearly so; the highest being 5.7%. When a similar dose of Krypton[85] was injected in the spleen and samples were taken from the radial artery thereafter, evidence for portal vein-pulmonary vein shunting was revealed as follows:

1. An equal or even a higher concentration of the Krypton[85] in the radial artery after splenic injection than when a corresponding dose was injected in the superior vena cava. (Fig. 3,4)

2. The persistence of Krypton[85] in the radial artery after the isotope had been exhausted from the pulmonary artery following the splenic injection. (Fig. 4)

The failure of the arterial oxygen saturation to be fully corrected on 100% oxygen inhalation is quite disturbing. The plasma is capable of carrying an extra 1.5 vols percent at 500 mm Hg. of oxygen tension in the alveolar air. This concentration should be capable of raising the oxygen saturation 8% if all the circulation crossed the pulmonary alveoli [3]. Cardiopulmonary bilharziasis is usually attended with hypervolemia even after correction of the anaemia [5]. Either the portal vein-pulmonary vein shunt is much greater than at present conceived or the hypoxia is due to some other factor which prevents the red cells from being

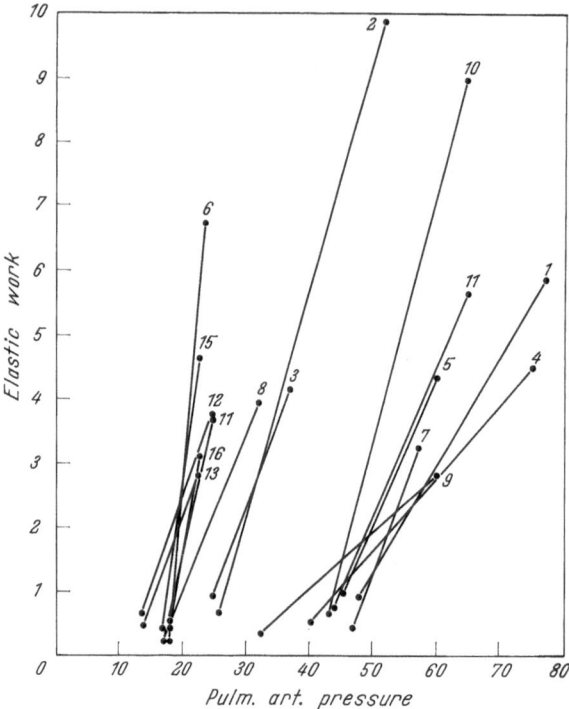

Fig. 5b. Elastic work at rest and during exercise in Bilharzial cor-pulmonale and in relation to mean pulmonary artery pressure

fully oxygenated in the brief interval in which they cross the capillary alveolar interface. Since patients with bilharzial hepato-splenomegaly exhibit low cholinesterase activity [10], atropine was injected i. v. and the blood was tested every minute for 5 minutes. It failed to improve but when it was exposed to room air it immediately rose to 100% saturation. Thus the problem of hypoxia remains to be solved.

Porto-pulmonary bilharziasis is a serious handicap to human energy. Patients as a rule hyperventilate at rest and exhibit a high ventilatory equivalent [1]. Furthermore, they experience severe dyspnea on effort which incapacitates them to a high degree. A study of pulmonary functions including hyperventilation and on exercise were undertaken and these were correlated with the prevailing pulmonary artery pressures at rest and on excersie [13].

At rest the tidal volume was relatively smaller than the average normal but the breathing was more rapid. This reduction in depth and increase in rate may have been selected as the most economical mechanism to compensate for the increased work of the ventilatory bellows under circumstances of diminshed lung compliance (consistently low in the group as a whole), irrespective of pulmonary artery pressures [13]. Vital capacity is undoubtedly decreased by the enlarged liver and spleen which are compressed and serrated against the lower ribs [1]. All of the cases showed a ratio of dead space to tidal volume of 1:2. The alveolar ventilation, however, either remained unaltered or was raised [13]. In this respect bilharzial ova deposition in the lungs resembles pulmonary micro-embolization from other sources, that is a state of hyperventilation without a corresponding perfusion [4]. This is further illustrated by an arterial-alveolar carbon dioxide gradient of 4—7 mm Hg. higher in the systemic artery [8]. The dyspnea of porto-pulmonary bilharziasis cannot be explained by an increase in the ammonia content of the blood as may be found in Laennec cirrhosis [9], since the ammonia levels are not raised in bilharziasis to stimulate the respiratory centre [11]. Furthermore, the low partial pressure of oxygen in the arterial blood is not of the order that excites the respiratory center and does not explain the dyspnea or the reduced tidal volume.

Table 1. *Percentage of the O_2 cost of breathing from total of O_2 uptake*

Case No.	1	2	3	4	5	6	7	8	9	Mean %
Cor-pulmonal	12	14	8	8	26	7	9			12 %
Non-cor-pulmonal	10	14	14	8	9	10	7	8	5	9.4 %

Normal values 1—3%.

The elastic work of breathing showed a definite increase at rest, as most of the cases revealed figures beyond 0.30 kg meter/minute [13]. This elastic work underwent a steep rise on effort irrespective of the pressures that obtained in the pulmonary artery either at rest or on exercise (Fig. 5a and b). The oxygen debt was about double the normal when the pulmonary artery pressure was physiological and more than triple that value with cor pulmonale [13]. The percent-

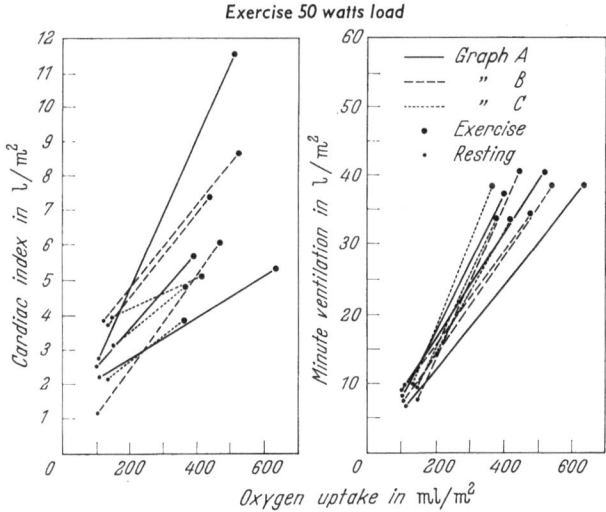

Fig. 6. Graph showing the relation between cardiac index, O_2 consumption and minute ventilation. Graph *A:* Normal pressures at rest and exercise; Graph *B:* Normal pressure at rest with high exercise; Graph *C:* High pressure at rest and higher exercise

3*

age of the total cost of breathing to the total oxygen uptake rises in the latter group to a level of 9--12% of the total oxygen consumed instead of a normal 1—3 % (Table 1). This obtains in the absence of obstructive airway disease. The relation between cardiac index, oxygen consumption and the corresponding in-

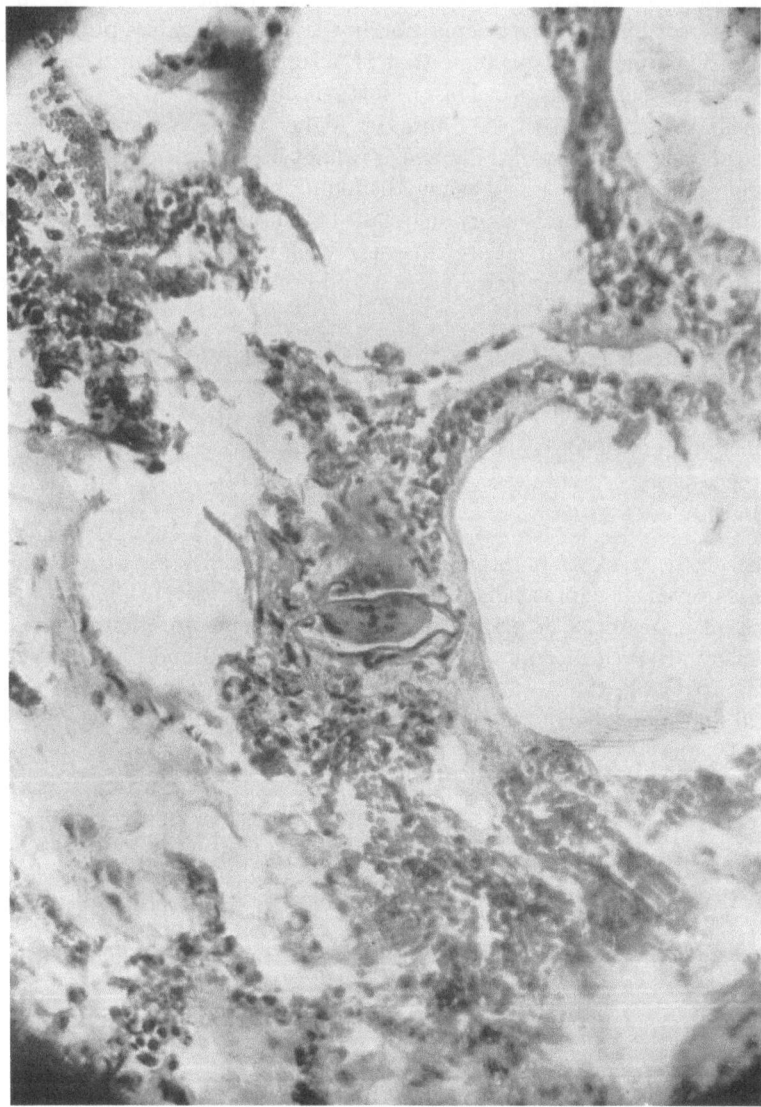

Fig. 7. Early bilharzial reaction with chronic inflammatory cells and fresh eggs

crease in ventilation is a very complex formula (Fig. 6). When the resting pulmonary artery pressure was initially high and was raised further on a standard exercise of 50 watts, the cardiac output was restricted to 5—6 l/minute but the ventilation increased enormously to 35 or 40 l/min at a relatively low oxygen consumption, in a range of 400—650 cc/minute [13]. Ordinarily an amount of

40 l/min ventilation in a normal person would have accounted for 2 litres or so of oxygen consumption/min on a much bigger load.

In this advanced group of bilharzial cor pulmonale the pulmonary compliance was particularly low at rest and it diminished further on exercise but the rate of

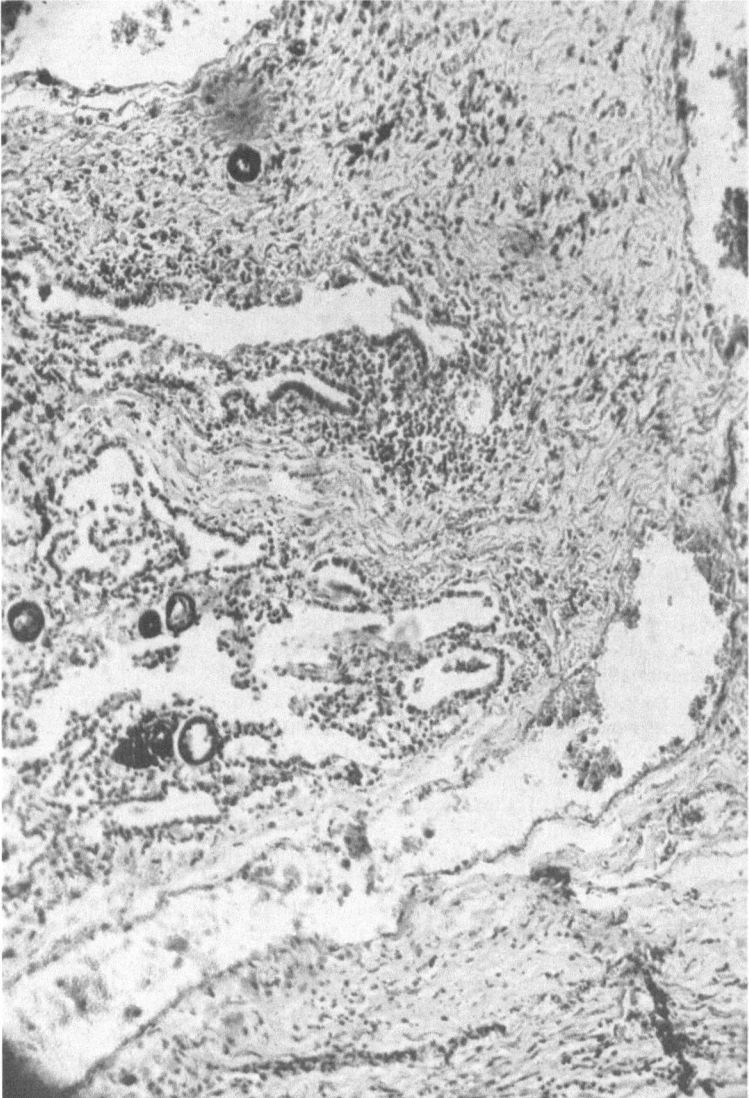

Fig. 8. Alveoli lined by cuboidal epithelium, note calcified eggs and marked interstitial fibrosis

fall of the compliance between the two states was insignificant if compared with another group in whom the pulmonary artery pressures were still normal. It seemed that the rigidity of the vascular and perivascular bed had already reached the limit, and was responsible for the reduced compliance of the lung as a whole. Since the vascular compliance was at its lowest, any increase in flow did not exert its usual widening effect in spite of the increase in the transluminal pressure [14]. The wedge pulmonary pressure is normal in cardiopulmonary bilharziasis and any change reflects only the arterial side of the pulmonary circulation and its vascular resistance [3]. My friend, Prof. Gazayerli kindly lent me Figs. 7 and 8. These show obvious pulmonary parenchymatous lesions of bilharziasis, which have not received due prominence before, but which do provide the anatomical basis for the uniform reduction of lung compliance in all forms of cardiopulmonary bilharziasis.

Bilharzia is a small parasite but it causes a serious widespread economic waste in many parts of the world. The efforts of the host to develop a multiplicity of self correcting mechanisms can simulate many congenital or acquired diseases of various etiologies. Man here is the subject of a natural experiment and it behooves us to study him and nature's methods in her attempt to preserve the integrated survival of the living whole.

References

[1] Ashba, J. K.: Pulmonary functions in cardiopulmonary schistosomiasis. M. D. thesis. Alexandria University (1959).

[2] Azmy, S., and S. Effat: Pulmonary arteriosclerosis of a bilharzial nature. J. Egypt. Med. Ass. 15, 87—90 (1932).

[3] Comroe, J. H. jr., R. E. Forster, A. B. Dubois, W. A. Briscoe, and E. Carlsen: The lung clinical physiology and pulmonary function tests. 2nd Ed. Chicago: Year Book Medical Publishers Inc. (1962).

[4] Cugell, D. W.: Measurement of alveolar ventilation, alveolar gas composition and pulmonary dead spaces. In: Advances in cardiopulmonary diseases. 1, 28—37. A. L. Banyai and B. L. Gorden (Eds.). Chicago. Year Book Medical Publishers Inc. 1963.

[5] Foda, M. T.: Haemodynamics in bilharzial cor-pulmonary. M. D. thesis. University of Alexandria (1959).

[6] —, and H. A. Zaki: Pulmonary haemodynamics in schistosoma cor-pulmonale before and after splenectomy. Egypt. J. Chest Dis. Tuberc. 2, 1 (1959).

[7] Fritts, H. W., A. Hardewig, D. F. Rochester, J. Durand, and A. Cournand: Estimation of pulmonary arteriovenous shunts flow using intravenous injections of T-1828 and Kr 85. J. Clin. Invest. 39, 1841—1850 (1960).

[8] Gemei, Y.: Unpublished data.

[9] Heinemann, H. O.: Respiration and circulation in patients with portal cirrhosis of the liver. Circulation 22, 154—159 (1960).

[10] Khalil, M.: Study of the nature of oxygen unsaturation in cases of bilharzial hepatosplenomegaly. M. D. thesis, University of Alexandria (1962).

[11] El Khanagry, H. A. Fahmy, M. H. Ghanem, and Y. Seddik: Ammonia tolerance in bilharzial hepato-splenomegaly. Alexandria Med. J. 7, 256—262 (1961).

[12] Shaw, A. F. B., and A. A. Ghareeb: The pathogenesis of pulmonary schistosomiasis in Egypt with special reference to Ayerza's disease. J. Path. Bact. 46, 401—424 (1938).

[13] Tarabeih, Ali A.: Mechanics of breathing in cardiopulmonary bilharziasis. M. D. thesis. Alexandria University (1965).

[14] Zaky, H. A.: Aneurysm of the pulmonary artery due to schistosomiasis. Dis. Chest 21, 194—204 (1952).

[15] —, El Heneidy, A. R. and M. T. Foda, Hemodynamic shunts in schistosomal cor pulmonale. Brit. Med J. 1, 367—369 (1962).

[16] — —, and M. Khalil: Use of Kr[85] in the study of hypoxia in portopulmonary bilharziasis (schistosomiasis). Brit. Med. J. 1, 1021—1024 (1964).

[17] — —, Tawfik, T. M.. Y. Gemei, and A. Khadr, Bronchopulmonary shunts in schistosomial cor-pulmonale. Dis. Chest 36: 164-172, (1959).

Pathological Aspects of Bilharziasis in Egypt

Anwar M. Elwi*

General incidence

The general incidence of bilharziasis in autopsy material is currently 44 to 45%. Examination of our autopsy records of the years 1903—1908 showed an incidence of 14%. The increased incidence of bilharziasis is attributed to the introduction and increased use of the perennial system of irrigation.

General pathology

The pathological lesions of bilharziasis are produced by cercariae, adult schistosomes of the mansoni and haematobium species and ova deposited by the latter and retained in the tissues of the host.

1. Cercariae

Cercariae are known to produce erythematous, petechial and even papular eruptions at their site of penetration through the skin. Such lesions are rarely noted in Egyptian patients.

2. Adult schistosomes

Adult schistosomes do not produce lesions in their vascular habitat. However, dead worms produce thrombophlebitis and necrosis of the surrounding tissues in the liver and the lungs.

3. Ova

Ova trapped into the tissues bring about the development of a granuloma which contain macrophages, foreign body giant cells, lymphocytes and plasma cells. Very often, eosinophils take a part in the tissue reaction. Necrosis of the cellular infiltrate or the parenchymatous cells may be noted rarely but such a feature is certainly insignificant. The ova which fail to be removed by the phagocytic action of macrophages undergo calcification and remain embedded in the fibrous tissue which replaces the granuloma. Fresh lesions continue to develop as long as the schistosomes live. Different stages of the bilharzial granuloma are often encountered simultaneously in one and the same lesion.

The extent of the damage to the tissues is proportional to the number of ova trapped inside them and this in turn depends on the number and species of the schistosomes. The ova laid by *S. haematobium* are twenty times more plentiful than those of *S. mansoni*.

Ova of *S. mansoni* produce lesions primarily in the intestine but those which fail to engage in the walls of the mesenteric vessels are carried by the blood as

---

* Department of Pathology, Cairo University, Cairo, Egypt, UAR.

emboli to the liver, gall bladder and pancreas where they produce lesions. Ova
of *S. haematobium* produce lesions primarily in the urinary bladder, ureters,
urethra, seminal vesicles, prostate, spermatic cord, testis, vulva, vagina, uterus,
uterine tubes and ovaries (Table 1). Embolic ova of *S. haematobium* are filtered
in the lungs but some of them may by-pass the lungs and reach different parts of
the body. The ectopic sites in which lesions produced by ova *S. haematobium*
may be found include the skin, conjunctivae, spinal cord, brain, heart, thyroid,
adrenals and vocal cords but all such lesions are exceedingly rare.

Table 1. *Common sites of bilharzial lesions and their incidence in autopsy material*

Organ	%
Intestine	60
Liver	22
Bladder	90
Ureters	44
Lungs	21

Intestinal bilharziasis

Bilharzial lesions of the intestine are caused by *Schistosoma mansoni* infection.
84% of the bilharzial intestines do not show significant gross changes and are
diagnosed by finding ova in paraffin sections of scrapings from the rectal mucosa.

Gross lesions in the form of sandy patches of the mucosa and induration of the
wall occurs in 16% of the bilharzial intestines and are found mostly in the rectum
which receives the largest number of ova.

Sandy patches develop in long standing cases when the submucosa becomes
densely thickened by fibrous tissue containing immense number of ova; the overlying mucosa become atrophic and thereby acquires a dirty yellowish colouration.
Ulceration of the atrophic epithelium occurs particularly on tops of the mucosal
folds.

Bilharzial polypi occur in half of the cases showing sandy patches. A rich mass
of bilharzial granuloma develops in the submucosa and gradually elevates the
mucosa. The latter develops adenomatoid hyperplasia and intense mucoid activity
in 44% of the polyps. Polyps of long duration show less hyperplasia and more
fibrosis of the supporting tissue.

Relation of intestinal bilharziasis to carcinoma: Carcinoma of the rectum is
associated with intestinal bilharziasis in 35% of the cases [5]. The possibility that
bilharziasis may be a factor in the development of rectal cancer has been raised
many workers. Our study of carcinoma of the recto-colon with and without bilharziasis showed no striking difference between the two groups apart from the
inclusion of ova in the neoplastic tissue [5].

Bilharziasis of the appendix: One-fifth of appendices removed at operation
showed evidence of bilharziasis. The bilharzial granuloma and fibrosis caused
stenosis of the appendicular lumen in about one-third of the bilharzial group.
Acute suppurative inflammation complicated 24% of the appendices of this group
[9]. The lumen of the appendix was markedly dilated distal to the stenosis indicating an increased intraluminal pressure of such a magnitude as to cause symptoms
of appendicular obstruction. Dense appendicular adhesions containing ova were

found in 30% of the bilharzial appendices. Appendicular adhesions are accepted as a cause of appendicular pain and thus their development in 30% of the bilharzial appendices appears to be significant.

Bilharziasis of the liver: Bilharzial lesions of the liver are encountered in 37% of cases of intestinal bilharziasis. Embolic ova escape into the intrahepatic radicles of the portal veins where they produce a granulomatous reaction followed by fibrosis. 55% of the bilharzial livers show no gross changes and the lesions are diagnosed by microscopic examination of tissue. 45% of the bilharzial livers show gross changes characteristic of bilharzial hepatic fibrosis or cirrhosis. Hepatic degeneration, necrosis, regeneration and disruption of the lobular architecture are absent and thus the term bilharzial hepatic fibrosis is preferable to that of cirrhosis. Bilharzial cases constitute 50% of current cases of cirrhosis at autopsy in contrast to only 26% in the years 1903—1908.

Bilharzial hepatic fibrosis is classified as coarse or fine type, depending on whether the large or the small portal tracts are mainly involved [11]. The ratio of the coarse to the fine type of bilharzial cirrhosis is 6 : 5.

The coarse type of bilharzial hepatic fibrosis, first described by SYMMERS [15], had long been considered to result from a very heavy intestinal infection but there had been always the difficulty in explaining how so many ova could pass through the walls of the large portal veins instead of passing along the blood stream to small portal veins. The recent work of ELIAS and POPPER [6] on the vasculature of the liver shows that marginal veins arise from the large veins and run parallel with them in the same portal canal. Small venules arise from these marginal veins and drain into adjacent liver lobules. Such a vascular pattern allows the embolism of heavy numbers of ova in and around the large portal tracts and the development of the coarse type of bilharzial hepatic fibrosis.

Some workers attributed the coarse bilharzial hepatic fibrosis to the death of a large number of worms following intensive antibilharzial treatment. The dead worms are carried to the intrahepatic portal veins where they produce thrombophlebitis which leads to fibrosis of the large portal tracts. This is not a common finding in our material and when it is seen, the portal tracts appear to have been markedly thickened by fibrous tissue containing many calcified ova long before the shift of dead schistosomes to the liver. Moreover, thrombophlebitis can hardly explain the uniform thickening of the whole course of the portal veins.

The fine type of bilharzial hepatic fibrosis was first described by DAY twenty years after the recognition of the coarse type [4]. Its pathogenesis was beset with some difficulty because of the scanty number of ova which can be recognized in the lesions. Many ova are certainly destroyed and removed and in many fields none may be seen in the residual fibrous tissue. The diagnosis of the coarse type of bilharzial fibrosis by needle biopsy is fairly easy but that of the fine type is difficult because of the scantiness of the ova.

Many portal veins are completely destroyed by the bilharzial granuloma. Small and medium sized veins may show intimal proliferation and subintimal thickening [2]. These lesions of the portal veins obstruct the intrahepatic flow of the portal blood and thereby portal hypertension becomes established in the late stages of both types. The resulting chronic venous congestion perpetuates the initial enlargement of the organ induced by bilharzial antigenic stimulation.

Chronic venous congestion of the spleen results in the formation of fibrosiderotic nodules and diffuse or focal subcapsular hemorrhages. Patches of perisplenitis develop over the hemorrhagic lesions and when healing occurs adhesions may bind the spleen to the diaphragm, liver, stomach, omentum, pancreas and other structures in the neighborhood.

The development of portal hypertension results in the opening and dilatation of many anastomotic vessels between the portal and systemic veins. Such collaterals compensate for the obstruction of the flow of the portal blood through the liver. Oesophageal varices are found in 40% of autopsies of bilharzial hepatic fibrosis. Eventually decompensation sets in and ascites develops. Patients die from hepatic failure or severe haematemesis. Such an event was noted in 20% of the cases only. Cor pulmonale due to pulmonary bilharziasis was responsible for the fatal outcome in 20% of cases of bilharzial hepatic fibrosis while 60% of the cases died from rheumatic heart disease, malignant tumors and pyelonephritis.

Bilharziasis of the urinary system

Bilharziasis of the bladder is mainly due to *Schistosoma haematobium* infection [13]. 31% of the bilharzial bladders do not show significant gross changes and are identified only after microscopic examination of paraffin sections.

Gross lesions in the form of sandy patches occur mostly in the postero-superior wall and near the ureteric openings. Bilharzial polyps of the urinary bladder have the same pathogenesis as their colonic analogues but they are fewer in number and are more restricted in distribution. Some polyps attain such a size that they are indistinguishable by the naked eye from tumors. Small superficial ulcers, not usually exceeding 1 cm in diameter, occur at the superior and posterosuperior parts of the bladder (3%). Extensive fibrosis of the whole wall of the bladder may lead to marked contraction of the organ (1%) whereas fibrosis of the neck obstructs the flow of urine and leads to the development of hydroureters and hydronephrosis (2%).

Table 2. *Incidence of bilharzial lesions of the urinary bladder and ureters*

Lesion	Urinary Bladder %	Ureter %
Sandy patches	69	27
Polyps	17	15
Cystic changes	6	9

Carcinoma develops in 9% of the bilharzial bladders. Bilharzial carcinoma of the bladder occurs at a relatively younger age and is seen on the lateral wall, posterior wall, anterior wall, vault and trigone, in that order of frequency [13]. Grossly, the tumor takes usually a polypoid (88%) or an ulcerative form (8%). Chronic inflammation of the bladder and the resulting metaplasia of the mucosa influence the histological picture which is that of squamous cell carcinoma (58.5%) transitional cell carcinoma (25.2%), anaplastic carcinoma (10.2%) or adenocarcinoma (4.6%). Lymphatic spread of the tumor occurs in 30% of the cases while haematogenous spread is exceedingly rare [8].

FERGUSON [10] was the first to point to the high frequency of carcinoma in Egypt and its causal relationship to urinary bilharziasis. Both assumptions have been the subject of many clinical and pathological studies which are summarized by GAZAYERLI [7]. Biochemical studies of the problem have yielded very interesting findings. ABUL-FADL and METWALLI [1] reported an elevated B-glucuronidase content in the living *Schistosoma haematobium* obtained from fresh infected urines, and they reported in 1963 [2] an increase in urinary B-glucuronidase enzyme activity in bilharzial infection and a more marked increase in bladder cancer. KHALAFALLAH and ABUL-FADL [12] studied the urinary excretion of tryptophan metabolites after giving a loading dose and concluded that the excretion pattern in cases of bilharzial bladder cancer appears so far to be close to that described by other workers for the industrial bladder cancer.

Bilharziasis of the lungs

Lesions produced by ova: The embolic ova produce acute necrotizing arteriolitis after which they escape outside the vessels and produce small parenchymatous lesions hardly visible to the naked eye. Ova from such lesions may reach the alveoli and appear in the sputum. The traumatized vessels heal by fibrocellular thickening of the intima and some vessels may become occluded. Widespread occlusion of the pulmonary vessels occurs in cases of heavy schistosomal infection; the fibrocellular tissue in their lumen is richly vascularized by newly formed capillaries "angiomatoids". Some angiomatoids may appear outside the vessels. Pulmonary hypertension results in dilation of the pulmonary artery and its main branches and hypertrophy of the right ventricles [14]; the dilation of the pulmonary artery may reach aneurysmal proportions. Congestive cardiac failure occured in 2% of all cases of bilharziasis and in 10% of the pulmonary group; half of the cases had advanced bilharzial hepatic fibrosis.

Lesions produced by adult Schistosomes: Dead schistosomes carried as emboli to the lungs produce necrosis of the pulmonary arteries and focal necrotizing pneumonia in the immediate vicinity (3% in all cases of bilharziasis and 14% of cases of pulmonary bilharziasis).

References

[1] ABUL-FADL, M. A. M., and O. M. METWALLI: The β-glucuronidase activity in the ova of human schistosomiasis. Proceedings of International Symposium on Bilharziasis. Cairo, U.A.R., 1962.
[2] — — Studies on certain urinary and blood serum enzymes in bilharziasis and their possible relation to bladder cancer in Egypt. Brit. J. Cancer 15, 137—141 (1963).
[3] AIDAROS, S. M., and A. M. SOLIMAN: Portal vascular changes in human bilharzial cirrhosis. J. Path. Bact. 82, 19—22 (1961).
[4] DAY, H. B.: The aetiology of Egyptian Splenomegaly and hepatic cirrhosis. Trans. Roy. Soc. Trop. Med. Hyg. 18, 121—130 (1924).
[5] DIMETTE, R. M., A. M. ELWI, and H. F. SPROAT: Relationship of schistosomiasis to polyposis and adenocarcinoma of large intestine. Amer. J. Clin. Path. 26, 266—276 (1956).
[6] ELIAS, H., and H. POPPER: Venous distributions. Livers. Arch. Path. 59, 332—340 (1955).
[7] EL-GAZAYERLI, M.: The relationship of environment to cancer in Egypt. Int. Path. 4, 37—40 (1963).
[8] EL-SIBAI, I.: Cancer of bladder in Egypt. Kasr-El-Aini J. Surg. 2, 183—241 (1961).

[9] Elwi, A. M., and I. El-Torai: Bilharziasis of the appendix. J. Egypt. Med. Ass. 38, 311—326 (1955).
[10] Ferguson, A. R.: Associated bilharziasis and primary malignant disease of the urinary bladder with observations on a series of forty cases. J. Path. Bact. 16, 76—94 (1911).
[11] Hashem, M.: The aetiology and pathogenesis of the endemic form of hepato-spleno-megaly: Egyptian splenomegaly. J. Egypt. Med. Ass. 30, 48—79 (1947).
[12] Khalafallah, A. S., and M. A. M. Abul-Fadl: Studies on the urinary excretion of certain tryptophan metabolites before and after tryptophan loading dose in bilhar-ziasis, bilharzial bladder cancer and certain other types of malignancies in Egypt. Brit. J. Cancer 18, 592—604 (1964).
[13] Makar, N.: Urological aspects of bilharziasis in Egypt, p. 208. Cairo: S.O.P. 1951.
[14] Shaw, A. F. B., and A. Ghareeb: The pathogenesis of pulmonary schistosomiasis in Egypt with special reference to ayerza's disease. J. Path. Bact. 46, 401—424 (1938).
[15] Symmers, W. St. C.: Note on a new form of liver cirrhosis due to the presence of the ova of bilharzia haematobia. J. Path. Bact. 9, 237—239 (1904).

Some Clinicopathological Aspects of Urinary Bilharziasis

N. MAKAR*

With 7 figures

Since BILHARZ [1] discovered Schistosoma worms in the portal veins of a young Egyptian cadaver, May 1851, bilharziasis, named in his honor, has been reported in almost every organ of the human body.

The manifestations of the disease in the urinary tract are mostly due to infection with the haematobial worms. The bladder and ureters are the organs which receive the brunt of bilharzial infestations in man; thus it seems plausible to focus one's present discussions on their clinical aspects, referring to some of their pathological backgrounds for further elucidation.

Incidence

According to SCOTT [16], "Schistosoma haematobium infests 60 percent of the people in the Delta and those parts of the Nile Valley under perennial irrigation, but only 5 percent of the people in the districts with basin irrigation".

At present, most of the agricultural land is under perennial irrigation and the aforementioned percentage is likely to be higher despite improvement in sanitation and hygienic equipment. At any rate, it is safe to say that about half the present inhabitants of Egypt are subject to urinary bilharziasis.

Age

No age is exempt from bilharziasis; children and adolescents are among its common victims; its highest incidence rate lies between 20 and 30 years of age. It is met with in the middle-aged as a recrudescence of previous infection and, less commonly, a primary one. In the old, it is rare; those who reach the age of 60 years have usually the landmarks of cured mild infestations.

Sex

The ratio of bilharzia incidence in the rural female to that of the male peasant is about 1 to 4, respectively, at all ages. As children, both sexes are equally exposed to infection.

During her adolescence and until her marriage, a period of a few years, the peasant girl is usually kept within doors and runs a smaller risk of infection than the peasant boy. As a wife, her chances of bilharzial infestation are somewhat mitigated by her frequent pregnancies and confinements; however, her daily visits to the village canal, paddling in its cercariae-infested water to fill her water vessels or bathe her children or wash the family linen, bring her in close contact with the source of bilharzial infestation.

* Department of Urology, Cairo University Cairo, Cairo, Egypt UAR

On the other hand, the male peasant (fellah), pursuing his field activities under all sorts of weather and for long hours with feet and arms immersed in contaminated water, is more exposed to repeated bilharzial infestation than his wife.

The incidence of the disease in towns is different, the ratio being 6.8% school girls to 93.2% school boys [3].

Symptoms and signs

The clinical picture of bilharziasis depends on the stage reached by the disease. It is uncommon to see its initial symptoms in Egyptians. FAIRLEY [4] described the early symptoms in the Australian troops who contracted bilharziasis in Egypt during the First World War. Severe itching at the site of cercarial skin penetration is the earliest symptom. About 3 weeks later the patient complains of urticaria, headaches, malaise, cough, pains in the abdomen, tenderness over the liver, spleen, intestines and also some joints. The evening temperature may rise from half a degree to 40 C. (104 F.), sometimes simulating that of typhoid fever; unusually, it may be normal. Blood examination reveals anemia (chlorosis), leucocytosis with a relatively high eosinophilia (50% or more). Such symptoms are due to toxemia [4], and are followed 2 to 4 months later, the time taken by the worms in migrating to the lower urinary organs, by those of bladder invasion, namely, haematuria, dysuria and painful frequent micturation.

1. Haematuria

Before the discovery of the worms, French authors and others had spoken of Egypt as the "Land of menstruating men"; and indeed, until recently, haematuria was considered by young bilharzial patients as a sign of virility.

This predominant sign varies in its severity and duration, being appreciable in the acute stages, less so in subacute ones, and dwindling, almost to disappearing, in chronic cases. It remains occult, detectable microscopically, for a long time. Opinions differ regarding its mode of production. The passage of innumerable bilharzial ova through a hyperaemic bladder mucous membrane has been suggested as the main cause of haematuria. The contractions of the bladder muscles on such a membrane together with its overlying granulomatous infiltrations seem to be also effective in its production. The fact that the haematuria is mostly terminal favors the latter explanation. The bleeding is usually slight unless aggravated by strenuous bodily exertion, riding on rough roads, or excessive heat or cold. Complications, due to secondary infection, ulceration or malignant changes occurring in the bladder mucosa, enhance the severity of haematuria and alter its terminal character into a total, more persistent and painful one.

2. Dysuria

Dysuria of varying intensity and duration is one of the chief complaints. In the early stages of the disease, the dysuria is brought about by spasm of the vesical sphincter and oedema of the covering mucous membrane; it is then mild and transient. In chronic cases dysuria may be due to bladder neck lesions obstructing the bladder outlet either by mechanical narrowing secondary to polypi, granulomata or fibrosis; or dynamic, due to functional impairment.

3. Pain

At first, a mere smarting towards the end of micturition pain is usually so insignificant that the patient may not complain of it; later, it varies in its intensity according to the occurrence of infection or other complications as mentioned before. Under these circumstances, the pain is felt throughout micturition and may be so severe as to lead the patient to assume different positions in trying to pass his urine. It is usually referred to the glans penis which is sometimes pinched by the patient in his endeavour to alleviate his suffering. It may also be felt over the bladder region or the rectum especially when these organs are not empty.

4. Pollakuria

Pollakuria occurs in the acute stage from congestion of the bladder and heigh-tened excitability of its mucosa. It is more marked at night. The prolonged, strong, muscular activity, which the peasant's or laborers' day work entails, reduces the vesical congestion and diminishes the pollakuria. In chronic cases, the degree of pollakuria depends on the conditions that obtain in the bladder

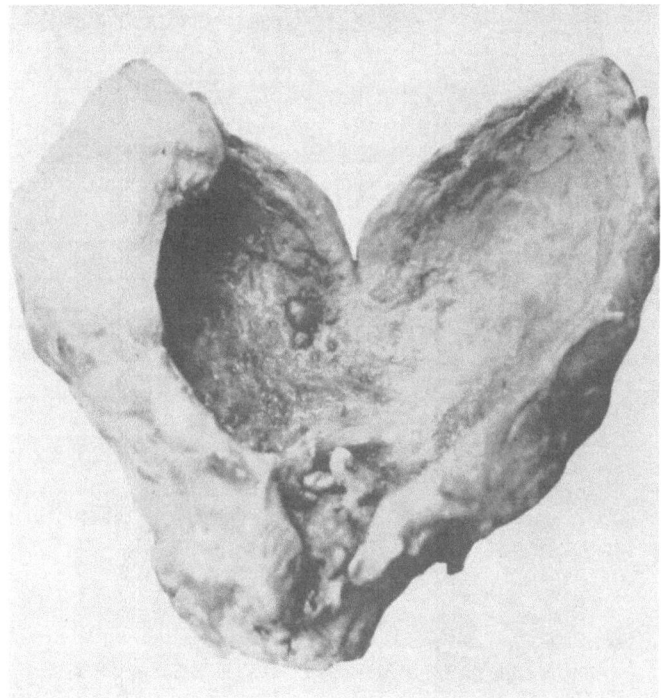

Fig. 1. A photograph of a postmortem specimen showing severe bilharzial fibrosis of the bladder wall and an atrophied mucosa covered with calcified bilharzial polypi and nodules causing obstruction at its neck

muscles and its mucosa. Generally speaking, fibrosis and sometimes also calcification affect the vesical muscles leading to reduction in the vesical capacity and consequently increased frequency of micturition. Sometimes, however, the involvement of the neck with chronic bilharzial infiltration, giving rise to urinary obstruction, is such that the fibrosed inelastic detrusor muscle stretches under

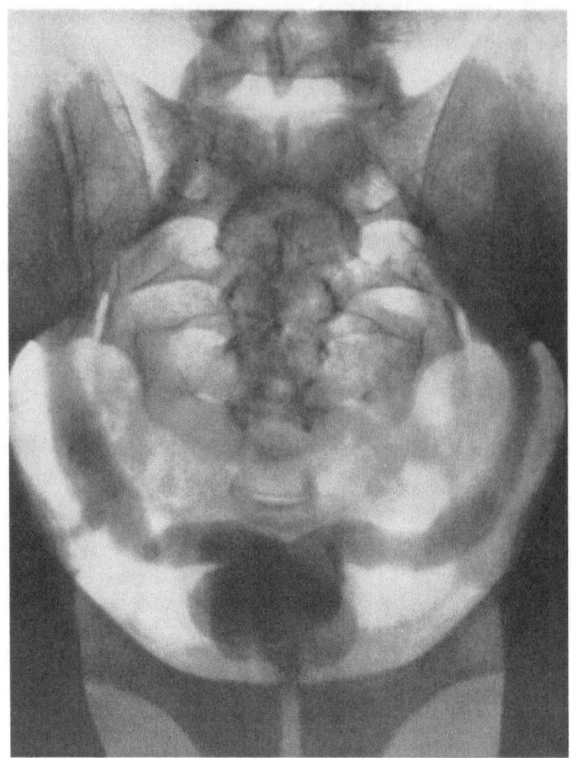

Fig. 2. Severe bilharzial fibrosis of the urinary bladder wall leading to marked reduction in its capacity and dilatation of the ureters which are also infiltrated with bilharziasis

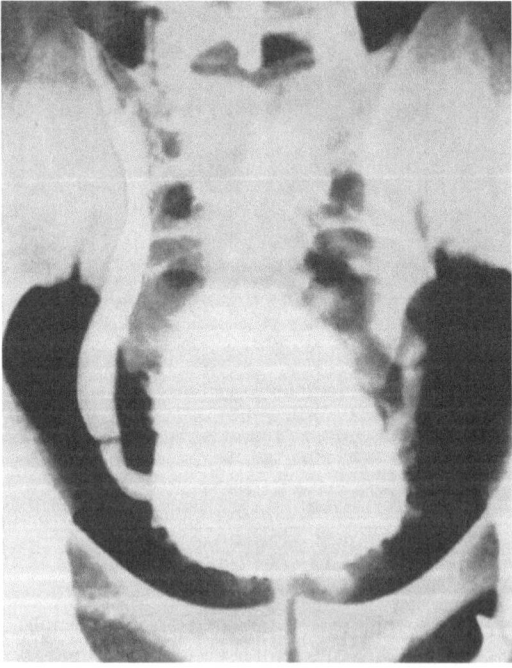

Fig. 3. Ascending cytograms showing crenations in the contour of the bladder wall and regurgitation of injected fluid into the dilated bilharzial ureters due to obstruction at the internal urinary meatus by bilharzial infiltration and fibrosis

the effects of back pressure and the atonic bladder distends on filling to reach higher levels than the normal. In such severe cases the clinical picture changes from pollakuria to the opposite, partial retention with dribbling (Figs. 1, 2 and 3).

Urine

The urine is at first acid, sterile and contains blood, ova and mucus. In later stages it becomes alkaline, turbid with pus, phosphates, blood cells and shreads of mucous membrane. Ova are few, mostly dead. In advanced cases, the urine acquires a strongly fishy or ammoniacal odor and contains a heavy deposit of pus and bilharzial debris. Secondary infection of the bilharzial bladder is a common complication in Egypt. The responsible micro-organisms are variable; E. coli predominating in early stages, streptococcus faecalis, staphylococcus and B. proteus in later ones. They reach the viscus through instrumentation or via blood and lymph channels from neighboring infected organs.

Cystoscopic appearances

Most of the signs of vesical bilharzial lesions can be detected by cytoscopy, particularly those that involve the submucosa and mucosa. The earliest is hyperemia of the mucous membrane which is not characteristic as it stimulates that of acute simple cystitis.

1. Bilharzial papules or tubercles mark the beginning of active invasion of the substantia propria and mucous membrane by the parasites. Pin-point, shiny vesicle-like tubercles surrounded by leashes or fine capillaries appear in different areas of the bladder mucosa, the base, trigone, especially in the vicinity of the ureteral orifices, the lateral walls and summit of the organ in this order of frequency.

Tubercles represent the smallest grouping of bilharzial elements and can be considered as a sure sign of activity of the disease.

2. Bilharzial nodules, bigger aggregations of bilharziomata, occur at about the same regions of the bladder as mentioned for tubercles but are not so shiny or vascular and are more lasting than these; unlike them, they are not affected by anti-bilharzial treatment but tend to undergo fibrosis and sometimes calcification (Fig. 4).

3. In advanced cases, the mucous membrane acquires a dull hazy ground-glass-like appearance which is due to its dimished vascularity brought about by peri-vascular fibrosis and endarteritis in the submucosa. The resulting atrophy of the mucous membrane may eventually convert it into a thin fibrous semi-transparent layer. Trauma or infection may lead to its ulceration.

4. Sandy patches. In very chronic bilharzial bladders, it is quite common to see cystoscopically, and also by the naked eye, through the thinned-out mucosa some calcified bilharzia ova lying beneath it, looking like "sand under water". This appearance of "sandy patches" is pathognomonic of bilharziasis wherever it is found, in the bladder, commonly, or elsewhere (Fig. 4).

5. Ulcers appear in the bilharzial bladder mucosa in different stages. In the acute stage, the occurrence of a small sized ulcer with thin margins, shallow pale-pink floor, lying in the vicinity of tubercles is not rare. As in the case of tubercles,

4 Bilharziasis

such superficial acute ulcers heal by appropriate medical treatment. The second more common, more distinct type of ulcer is the chronic one which develops later

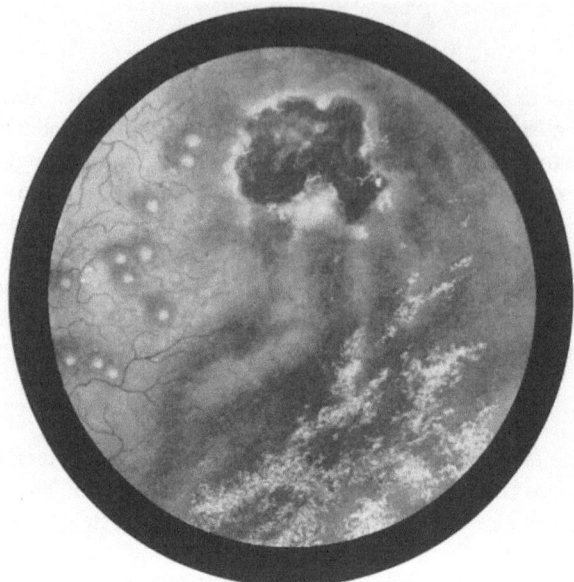

Fig. 4. Bilharzial nodules. Chronic bilharzial ulcer with densely fibrosed margin and calcific base. Sandy patch (on the right)

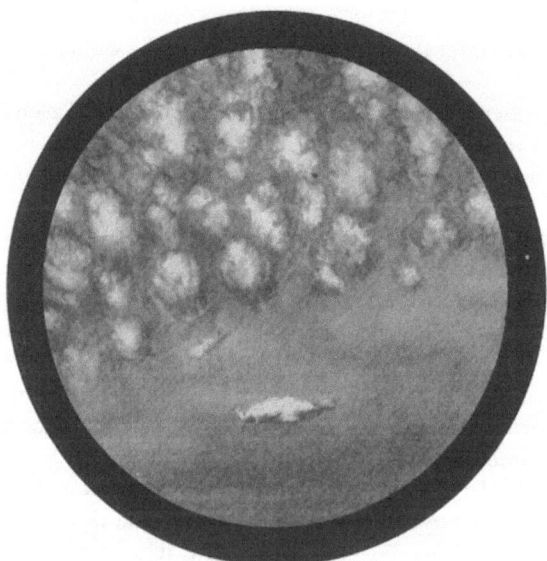

Fig. 5. Cystoscopic view of cystitis glandularis

in cases of severe bilharzial cystitis. Its usual site is the bladder-bas-fond slightly above its horizontal diameter to one side of the middle line (Fig. 4). Urinary stasis mostly brought about by bilharzial bladder-neck obstruction and resistant infection are the important etiological factors in its production. Varieties of forms and subdivisions have been mentioned by different authors in describing the chronic ulcerative processes found in the bilharzial bladder. Generally speaking, however, it may be said that this process is progressive and as long as the underlying causes remain untreated, it continues to extend in all directions, burrowing through the greater part of the muscular wall and also spreading at the expense of the mucosa. Fibrosis and sometimes calcification at its base are other factors which prevent healing. The presence of such ulcers aggravates all the symptoms of the disease. Haematuria and pain, intermittent, but of a severe nature occur in bouts. The urine contains bright red, sometimes clotted blood, and a lot of debris. Their persistence is an additional factor in chronic bladder epithelial irritation as can be deduced from the frequent occurrence of cystitis glandularis and cystica in the same bladder, and less commonly from that of squamous metaplasia, or carcinoma in the mucous membrane near the ulcers.

6. On the other hand, the bladder mucosa may respond to the invading parasites by hyperplasia. The submucous bilharziomata push on the mucous membrane until they protrude as polypi inside the vesical cavity. The covering epithelium undergoes hyperplastic changes resulting in thickening or infolding of some parts. The common sites for polypi are the relatively vascular regions of the bladder, e.g., those neighboring the ureteral orifices and internal meatus. In the fresh state, they are vascular, rosy looking buds. Later, they assume a dull brownish coloration and a more coarsely granular strawberry-like surface which may be spotted over with calcareous deposits. They vary in number and size, may be single or so numerous as to cover a wide area of the vesical cavity and as small as a pea, or as large as an almond. The consistency varies, at first somewhat elastic or fleshy, bleeding on cystoscopic touch, in time they shrivel into smaller friable mulberry-like bodies. Bilharzial polypi or papillomata rarely undergo malignant changes, thus differing remarkably from the non bilharzial variety. Situated at ureteral orifice or the vesical outlet they may cause obstruction to the outflow of urine. Sometimes they slough due to heavy infection leaving behind superficial ulcers; portions may break off to be later incorporated within phosphatic calculi. An old polyp may become encrusted, simulating a stone in appearance and showing signs of mucosal irritation in its vicinity.

7. The hyperplastic epithelium sometimes invaginates its deep layers into the submucosal strata as tubular processes or epithelial "cell nests" or it forms acinar-like pseudoglandular structures – "cystitis glandularis". These appear under the cysto scope as small fleshy-looking mamellated infiltrations embedded in the mucosa with their summits slightly raised above the surface (Fig. 5). Intermingled with these, more bouyant, shiny cysts "cystitis cystica" can be seen perching on the mucous membrane of the trigone and, less frequently, the posterior bladder wall.

Cystitis glandularis, benign per se, is indicative of severe epithelial irritation of the mucosa in which it lies, caused by chronic bilharziasis and infection often aggravated by concomitant urinary stasis. Cystitis glandularis is apt to regress or even disappear on appropriate therapy (Fig. 7). It is regarded by some as precancerous [9, 12, 18]; others accord it a transitory reparative function [13]. Its association with bladder cancer is fairly common in bilharzial cases (30%

4*

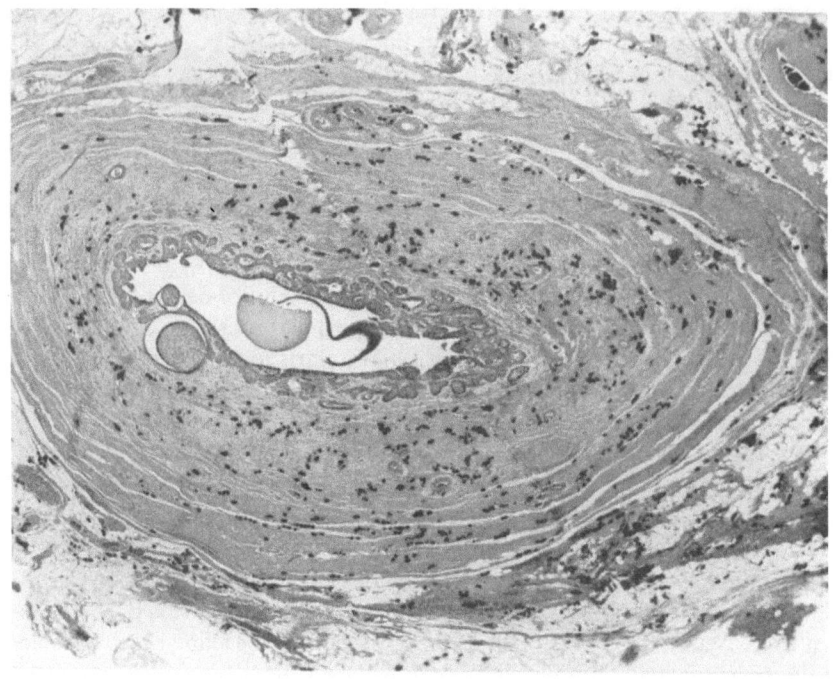

Fig. 6. Section of a bilharzial ureter showing pseudoglandular proliferation and invagination of its epithelium "ureteritis Glandularis"

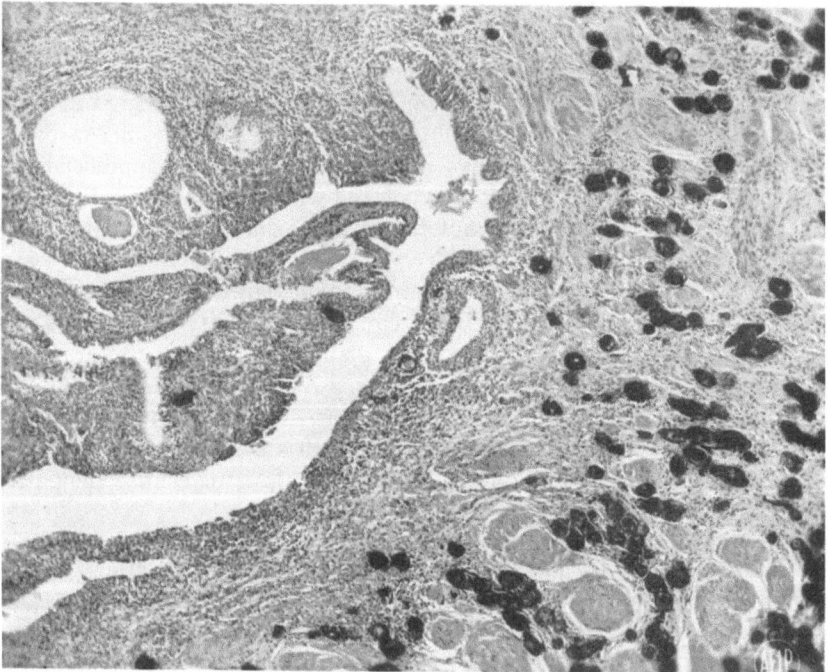

Fig. 7. From same section as that of Fig. 6, showing bilharzia ova and histyocytic infiltration of the ureteral submucosa

[17]. It has been observed accompanying the very rare carcinomas of bilharzial ureters (Figs. 6 and 7).

Such findings indicate a potentiality more complex than that required for simple repair. Clinically, the disease differs in its age incidence according to whether it is associated with bilharziasis or not. If it is so associated, the age is younger, 20—50 years old [11]. If not, the incidence is greater in the middle to old age. The sex ratios are also dissimilar — 5 females to 34 males in bilharzial cases [11] against 10 females to 9 males, respectively, in simple chronic cystitis [19]. The symptomatology of the latter differs from bilharzial cystitis in that a lot of mucus is passed with the urine.

8. *Carcinoma* in the bilharzial bladder is still of frequent occurrence in Egypt. Severity and repetition of infestations, lack of proper nourishment and of sanitary and hygienic conditions are probably among the factors responsible for the higher incidence of the disease than in other countries.

The exact relationship between cancer and bilharziasis is a difficult problem which is still under investigation. In this connection, the following facts may be of some interest:

a) The highest age incidence of cancer in bilharzial cases is 30—40 years of age, about two to three decades younger than in non bilharzial bladders.

b) Cancer in bilharzial bladders is the most frequent type of cancer in Egypt. The incidence rate of ordinary vesical cancer is lower than that reported in Europe and America.

c) In bilharzial bladder, cancer occurs as 50—60% squamous cell carcinoma and 7% adenocarcinoma [2]. These figures are much higher than those reported for non bilharzial cases in which the transitional cell neoplasm predominates. Typically, the patient has had chronic bilharziasis for 10 years or more. During this period he may have had exacerbations of symptoms, possibly synchronously with each fresh bilharzial reinfection.

The onset of malignant symptoms is usually insidious, though they may be sometimes initiated by an attack of severe hematuria. Instead of gradually abating as in previous bouts, they may persist and progress. The haematuria is total, copious, the blood is bright red, fluid or clotted; micturition is urgent, frequent and painful, sometimes advancing to strangury.

Dysuria is marked and may progress to retention with overflow. The patient looks anemic with haggard, pinched features expressing helpless suffering and anxiety.

Examination reveals a tender, distended bladder and, bimanually, a hard unlimited infiltration of its base with little or no mobility within the pelvic cavity; perivesical or parasacral glands, prostate, seminal vesicles or rectum may be involved; secondaries in the bones of the pelvis or vertebrae, in liver, lungs or heart may be present. Thus, the symptomatology of cancer in bilharzial bladders is, on the whole, similar to that of non bilharzial cases. But whereas in the latter, malignancy not uncommonly occurs in previously healthy organs, in the former, neoplasia often supervenes on the old ruins of chronic bilharzial cystitis.

Elaboration on this and other pertinent clinical points, though of great interest is not feasible here.

So far there are no grounds for considering bilharziasis as carcinogenic but its presence in the bladders of Egyptians, in particular, seems strongly to contribute towards the evolution of malignancy in them.

The bilharzial ureter: Bilharzial infiltrations effect the intravesical segments of the ureters mostly by extension from neighboring vesical bilharziomata, particularly those lying in its submucosa near the ureteral orifices. Here the ureteral infiltrations are greater in terms of density of fibrosis and consequent stenosis of the tubes.

The segment of the ureter, proximal to the bladder, is probably invaded by the bilharzial parasites through the plexus of veins surrounding it. It is not uncommon to find infiltrations localized to the ureteral submucosa and muscles about the 3rd or 4th lumbar vertebrae.

There is some experimental evidence to show that the worms probably reach these sites via anastomoses between the superior and inferior mesenteric veins and those of the right and left ureter, respectively [10].

Here and also in the juxta vesical portions of the ureter, the bilharzial manifestations, as met with during operations, appear as small nodules, superficial small ulcers, sandy patches and cysts. These last are bigger, darker in color, more prominent and numerous than in the bladder; they often cause some obstruction to the passage of catheters.

On cystoscopy, the ureteral orifices may look normal. More commonly, however, they are deformed and patulous, with lips freckled with nodules or covered by overhanging polypi. In chronic severe cases, the orifices may be hidden behind folds of thickened mucosa. The efflux is weak and irregular, the urine welling slowly and rather imperceptibly through two somewhat tubular swellings.

The rigidity and muscular atrophy of the walls weaken or abolish the valvular action which normally takes place at the orifices and in such cases reflux of fluids injected into the bladder, as in ascending cystography, may occur (Figs. 2 and 3). On the other hand, the deformities of the orifices and the intramural segments of the ureters, already alluded to, may be such that ureteral catheterization becomes very tedious or impractical. The juxtavesical segment, proximal to the stenosed distal part, at first undergoes compensatory muscular hypertrophy to cope, for some time, with the impediment in the outflow of urine. Later on, the effects of urinary stasis and back pressure lead to atony and dilatation in the ureteral muscle wall. This takes an ampullary or fusiform appearance, rather common in bilharzial cases, but not pathognomonic. In more advanced conditions, dilatation extends centripetally, the dilated tube assuming more and more a cylindrical pattern. Gradual lengthening and widening of the ureteral dimensions occurs later resulting in tortuosity and kinking of the tube, which in severe cases becomes also coiled up into loops simulating the small intestines. Such a megaureter possesses a pseudomesentery including blood vessels of appreciable size which cannot be ignored during operative manipulations of the ureter. Owing to the kinking and incurvations in the vall, the passage of catheters or even fluids through them may be difficult until the ureters are straightened out by cutting through the adhesions and fibrous bands that bind the loops together. Appreciable lengthening of the ureter then takes place, a fact which may be taken advantage of in neovesicoureterostomy and other operations, after excising damaged bilharzial ureteral portions. Less commonly, a mild uniform dilatation of the ureter may be found without evidence of any obstructing distal lesion. In some of these cases, a reduction in the capacity of the bladder or in its contractile power, as stressed by GELFAND [5] and EL SADR [14], is responsible; in others, the underlying factor seems to be inflammation of the bladder neck probably secondary to chronic prostatitis or vesiculitis.

Symptomatology. The incidence of the disease is about the same in both bladder and ureters. It is rare to see a bilharzial ureter without concomitant bladder bilharziasis [7, 15]. In the acute stage the symptoms of bilharzial ureteritis are vague, eclipsed by the more prominent bladder symptoms. Ureteral colicky pains, tenderness along the course of the tube and the passage of fibrinous filaments (ureteric casts) blood cells and ova in the urine may be observed.

The late symptoms, mainly due to chronic ureteral obstruction, are more outstanding and serious. The patient suffers from a persistent dull ache in the loins aggravated now and then by attacks of renal colic which resemble those produced by calculi, though the pain is usually less severe or durable and the attacks are not so frequent. They may be followed by the passage of blood, debris and phosphatic "mud" in the urine. The late symptoms are those of hydronephrosis or pyonephrosis as from other causes but in bilharziasis, owing to the high percentage of bilateral ureteral lesions (about 80%), the renal manifestations often take a definite course peculiar to this disease. On the side of the more serious lesion, the kidney is, to begin with, tender and slightly palpable; then it becomes less and less tender as it grows bigger and more palpable. Later still, the same kidney shrinks, feels firmer and more sensitive. Meanwhile, the other kidney is passing through similar phases and the larger and less tender kidney has the better function [8].

Such a sequence of pathological changes is of diagnostic importance. Before the days of pyelography, the smaller, firmer, more tender and painful but more damaged organ was mistaken for the better functioning one and futile surgical intervention was carried out on it by preference. One should remember that a kidney involved in bilharziasis, however good may be its present condition, is apt to deteriorate.

For these reasons, one should refrain from doing nephrectomies on hydronephroses due to ureteral bilharziasis unless they be irreparably disorganized. Radical shortcut interventions may be easier to undertake, may give prompt relief and immediate brighter aspects than more lengthy tedious constructive operations but their benefits are not durable and their prospects not equally satisfactory.

Stones. These are still more common in bilharzial bladders and ureters than in others. Apart from infection, which, as GELFAND [5] pointed out, is an important causative factor, the bilharzial matrix itself expedites their formation. The mucous membrane is roughened or ulcerated by disease; bilharzial detritus, fragments of calcified or encrusted polypi, rarely dead ova are available as nuclei. Obstruction to the free passage of urine, i.e., urinary stasis occurs only too frequently in bilharzial ureters due to the presence of cysts, polypi, intramural fibrosis. It is also seen in the bladder from similar conditions occurring at the vesical neck. Obstruction and muscular weakening of both organs by disease are important factors which may contribute to stone formation even in the absence of secondary infection.

Small concretions composed of calcium oxalate or phosphates may be formed "in loco" in the dilated segment of a stenosed ureter. They are grain-like bodies which dip into the mucosa, sometimes plugging the mouths of more deeply situated cysts [6].

In secondarily infected cases, bigger stones, mainly phosphatic, may be found incarcerated or migrating in the obstructed tube. In the bladder, concretions are rare, the larger stones are still common though not so common at the present time as they used to be before the advent of antibiotics and prevalence of bilharzial centers in Egypt for combatting bilharziasis.

The late stages of the disease present a sad clinical picture. The patient is profoundly anemic (hemoglobin sometimes as low as 30%), emaciated from indigestion and lack of nutrition. He complains of insomnia, his sleep being interrupted by an incessant frequency and urgency of micturition. His purulent urine hurts to the degree of strangury in its passage or rather dribbling through his weak sphincters. Uremia, the final inevitable complication, supervenes, sometimes acutely but usually insidiously over weeks or months. Some of these cases of advanced urinary bilharziasis with bilharzial uretero-renal lesions are subject to a chronic progressive type of toxic uremia which does not prevent them from carrying on with some light routine work until an accident, fever or minor operation upsets the balance between life and death. The patient then passes into deep and terminal uremia.

Summary

The main features of vesical and ureteral bilharzial disease, as seen in the mucous and submucous strata on cystoscopy and during operations, have been described.

In the case of the more deeply situated muscular infiltrations, radiologic as well as operative exposures have been taken into consideration in giving an outline of the clinicopathological pictures of the disease.

Lack of space and time have prevented discussing the carcinomatous traits of the subject, hoping for a more opportune circumstance.

An attempt has been made to stress the relationship between cystitis glandularis and other pathological changes, malignancy in particular.

References

[1] Bilharz, T.: Lettre de Bilharz à Siebold ler Mai 1851. Z. Wiss. Zool. 4, 59; Wiener Med. Wschr. 4 u. 5 (1856).

[2] Dimmette, R. M., H. F. Sproat, and E. S. Sayegh: The classification of carcinoma of the urinary bladder associated with schistosomiasis and metaplasia. J. Urol. 75, 680—686 (1956).

[3] Elgood, B. S.: Bilharziasis among women and girls in Egypt. Brit. Med. J. 2, 1355—1357 (1908).

[4] Fairley, N. H.: Observations on the clinical appearance of bilharziasis in Australian troops and the significance of symptoms noted. Quart. J. Med. 12, 391—403 (1919).

[5] Gelfand, M.: Schistosomiasis in South Central Africa. A clinicopathological study. Capetown: Juta & Co. 1950.

[6] Ghorab, M. M.: Ureteritis calcinosis. Proc. Int. Symposium on bilharziasis. Cairo, 1, 557—558 (1962).

[7] HONEY, R. M., and M. GELFAND: The urological aspects of bilharziasis in Rhodesia. Edinburgh: E. & S. Livingstone 1960.

[8] IBRAHIM, A.: Surgical conditions of bilharziasis. Proc. Congress of Int. Surg. Soc. Cairo 1936.

[9] LOWSLEY, O. S., and I. J. KIRWIN: Clinical Urology. 2nd Ed., 2 vol. Baltimore: Williams & Wilkins 1944.

[10] MAKAR, N.: Urological aspects of bilharziasis in Egypt. Cairo, Egypt: Société Orientale de Publicite Press 1955.

[11] MOHAMED, A. SH.: The association of bilharziasis and malignant disease in the urinary bladder. Pathogenesis of bilharzial cancer in the urinary bladder. J. Egypt. Med. Ass. 37, 1066—1085 (1954).

[12] PATCH, F. S., and L. J. RHEA: The genesis of and development of Brunn's nests and their relation to cystitis cystica, cystitis glandularis and primary adenocarcinoma of bladder. Canad. Med. Ass. J. 33, 597—606 (1945).

[13] PRATES, M., and J. GILLMAN: Carcinoma of the urinary bladder in the Portuguese East African with speical references to bilharzial cystitis and pre-neoplastic reaction. S. Afr. J. Med. Sci. 24, 13—40 (1959).

[14] SADR, A. R. EL.: Surgical aspects of bilharziasis of the ureter. Med. Lab. Prog. 10, 231—245 (1949).

[15] SAYEGH, E. S.: Late complications of urinary bilharziasis. J. Urol. 63, 353—371 (1950).

[16] SCOTT, L. S., and E. C. SORBIE: Development of carcinoma in an ectopic bladder. Brit. J. Urol. 28, 264—267 (1956).

[17] SEBAII, I. EL.: Tumors of the bladder. In: Gynecological urology. YOUSSEF, A. F. (Ed.). Springfield, Illinosis: Charles C. Thomas 1960.

[18] STOERCK, O., and O. ZUCKERKANDL: Über Cystitis glandularis und den Drüsenkrebs der Harnblase. Z. Urol. 1, 133—145 (1907).

[19] WARRICK, W. D.: Cystitis cystica. Bacteriological studies in a series of 28 cases. J. Urol. 45, 835—843 (1941).

Malignant Bladder Tumors associated with Schistosomiasis.
A Gross and Microscopic Study*

Kamal G. Ishak**, Paul C. Le Golvan***, and Ismail El-Sebai[+]

With 25 figures

This is a study of 91 cases of malignancy of the bladder associated with schistosomiasis. These cases were all from Egypt, U.A.R., and were treated by radical cystectomy. The surgery was performed by one surgeon (Dr. El-Sibai). The clinical features and follow-up will be reported separately. The value of this study lies in the uniformity of the material and the availability of the physician who had performed the surgery to assist in the gross description, dissection, study, selection and cutting of the sections.

The ages of the patients in this study ranged from 25 to 60 years. The great majority of patients were between 30 and 50 years of age. There were 77 males and 14 females.

All of the material was fixed in formalin. Representative sections were taken depending on the findings. Hematoxylin and eosin was used as a routine stain. Special stains were utilized in selected cases.

The following plan of study was used and charted: (1) Gross description, (2) Classification of tumor and degree of differentiation, (3) Extent of invasion in bladder wall, (4) Extravesical extension other than lymph nodes, (5) Lymph node metastases and lymph node changes, (6) Metaplasia in bladder mucosa, (7) Schistosome infection of bladder wall, (8) Inflammation and secondary changes in bladder, (9) Bladder neck changes, (10) Ureteric alterations, (11) Prostate, seminal vesicles and vas deferens, changes noted, (12) Uterus, fallopian tubes, ovaries and vagina, changes noted.

This plan was followed in detail by charting and utilizing a plus-minus system and with gradation of 0 to 4 + for severity. The sections were reviewed independently by two pathologists (P. C. L. and K. G. I.) and, if any differences in grading or interpretation were noted, the sections in question were re-evaluated in order to resolve these differences.

Gross findings

The tumors were classified according to the most striking gross appearance (see Table 1). It can be seen from this table that most of the tumors were classified as "fungating". This term was used for tumors with a broad base, either cauliflower-like in appearance, or simply for a heaped-up mass projecting into the

* This study was initiated at the U.S. Naval Medical Research Unit-3, Cairo, Egypt (U.A.R) and completed at the Armed Forces Institute of Pathology, Washington, D.C.
** Hepatic Branch, Armed Forces Institute of Pathology, Washington, D.C., U.S.A.
*** Pathology and Allied Sciences Service, Veterans Administration Central Office, Washington, D.C., U.S.A.
[+] Cancer Institute, Cairo University, Cairo, Egypt, U.A.R.

cavity of the bladder. The term "infiltrative" was used for those tumors forming a mass in the bladder wall without much distortion or disturbance of the mucosa, and with very little projection into the bladder cavity. The term "ulcerative" was reserved for those cases which presented a distinct well-circumscribed crater,

Table 1. *Gross classification*

	Fungating	Infiltrative	Ulcerative	Total
No. cases	79	9	3	91

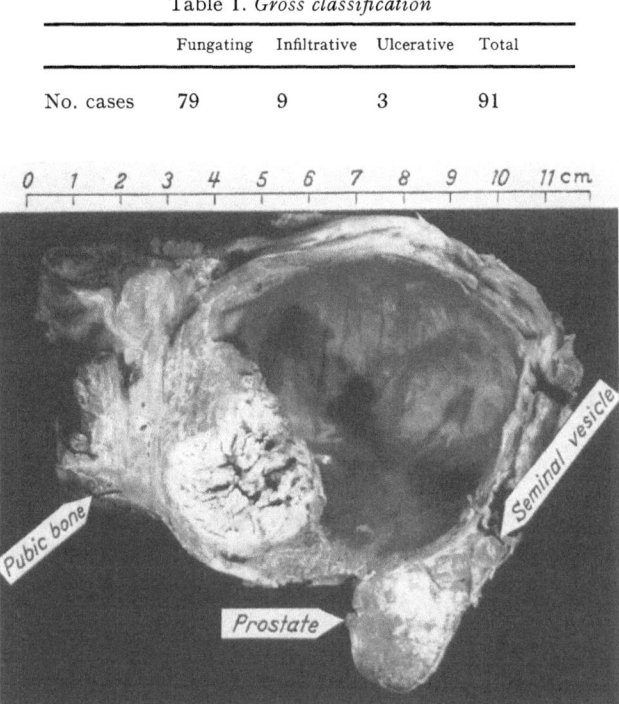

Fig. 1. Gross photograph of squamous cell carcinoma arising from anterior wall, with extension through the entire thickness of the bladder wall and invasion of the anterior abdominal wall (left)

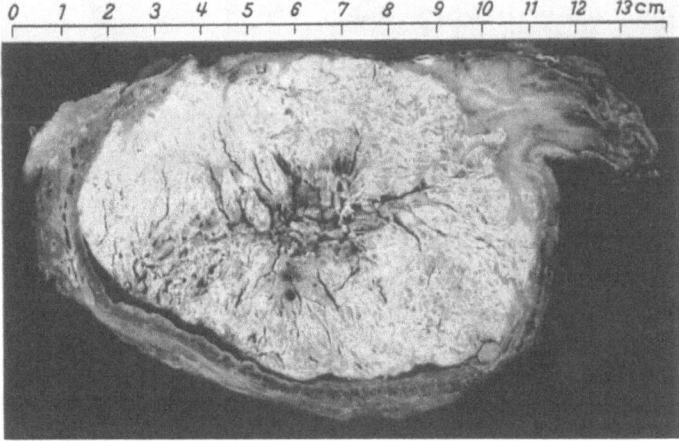

Fig. 2. Gross photograph of a section through a squamous cell carcinoma involving anterior (top) and superior (right) walls of the urinary bladder

such as in a chronic gastric ulcer, and in which the presence or absence of malignancy would not easily be judged by gross examination.

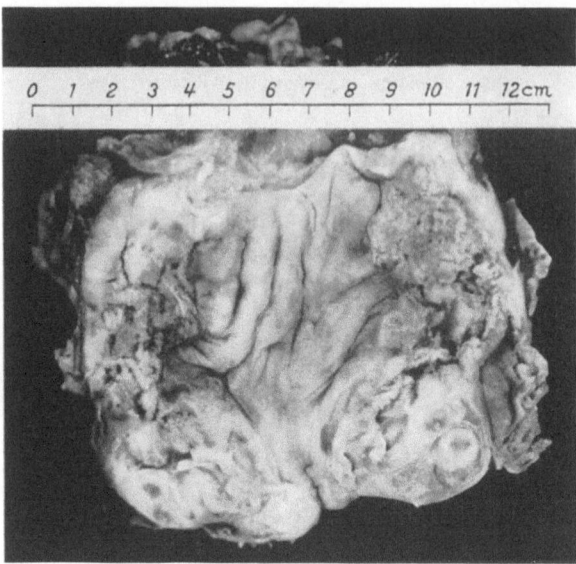

Fig. 3. Gross photograph of fungating transitional cell carcinoma involving posterior wall of urinary bladder. The bladder has been opened through the tumor posteriorly. The internal meatus is seen at the bottom of the photograph

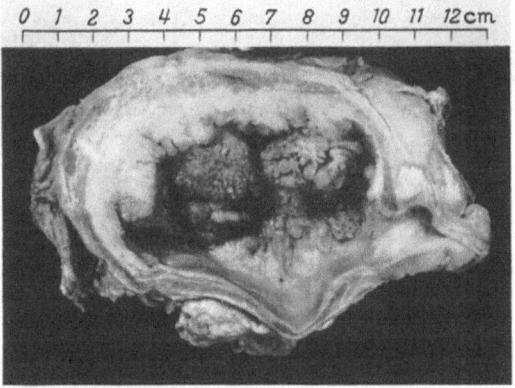

Fig. 4. Gross photograph of mucinous adenocarcinoma involving the posterior and superior walls. with invasion of two thirds of the muscle coat of the bladder. The internal meatus is seen on the right side of the photograph

    The gross description was arbitrary. The "fungating" tumors were very often "infiltrative". As can be noted, we did not use the term "papillary". Most of these cases were far advanced, otherwise, less radical surgery might have been indicated. The lack of such less advanced cases, of course, indicates a certain selectivity which must be taken into account in evaluating the results and findings.

    For the site of origin of the tumors (Table 2), we used the areas trigone, anterior, posterior, superior-apical and diffuse-multiple. These areas of origin are self-explanatory. The central area of the tumor mass was used as the site of origin. Very few cases arose from the trigone, but, of course, some of the cases classified as diffuse-multiple may have arisen from this area. We were amazed, however, at the lack of involvement of the trigone area and the ureteral orifices by neoplasia. As can be noted in Table 2, at least one half of the cases arose from the anterior or posterior walls and were well-defined in these areas.

Table 2. *Site of origin of tumors*

	Trigone	Anterior	Posterior	Superior-apical	Diffuse-multiple	Total
Female	1	5	4	1	3	14
Male	1	23	20	8	25	77
Recap	2	28	24	9	28	91

For the tumor size, we used the three-dimensional measurement in centimeters. The smallest tumor measured $2 \times 2 \times 2$ centimeters (8 cubic centimeters) and the largest about $10 \times 10 \times 10$ centimeters (1,000 cubic centimeters). The average size was about $6 \times 5 \times 6$ (about 180 cubic centimeters). Upon cutting through the tumors, we described the surfaces with the terms "homogenous", "variegated", or "papillary". Most of the tumors fell into the "variegated" classification, followed by "homogenous"; very few of the neoplasms were "papillary". The tumors were generally large and, therefore, the lack of the "papillary" pattern is easy to understand. Many of the tumors also had secondary changes of hemorrhages, necrosis and ulceration, which changes were recorded separately.

Microscopic findings

The tumors were classified as squamous, transitional or adenocarcinomas (see Table 3). They were further subdivided into "well-differentiated", "moderately well-differentiated", and "poorly differentiated" types (see Table 4). We did not

Table 3. *Histologic classification of tumors*

	Squamous	Transitional	Adenocarcinoma	Sarcoma	Total
Cases	49	35	4	3	91

Table 4. *Degree of differentiation*

	Squamous	Transitional	Adenocarcinoma	Sarcoma	Total
Well differentiated	18	0	0	3	21
Moderately well differentiated	25	18	2	n/a*	45
Poorly differentiated	6	17	2	n/a*	25
Total	49	35	4	3	91

* n/a = not applicable

attempt any further classification of the sarcomata. The adenocarcinomas were rather straightforward and no great difficulty was encountered. We realized that certain arbitrary decisions had to be made with the squamous and transitional groups. Some of the tumors which we classified as squamous would probably be classified as transitional with squamous features by others. Generally speaking, the interpretation and classification was not too difficult.

In comparing the histologic classification with the gross types, we found that we could not predict with any degree of certainty the histologic type from the

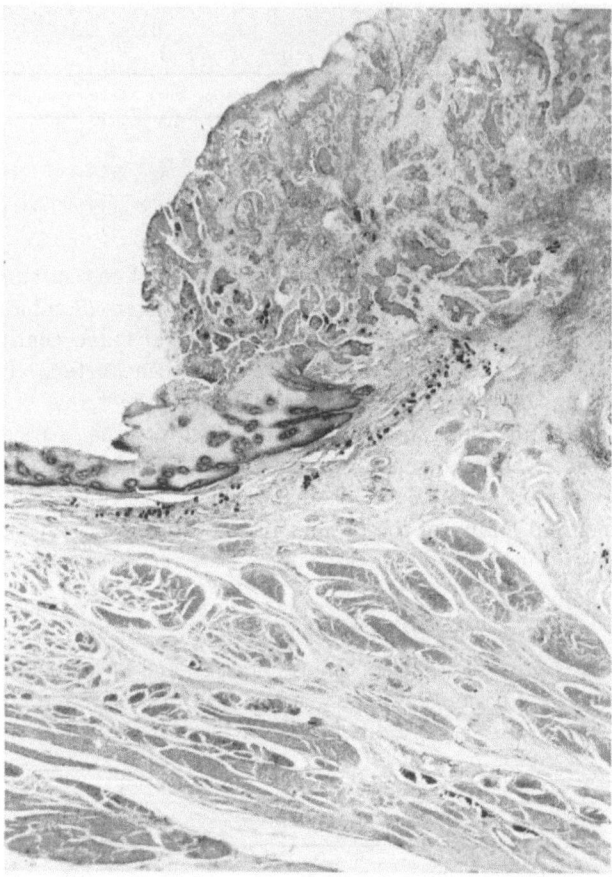

Fig. 5. Transition from squamous metaplasia (left) to invasive squamous cell carcinoma (right). A few schistosome eggs are noted in the lamina propria. H & E, X 14. AFIP Neg. 65-6612

gross appearance. We did note the mucoid appearance on cut surface in some of the adenocarcinomas. We did not classify any of the transitional carcinomas as "well differentiated" because most were either at least grade III or IV by the conventional grading (Broder's) system.

In ten of the cases satellite tumors were found. These were smaller tumors independent of the main tumor mass, which could have arisen by lymphatic spread, implantation or "de novo" (multicentric origin). These satellite tumors were present in 3 of the squamous, 4 of the transitional and 2 of the adenocarcinomas; one of the sarcomas also showed satellite nodules.

The extent of invasion of the bladder wall was classified after both gross and microscopic examination (Table 5). On comparison of the gross and microscopic findings, we were able to determine quite well by gross examination alone the degree of involvement by tumor. As can be noted from the table, most of the tumors were well advanced. In the *three* cases in which there was only involvement of the mucosa and submucosa, one was an adenocarcinoma arising from the superior apical region of the bladder. There were no metastases and no evidence of extra-

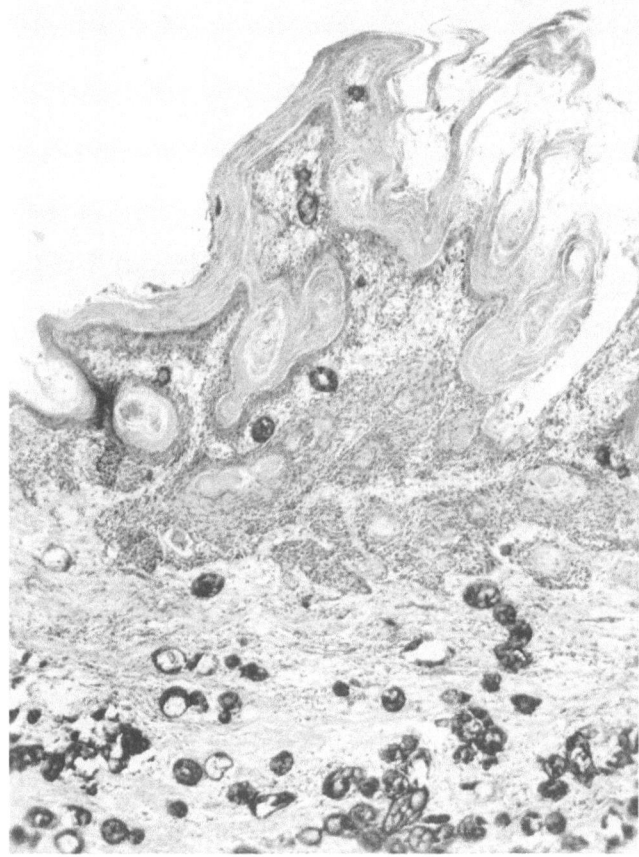

Fig. 6. Edge of keratinizing squamous cell carcinoma. A few schistosome eggs are present within the tumor and a moderate number of calcified eggs are seen in the fibrotic tunica propria. H & E, X 70. AFIP Neg. 65-6779

vesical extension. The second case was a small ($2 \times 2 \times 2$ cm) poorly-differentiated transitional carcinoma arising from the vault of the bladder with no evidence of

Table 5. *Extent of invasion of bladder wall*

Mucosa/submucosa	Muscle 1/3	Muscle 2/3	Muscle 3/3	Beyond	Total
3	8	5	8	68	91

extravesical extension. The third case was a well-differentiated squamous carcinoma arising from the posterior wall and measuring 4.5×3.5 cm; in this case too extravesical extension or metastases had not occurred.

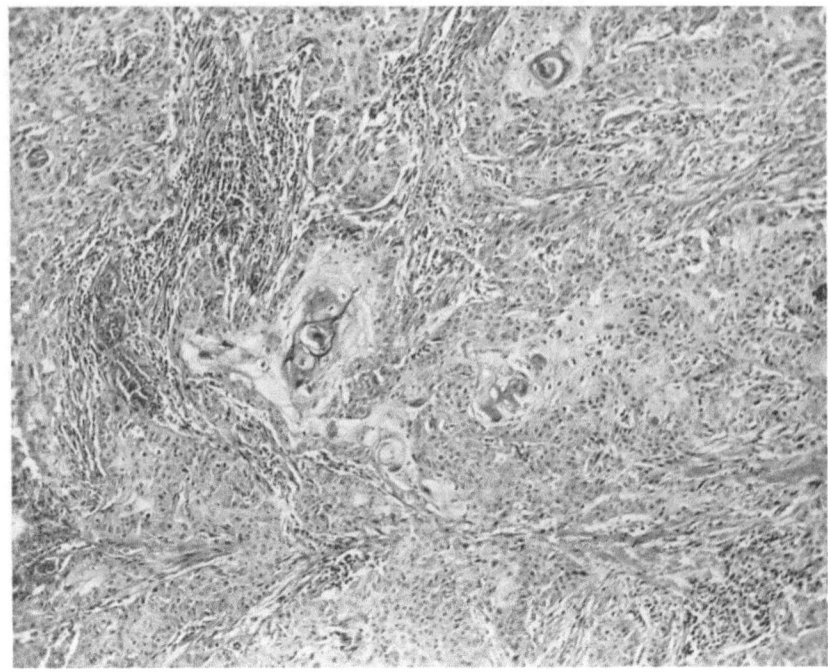

Fig. 7. Squamous cell carcinoma, moderately well-differentiated, with epithelial pearl formation. H & E, X 75. AFIP Neg. 65-6760

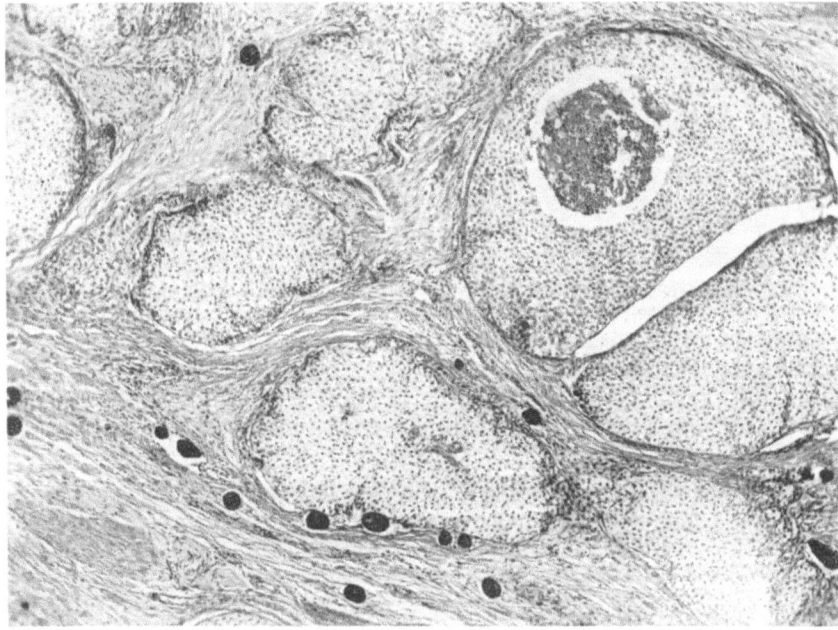

Fig. 8. Transitional cell carcinoma, moderately well-differentiated. A few calcified schistosome eggs are present in the supporting stroma. H & E, X 6. AFIP Neg. 65-6614

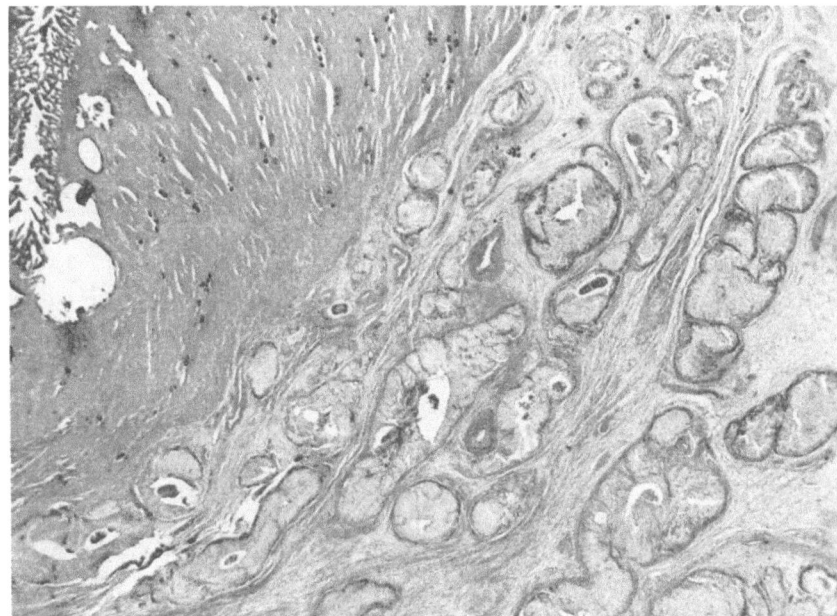

Fig. 9. Transitional cell carcinoma invading perivesical tissues in region of seminal vesicle. H & E, X 50. AFIP Neg. 65-6613

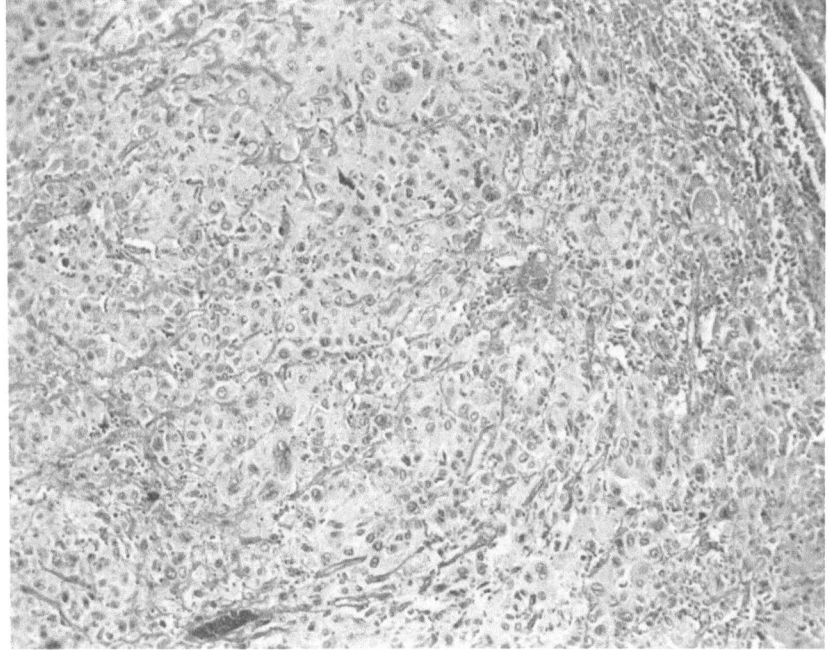

Fig. 10. Transitional cell carcinoma, poorly differentiated. H & E X 80. AFIP Neg. 65-6772

5   Bilharziasis

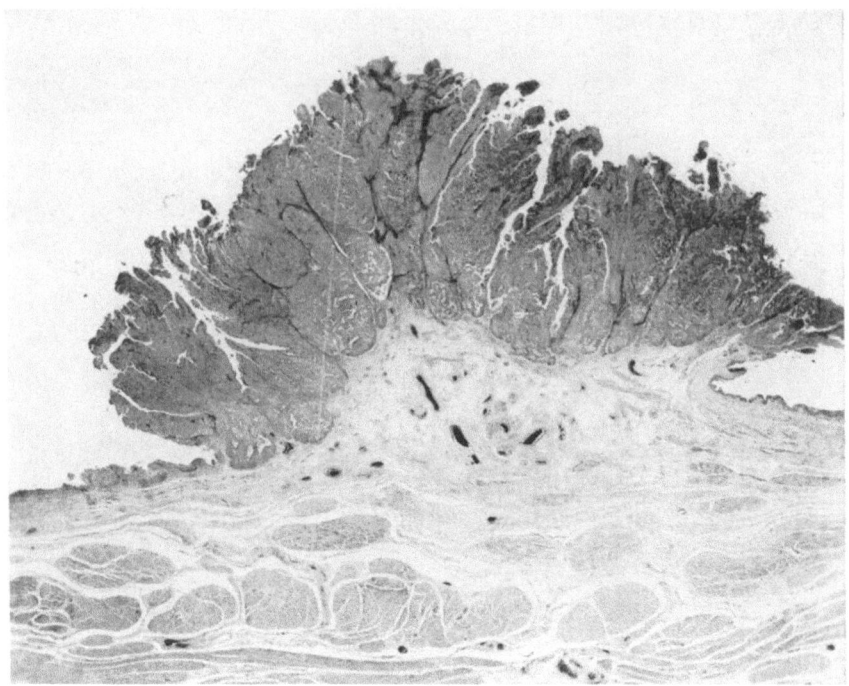

Fig. 11. Transitional cell carcinoma, satellite nodule. H & E, X 7. AFIP Neg. 65-6611

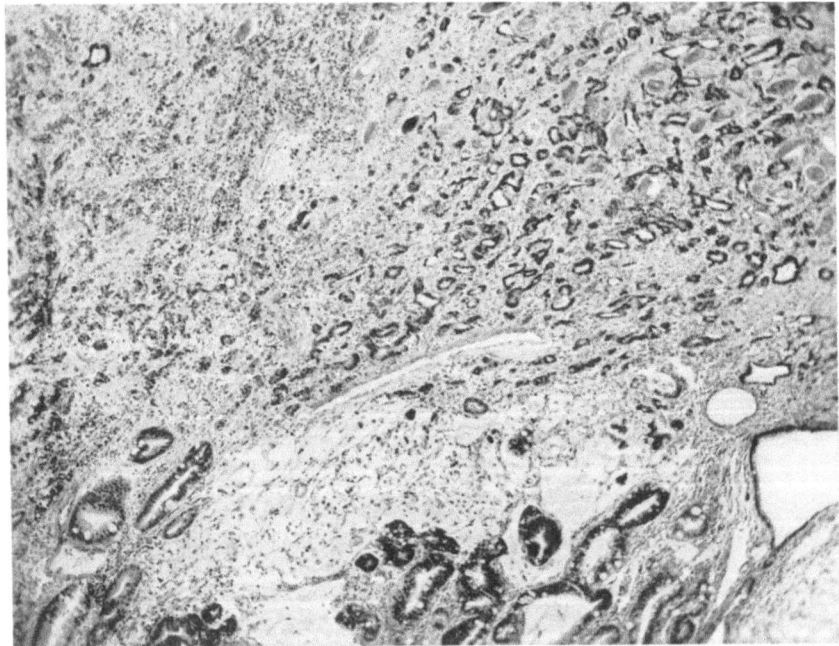

Fig. 12. Mucinous adenocarcinoma. Many signet-ring cells are seen near the top of the section. Schistosome eggs are present in the lower part of the tumor. H & E, X 50. AFIP Neg. 65-6777

Of the eight cases that extended only through 1/3 of the muscle layer, three were transitional, four squamous and one an adenocarcinoma. None of these cases demonstrated any evidence of extravesical extension or lymph node metastases.

Of the *five* cases that extended only through 2/3 of the muscle wall, four were squamous and one was transitional. Only one of the cases had extravesical extension and this was into the uterine cervix. In this case we obviously had not noted the correct extension into the bladder either grossly or with our sections.

Of the *eight* cases extending only through 3/3 of the muscle, five were classified squamous and three transitional. One case involved the prostate and seminal vesicles, but no metastases to lymph nodes were found.

In the sixty-eight cases that extended beyond the muscularis (see Table 6), twenty-five had lymph node metastases and twenty-two had other extravesical extension. Thirty-eight cases had involvement of lymph nodes, other tissues or both.

Table 6. *Extravesical tumor extension — 38 cases*

Organ	No. of cases
Lymph node metastases	25
Prostate	10
Seminal vesicles	10
Vas deferens	3
Ureters	5
Uterus	1
Small intestine	1
Omentum	1
Pubic bone	2
Anterior abdominal wall	2

Associated metaplastic changes

The metaplastic changes in the bladder mucosa are recorded in detail in Tables 7 and 8. The various types of metaplasia occurring in the 91 cases of carcinoma of the bladder are listed in Table 8; the three sarcomas were not accompanied by metaplasia. These metaplastic changes are further broken down according to the histologic classification of the carcinomas in Table 8.

Table 7. *Metaplastic changes in bladder mucosa*

	Squamous metaplasia	Leuko-plakia	Ca-in-situ	Cystitis glandularis	Cystitis cystica	None	Total
No. cases	47	45	21	29	12	24	67
Percentage	52	50	23	32	13	26	74

By cystitis glandularis is meant the downward proliferation of the lining epithelium into the lamina propria, with formation of von Brunn's nests with or without a central lumen; the cells lining the lumina were often columnar in type. Occasionally, filiform projections into the bladder lumen were noted. Where the lumina were dilated by accumulation of secretion to form microscopic or grossly visible "cysts" lined by a single layer of cells, the term cystitis cystica was used. In 6 of the cases columnar cells lining the cavities in von Brunn's nests were

5*

Table 8. *Metaplastic changes in relation to type of vesical carcinoma*

	Squamous carcinoma	Leuko-plakia	Ca-in-situ	Cystitis glandularis	Cystitis cystica	None	Total
Squamous carcinoma (49 cases)							
No. cases	36	33	15	15	6	5	44
Percentage	73	67	31	31	12	10	90
Transitional carcinoma (35 cases)							
No. cases	10	11	5	11	4	15	20
Percentage	28	31	14	31	11	43	57
Adenocarcinoma (4 cases)							
No. cases	1	1	1	3	2	1	3

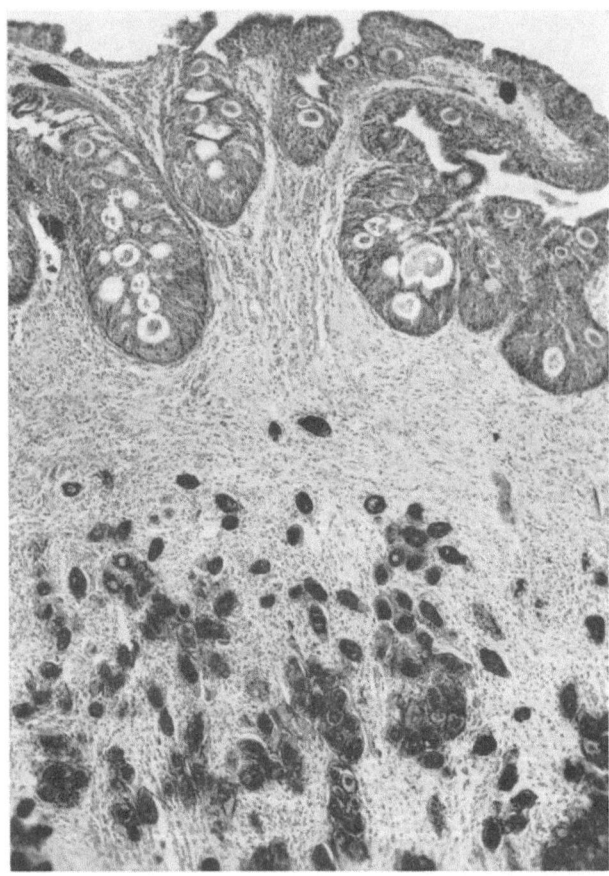

Fig. 13. Cystitis glandularis. Numerous calcified schistosome eggs, with a moderate inflammatory response, are noted in the tunica propria. H & E, X 55. AFIP Neg. 65-6595

mucinous producing, and resembled intestinal goblet cells. This intestinalization was always seen in areas of cystitis glandularis and was present in 3 of the squamous, one of the transitional and one of the adenocarcinomas.

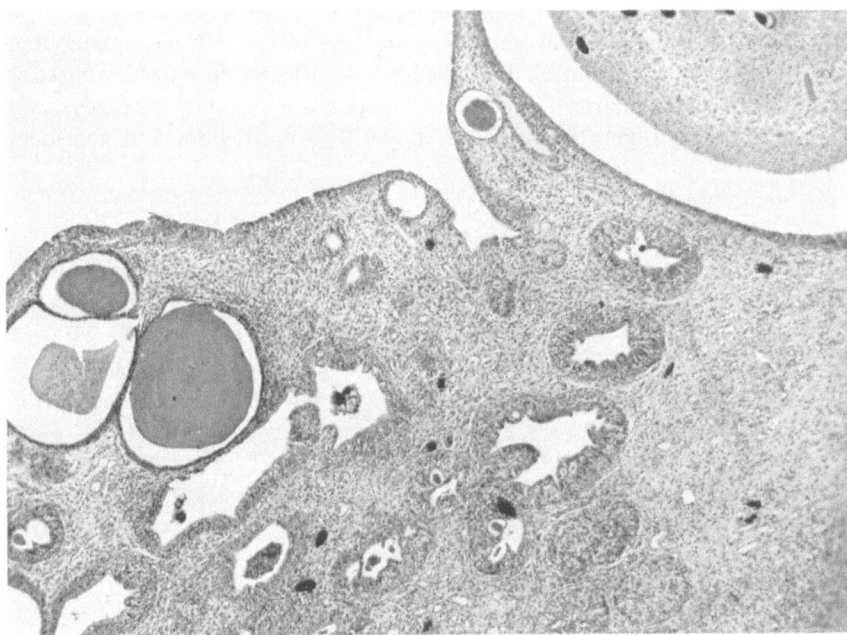

Fig. 14. Cystitis glandularis and cystica. H & E, X 40. AFIP Neg. 65-6594

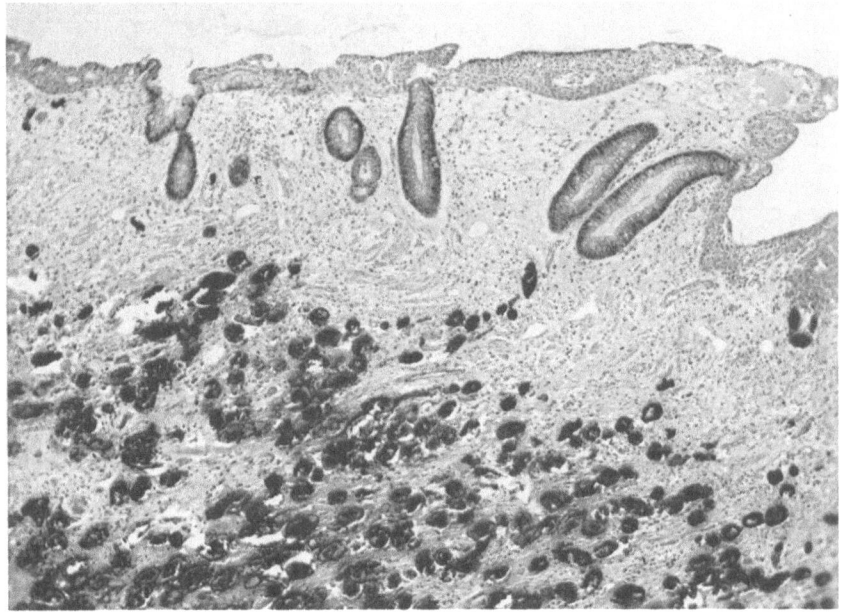

Fig. 15. Columnar cell metaplasia (intestinalization). Note placque-like deposit of calcified schistosome eggs with marked fibrosis and minimal inflammation. H & E, X 55. AFIP Neg. 65-6596

Squamous metaplasia was used for cases in which the transitional bladder epithelium was replaced by stratified squamous cells, with or without acanthosis and surface keratinization; in very occasional cases the surface squamous cells showed keratohyaline granules. This change was either diffuse or alternated with areas of cystitis glandularis. The term leukoplakia was reserved for cases in which there was extensive keratinization of the surface epithelium and considerable

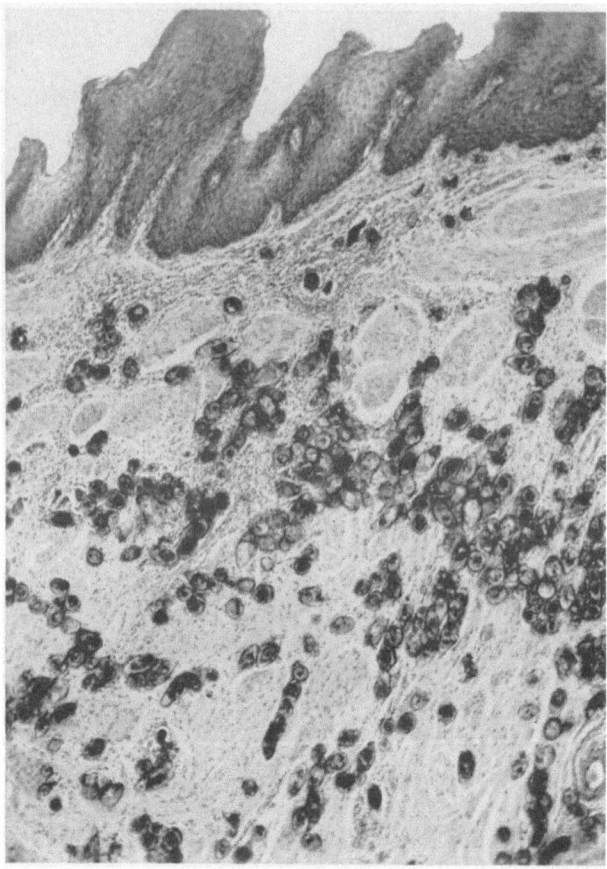

Fig. 16. Squamous metaplasia with acanthosis. Numerous calcified schistosome eggs seen in the section. H & E, X 50.
AFIP Neg. 65-6597

proliferation and activity of the basal cell layer. Areas of squamous metaplasia and leukoplakia were often seen to merge abruptly or gradually into invasive squamous cell carcinoma. Carcinoma in situ was usually seen in areas of squamous metaplasia. This term was reserved for those cases showing considerable variation in size and shape of the cells and nuclei, loss of polarity and mitotic activity. Ca-in-situ was usually seen focally, and was never present as a diffuse epithelial change.

The metaplastic changes were seen in areas of the bladder wall where egg deposition was very heavy, but they were also often seen in parts of the bladder wall showing few or no eggs. This was especially noticeable in some of the cases in which squamatization of the entire urinary bladder, lower ureters and prostatic urethra was present, though very few eggs were seen in the tunica propria. In view of this the possibility of co-existing vitamin A deficiency in patients with schisto-somiasis should always be sought after and ruled out.

Metaplastic changes similar to those in the urinary bladder were also seen in the bladder neck, prostatic urethra and in the lower ends of the ureters.

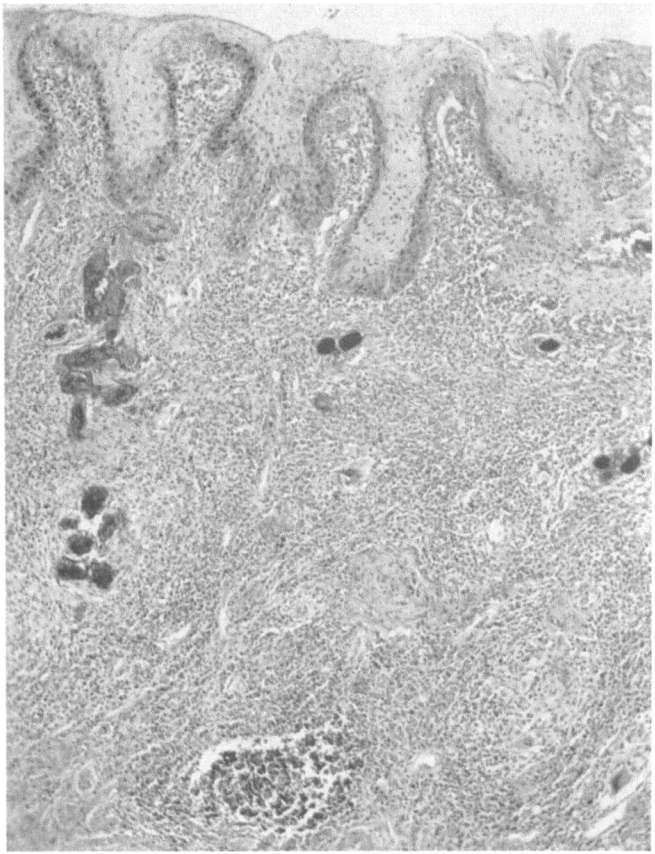

Fig. 17. Squamous metaplasia with marked acanthosis. The inflammatory response is greatly out of proportion to the number of eggs present in tunica propria. H & E, X 70. AFIP Neg. 65-6775

From the analysis of the data on metaplastic changes, it can be seen that these changes were recorded more often in those cases classified as squamous. In 90% of these cases, some changes were noted. Carcinoma-in-situ and leukoplakia (precancerous changes) were considerably greater in the squamous than in the transitional carcinomas. It is interesting that in 43% of the transitional carcinoma cases *no* metaplastic changes were present. This is in contrast to 10% for the squamous carcinoma cases. Cystitis glandularis and cystitis cystica were roughly equal in percentage in both groups. The small number of cases in the adeno-carcinoma and sarcoma groups, of course, precludes the use of these for any significant interpretation.

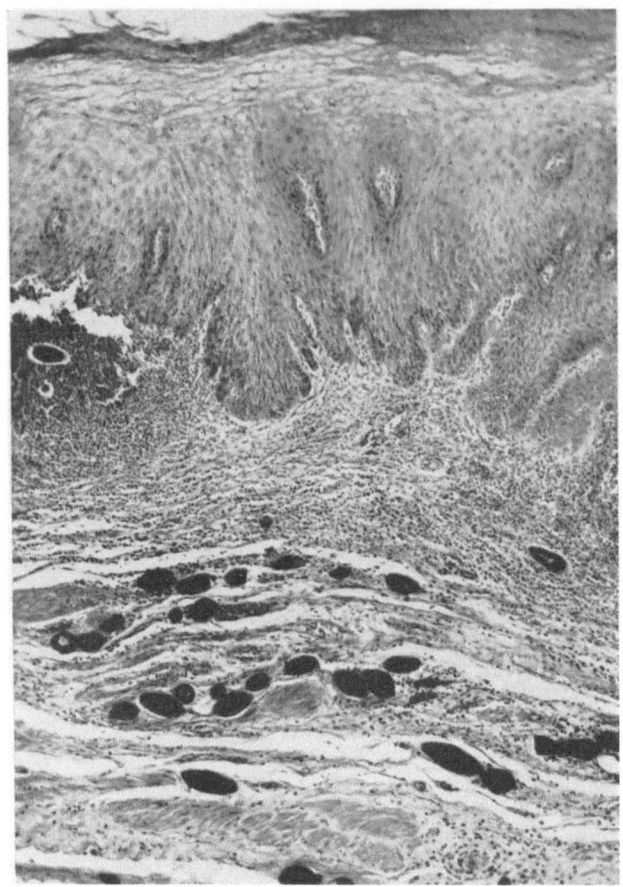

Fig. 18. Leukoplakia associated with schistosomiasis. H & E, X 70. AFIP Neg. 65-6603

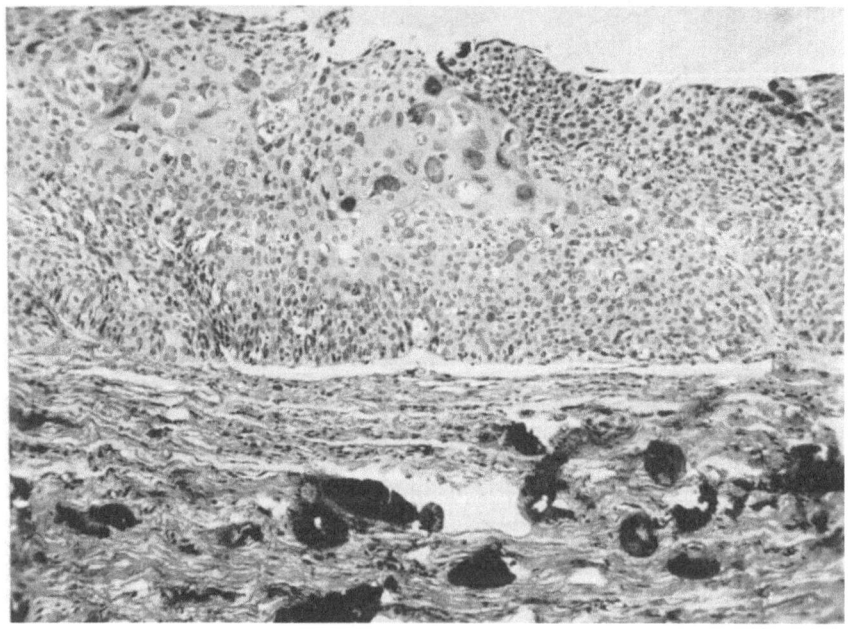

Fig. 19. Carcinoma in situ associated with schistosomiasis. The tumor in this case was a squamous cell carcinoma. H & E, X 120. AFIP Neg. 65-6580

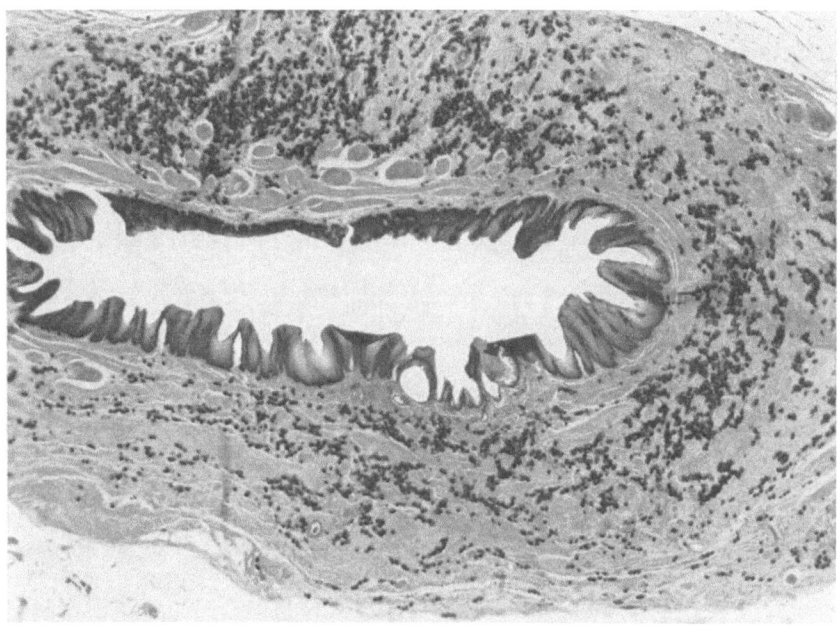

Fig. 20. Ureter, lower third, showing extensive squamous metaplasia and a marked deposition of eggs throughout the wall. The urinary bladder showed squamous metaplasia, leukoplakia, carcinoma in situ and a squamous cell carcinoma. H & E, X 12. AFIP Neg. 65-6623

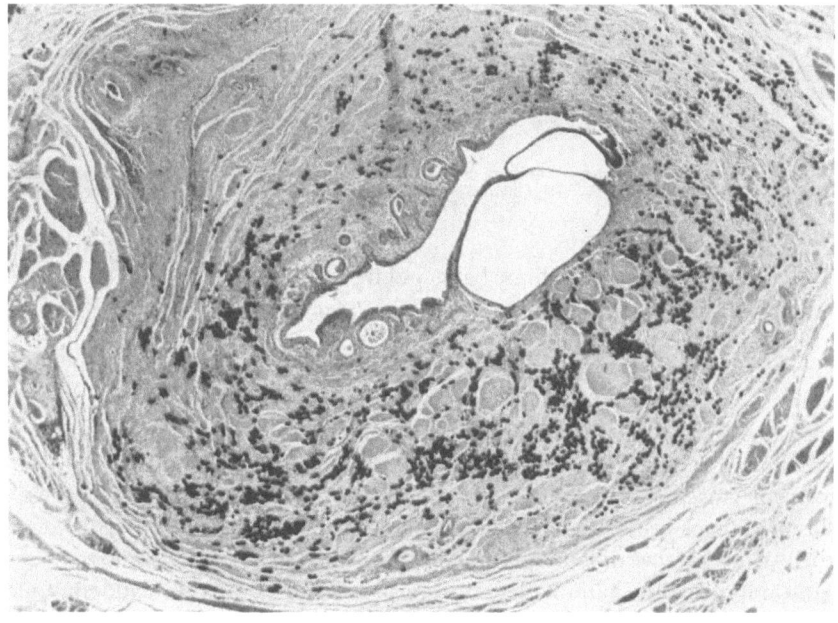

Fig. 21. Ureter, lower third, showing ureteritis glandularis and cystica and a heavy deposition of schistosome eggs. H & E X 12. AFIP Neg. 65-6613

Associated schistosomiasis

It is not the purpose of this presentation to describe in detail the gross and microscopic alterations resulting from schistosomal infection. These changes have been repeatedly described in the past by many workers; they were not significantly different from those occurring in the urinary tracts of patients without vesical carcinoma. The reader is referred to the monograph of MAKAR [17] and the recent publications of ABOUL FADL and co-workers [1] and GILLMAN and

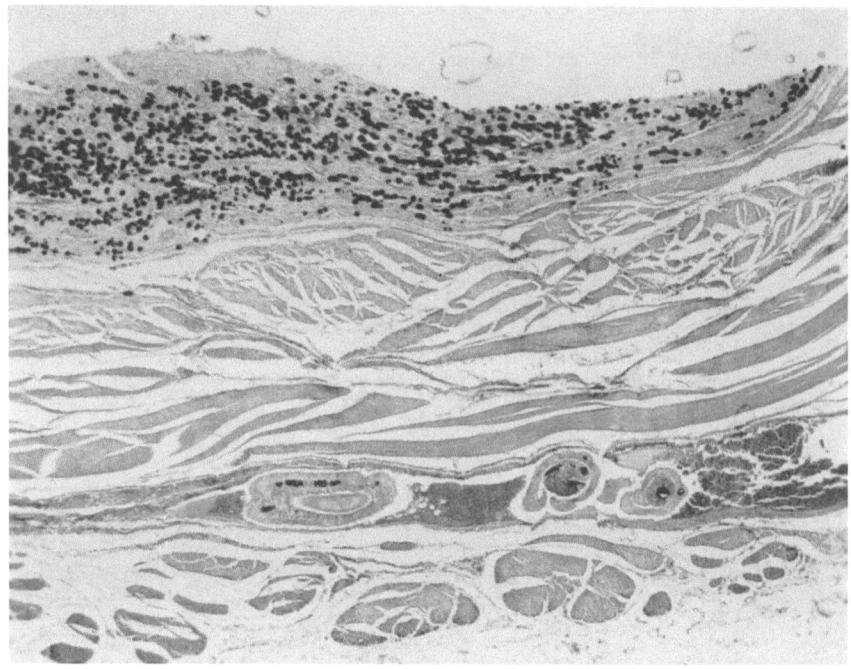

Fig. 22. Urinary bladder showing extensive mucosal ulceration, heavy deposition of calcified eggs in the lamina propria, with a minimal inflammatory response. Several adult worms seen are in a large vein between the muscle bundles. H & E, X 18. AFIP Neg. 65-6605

PRATES [12]. The latter authors have published excellent schematic representations of the connective tissue and epithelial reactions in vesical schistosomiasis in relation to cancer.

Grossly, the bladder mucosa not involved by carcinoma showed the gamut of well-recognized schistosomal lesions. "Sandy patches" were observed in 55 of the 91 cases in this series. Bilharzial (schistosomal) nodules were noted in 25 cases; microscopically these were composed of granulation tissue around the eggs, either with an ulcerated surface or covered by intact epithelium. In five of the cases small papillomas were seen. Twelve of the bladders showed cystitis cystica. Greyish-white patches of leukoplakia were identified in 24 of the bladders. Grossly recognizable, usually shallow ulcers, were present in 10 of the bladders. Calcific deposits (concretions) usually overlying areas of ulceration, were seen in 10 of the cases. Visible superficial or deep hemorrhages were found in 14 of the cases.

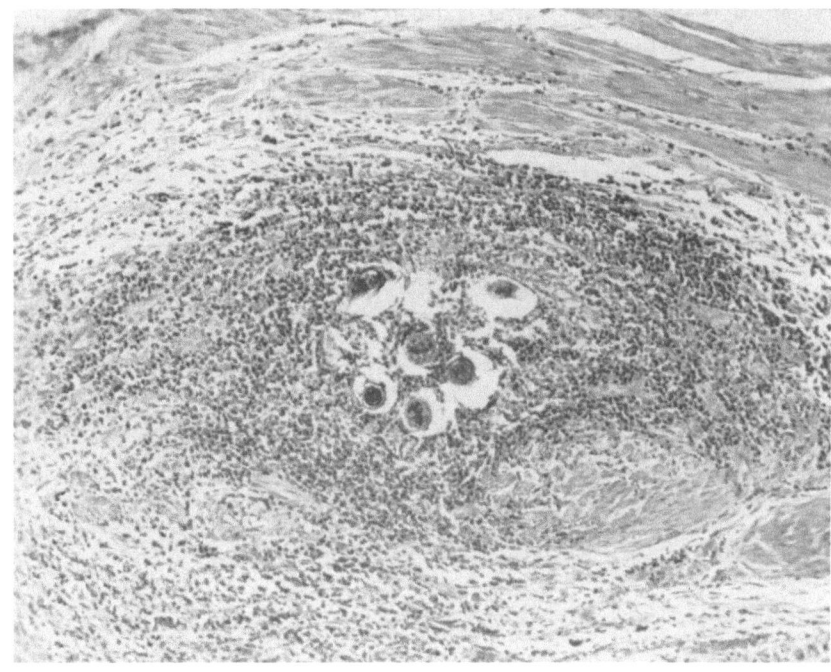

Fig. 23. Intensive inflammatory reaction in the vicinity of a group of viable schistosome eggs. H & E, X 110. AFIP Neg. 65-6581

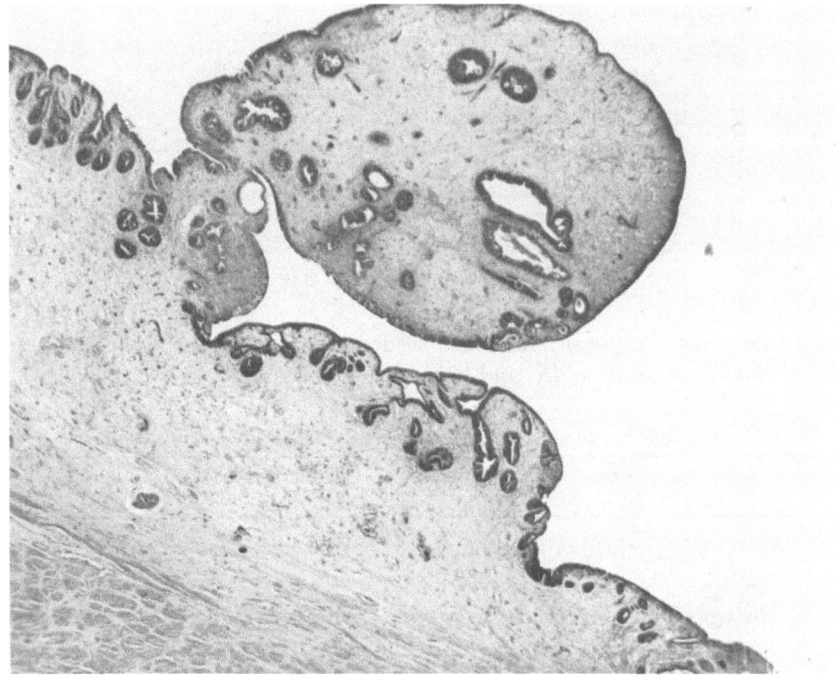

Fig. 24. Schistosomal (bilharzial) polyp. H & E, X 18. AFIP Neg. 65-6610

Sixteen of the bladders showed trabeculation or fasciculation indicating some degree of obstruction; in 13 of these cases bladder neck contraction was present.

The schistosomal involvement of the bladder wall is recorded in Table 9. The degree of egg deposition in the bladder wall was graded from zero (0) to four (4 +).

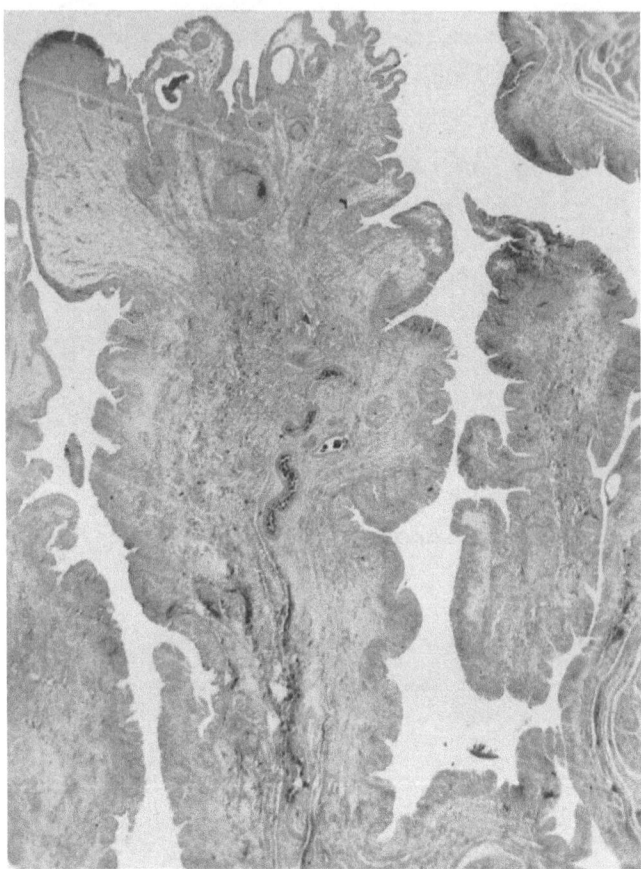

Fig. 25. Schistosomal papilloma. H & E, X 13. AFIP Neg. 65-6781

The various areas of oviposition in the bladder were separated into layers such as mucosa, submucosa, muscularis and beyond the muscularis. As is well recognized,

Table 9. *Schistosome egg deposition in bladder submucosa*

	Degree 1+	2+	3+	4+	Calcified egg	Viable egg	Adult worms	Total
Cases	22	46	13	10	80	11	6	91

most of the egg deposition is in the submucosa. Most of the eggs were those of *Schistosoma hematobium*, nonviable and calcified, although we did record viable eggs in eleven cases. Adult worms were found in six cases.

Most of the eggs were calcified, and in those cases with the heaviest (four plus) deposition, this amounted to plaque-like formation. The reaction noted varied considerably but, in general, with calcification the intensity of the inflammatory response considerably diminished. Several samples of bladder wall were taken from various areas not involved by tumor, in addition to multiple sections though the tumor (s). In general, there were relatively few eggs deposited in the bladder neck area.

Microscopically, in addition to the egg deposition which is recorded in Table 9, the bladder wall showed varying degrees of chronic inflammation. Most of the cells were mononuclear in type (lymphocytes and plasma cells) but varying numbers of eosinophils were also present; the latter cells were most noticeable in relation to the viable non-calcified eggs. Occasional lymphoid follicles with or without germinal centers, were sometimes seen deep in the muscle wall or adventitia, apparently not related to egg deposits. Active schistosomal granulomas were only noted occasionally in 17 of the cases.

In our opinion there was no correlation between the inflammatory response and intensity of egg deposition on the one hand, and the type of carcinoma on the other.

Microscopic evidence of some degree of mucosal ulceration, most often over calcified egg placques (sandy patches), was present in most (eighty) of the bladders. Varying degrees of fibrosis, with or without atrophy of the muscle bundles, were also seen in the great majority of the cases. In the areas of scarring, sclerosed and hyalinized vessels were frequently observed.

In addition to the inflammatory response around the eggs, most of the tumors, usually at the periphery, showed a varying inflammatory reaction, which we interpreted as a host response to the neoplasm. This was particularly noticeable with the squamous carcinomas, and many of these showed a foreign-body granulomatous response to keratin and other neoplastic debris.

The lower ureters generally paralleled the bladder in the deposition of eggs, and, as our sections were usually taken within one or two centimeters from the orifices, this gave a fairly representative idea of the deposition within the distal ureter (see Table 10).

Table 10. *Egg deposition in ureters, seminal vesicle, vasa deferentia, prostate and pelvic lymph nodes degree*

Site	1+	2+	3+	4+	None	Total No. cases
Ureters	21	30	15	12	13	91
Seminal vesicles	16	30	16	8	7	77
Vasa deferentia	30	8	0	0	39	77
Prostate	17	10	3	0	47	77
Lymph nodes	31	12	3	1	44	91

Of the thirteen cases in which no eggs were present in the ureters, seven had a 2 + bladder deposition and six cases had only a 1 + deposition. In twelve cases with 4 + egg deposition in the ureters, six of the bladders had a 4 +, three had 3 + and three had 2 + egg deposition; this is what one would expect. There was little variation in deposition between the right and left ureters.

Egg deposition in the seminal vesicles is also listed in Table 10. This again generally paralleled the deposition in the ureters and the bladder, and again there was only very slight variation in oviposition between the right and left seminal vesicles.

The vasa deferentia were generally much less involved than the seminal vesicles. The egg deposition in these is recorded in Table 10. This relative immunity of the vas to egg deposition is easily understood because it is a very small structure, the venules are extremely small and the wall is very thick, compact and muscular. The prostate, as noted previously, was relatively free of egg deposition; the involvement of this organ is listed in Table 10.

Schistosome egg deposition in the lymph nodes was not spectacular and again generally coincided with the degree of involvement of other areas of the pelvis (see Table 10).

Egg deposition was also noted in other surgically-excised tissues such as the uterus, cervix, vagina, fallopian tubes, ovaries, sections of small and large bowel, appendices, etc. This deposition was not great and was quantitatively overshadowed by the extensive deposits in the bladder.

In conclusion the greatest egg deposition was present in the submucosa of the bladder, in areas away from the trigone. The ureters were probably next in severity of involvement, followed by the seminal vesicles, lymph nodes, vasa deferentia, prostate and other tissues.

Discussion

For many years a high incidence of malignant bladder neoplasms has been reported from Egypt. There has been considerable variation in the incidence of carcinoma of the bladder in relation to other malignant neoplasms and the reader is referred to MAKAR's monograph [17] for a review of most of the published reports. Some of these series are listed in Table 11. The lowest figure of 4.1% was

Table 11. *Incidence of vesical carcinoma in relation to other malignant neoplasms in Egypt*

Authors	Year	Reference number	All cancers (No. of cases)	Carcinoma of bladder (%)
DOLBEY and MOORO	1924	8	222	23.0
SOROUR	1928	26	365	22.0
BARSOUM	1939	4	—	19.0
BARSOUM	1953	5	292	4.1
MAKAR	1955	17	3872	43.0
HASHEM	1961	13	—	19.0
ABOUL NASR et al.	1962	1	484	11.3

that of BARSOUM [5] and the highest figure of 43% was that of MAKAR [17]. The reasons for some of the discrepancies were discussed by ABOUL NASR et al. [1] and will not be dwelt upon here. The incidence of cancer of the bladder reported by these latter authors from Egypt was 11%, a much more realistic figure; this figure is comparable to the 9% incidence reported by SHAMMA [25] from Iraq.

The relationship of carcinoma of the bladder to schistosomiasis of the urinary tract has been the subject of lengthy debates for decades. Most of the cases studied by Egyptian workers have shown a high incidence of schistosomal infection in association with bladder carcinoma. In the series of 652 cases of cancer of the bladder collected by ABOUL NASR and his co-workers [1] in Egypt, 97% showed evidence of associated vesical schistosomiasis. The smaller series reported by LEGOLVAN et al. [16] showed an incidence of associated schistosomiasis of 91.7%.

HASHEM [13] reported an incidence of 83.1% in 1961. The differences between these figures may be related to the nature of the material studied, whether surgical or autopsy, or both. In the cases reported by SHAMMA [25] from Iraq 44% of the bladder carcinoma patients had associated schistosomiasis.

Very few studies comparing the incidence of carcinoma of the bladder in Egyptians and in non-Egyptians residing in Egypt have appeared in the literature. MAKAR [17] analyzed 3 such series from Cairo Hospitals and found the frequency of carcinoma of the bladder to other cancers to be 43% for Egyptians, and 3% and 11% for non-Egyptians. Although ABOUL NASR et al. [1] have criticized these figures, because carcinoma of the bladder was compared only to cancers arising in five other sites, the fact remains that the incidence of bladder carcinoma was much higher in Egyptians than in non-Egyptians over a given period of time.

Although a relationship between urinary schistosomiasis and vesical carcinoma has been accepted by most workers in Egypt since the work of FERGUSON [1] was published this has not been true for all other parts of Africa in which schistosomiasis is endemic. A high incidence of carcinoma of the bladder has been reported from Portuguese East Africa [12, 23]. GELFAND [11], DODGE [7] and PAYET [22], on the other hand could find no such increased incidence in South Central Africa, in Uganda, or in French West Africa respectively. According to HIGGINSON and OETTLE [15] schistosomiasis is the major etiological factor in relation to cancer of the bladder among the South African Bantu. EDINGTON [9] is of the opinion that schistosomiasis cannot be discounted as a factor in cancer of the bladder in Africans from the Gold Coast. GILMAN and PRATES [12] have compared carcinoma of the bladder in Egypt with that occurring in Portuguese East Africa; the incidence was 2—3 times greater in Egypt than in the latter country. Bladder calculi, encrusted vesical ulcers and cystitis glandularis were much less frequently seen in Portuguese East Africa than in Egypt. These authors also noted that carcinoma of the liver was rare in Egypt but common in Portuguese East Africa. They felt that comparative studies between Egyptians and Africans living in Portuguese East Africa and other parts of Africa were long overdue.

The clinical and surgical aspects of carcinoma of the bladder associated with schistosomiasis will not be dwelt upon in this presentation. The reader is referred to the publications of SAYEGH [24], GELFAND [11], MAKAR [17], and ABOUL NASR et al. [1]. In general, the age incidence for carcinoma of the bladder associated with schistosomiasis is between the third and fifth decades of life [1, 16, 17]. 40% of the patients in the series published by ABOUL NASR et al. [1] were in the fifth decade of life; 73% were below 50 years of age. In the experience of MAKAR [17] a history of schistosomiasis precedes the onset of cancer by ten years and more. The preponderance of vesical carcinoma in males is also striking, though different figures have been published by various authors. Thus MAKAR [17] gave a male to female ratio of 9 : 1, which agrees with the data of LEGOLVAN et al. [16]. ABOUL NASR et al. [1] on the other hand, reported a male to female ratio of 5 : 1, which corresponds to the ratio in the present series of cases.

The metaplastic alterations which complicate urinary schistosomiasis and are so frequently present in the patients who have vesical carcinoma need no elaboration. They have been commented upon by all workers who have studied the pathologic changes in the urinary tracts of such patients [1, 6, 12, 13, 15, 17]. About 90% of the cases in the present series showed metaplastic changes. Carcinoma-in-situ and leukoplakia (in addition to squamous metaplasia) occurred with greater frequency in the squamous cell carcinomas. It is of interest that 43% of the transitional carcinomas were not accompanied by any metaplastic changes; this has also been the experience of DIMMETTE et al. [6]. The types of metaplasia seen in vesical carcinoma associated with urinary schistosomiasis are no different from those seen in non-schistosomal bladder cancers; the latter are reviewed by MOSTOFI [19]. The pathogenetic mechanisms of metaplasia of the urinary bladder in schistosomiasis are poorly understood; they will only be resolved by further experimental research, and by application and correlation of the findings with human material.

The high incidence of squamous cell carcinoma in the series of bladder carcinoma published from Egypt has been noted for a long time. Table 12 lists these

Table 12. *Types of malignant neoplasms of the urinary bladder associated with schistosomiasis in Egypt*

Authors and year	Reference number	No. of cases	Squamous carcinoma	Transitional carcinoma	Adeno-carcinoma	Other
MAKAR (1955)	17	300	40.0	30.0	10.0	20.0
DIMETTE et al. (1956)	6	90	55.5	37.9	6.6	—
LEGOLVAN et al. (1958)	16	73	42.5	46.6	8.9	4.1
HASHEM (1961)	13	261	62.3	33.3	1.8	2.6
ABOUL NASR et al. (1962)	1	299	60.75	33.75	4.75	0.75
ISHAK et al. (1966)	Present series	91	53.8	38.5	4.4	3.3

series of cases as classified by the reporting authors. This high incidence of squamous carcinoma has also been observed in the series of vesical carcinoma in Africans from South Africa [15, 21] and from Portuguese East Africa [12]. GILLMAN and PRATES [12] have compared some of the series from Africa (including Egypt) with series published from India, Europe and the United States. The reason for the higher incidence of squamous carcinoma in association with schistosomiasis is not known. Reference has already been made to the fact that in the present series and in most of the published series, squamous metaplasia and/or leukoplakia were found to be proportionately greater in association with squamous carcinoma than with other types of vesical carcinoma [1, 6, 12, 13, 16]. The series published by DIMMETTE et al. [6] shows the closest agreement to the present series in the relative frequency of the various types of vesical carcinoma.

It should be emphasized that in the present series of cases there was no direct relationship between the degree of oviposition in the bladder wall, or of the associated cellular reaction, and the type of carcinoma present. GILLMAN and PRATES [12] also found that the number of eggs in the bladder alone was no measure of carcinogenicity, nor was the presence of a few eggs adequate to exclude the potential importance of schistosomiasis as a factor in the etiology of cancer of the bladder.

These authors felt that whatever role schistosomiasis may play in promoting vesical cancer, this role is by no means direct, and that it will be necessary to take into account other factors in the environment, as well as in the members of the population, before the importance of schistosomiasis can be assessed as a cause of morbidity in general and of cancer in particular.

Many theories have been propounded to account for the high incidence of carcinoma of the bladder associated with schistosomiasis. These various theories have been reviewed by MOHAMED [18], MAKAR [17] and GILLMAN and PRATES [12]. Very little information has been forthcoming to take into account the multiplicity of factors which may be involved, such as the severity of the schistosomal infections, the effect of repeated infections (treated and untreated), the superimposition of urinary stasis, secondary infection and calculi, the excretion of various metabolites in the urine, dietary factors, the effect of smoking, sex differences, and possible racial and genetic factors.

Attention has recently been focused on the excretion of tryptophan metabolites in schistosomiasis. Thus, ABUL-FADL and KHALAFALLAH [2] showed an increase of 3-hydroxy-anthranilic acid to twice the normal level in Egyptian patients with schistosomiasis, whilst patients with cancer of the bladder associated with schistosomiasis had a four-fold increase of this metabolite. Serotonin excretion was increased threefold and tenfold respectively. An increase in urinary B-glucuronidase enzyme activity in schistosomiasis, and a more marked increase in cases associated with bladder carcinoma, was subsequently reported by the same authors [3]. TROUT and associates [27], however, did not find a significant excretion of 3-hydroxyanthranilic acid, 3-hydroxy-kynurenine nor 2-amino-3-hydroxy-acetophenone in the urine of patients with schistosomiasis from Portuguese East Africa. Experimental work by HASHEM and BOUTROS [14] has shown that the administration of a carcinogen, 2-acetylamino-fleurine to mice infected with *Schistosoma hematobium* leads to the induction of both benign and malignant neoplasms of the urinary bladder. Although the investigations of ABUL-FADL and associates [2, 3], TROUT et al. [27] and HASHEM and BOUTROS [14] are interesting and worthwhile much additional work requires to be done, in order to take into account the role of the aforementioned multiple factors which may be involved in the induction of cancer of the bladder in man. As MOSTOFI [20] has pointed out an international approach is needed, and cooperation between urologists, pathologists, biochemists, epidemiologists and biostatisticians is essential. More basic research on schistosomiasis is urgently needed.

Summary

1. The gross and microscopic changes in 91 cases of carcinoma of the bladder associated with schistosomiasis have been presented. The ratio of males to females in this study was about 5 : 1. The age incidence ranged from 25 to 60 years; most of the patients were in the third, fourth and fifth decades of life.

2. Seventy-nine of the tumors were grossly classified as fungating, 9 as infiltrative and 3 as ulcerative in type.

3. Only two of the neoplasms were located in the region of the trigone. The remaining tumors were in the anterior wall (28 cases), posterior wall (24 cases)

and superior-apical region [9]. In twenty-eight of the cases the bladder was diffusely involved by multiple tumors.

4. Forty-nine (53.8%) of the neoplasms were classified histologically as squamous, 35 (38.5%) as transitional and 4 (4.4%) as adenocarcinoma. There were
3 sarcomas in this series. Satellite nodules were found in ten of the bladders.

5. The extent of invasion of the bladder wall is presented. Sixty-eight of the
carcinomas extended beyond the muscularis. Twenty-five of these also showed
lymph node metastases, whilst 22 showed extension to the pelvic viscera and other
structures.

6. The metaplastic alterations in the bladder mucosa are analyzed. Seventy-
four of the 91 cases were accompanied by metaplastic changes. 90% of squamous
carcinomas and 57% of the transitional carcinomas showed metaplastic changes.
Squamous metaplasia was more frequently noted in the squamous (73%) than in
the transitional (28%) carcinomas. Leukoplakia also occurred with greater frequency in the squamous (67%) than in the transitional (31%) carcinomas. Carcinoma-in-situ was found in 31% of the squamous and in 14% of the transitional
carcinomas. Cystitis glandularis was present in an equal number of squamous
and transitional carcinomas. It is interesting that 43% of the transitional carcinomas showed no associated metaplasia, but only 10% of the squamous carcinomas
were without metaplastic changes.

7. The associated schistosomal infection is reported in detail.

References

[1] ABOUL NASR, A. L., M. E. GAZAYERLI, R. M. FAWZI, and I. EL-SIBAI: Epidemiology and
    pathology of cancer of the bladder in Egypt. Acta Un. Int. Cancr. 18, 528–537 (1962).
[2] ABUL-FADL, M. A. M., and A. S. KHALAFALLAH: Studies on the urinary excretion of
    certain tryptophan metabolites in bilharziasis and its possible relation to bladder
    cancer in Egypt. Brit. J. Cancer 15, 479–482 (1961).
[3] —, and O. M. METWALLI: Studies on certain urinary and blood serum enzymes in bil-
    harziasis and their possible relation to bladder cancer in Egypt. Brit. J. Cancer 17,
    137–141 (1963).
[4] BARSOUM, H.: Cancer of the bladder in Egypt. J. Trop. Med. Hyg. 43, 342–343 (1939).
[5] — Cancer in Egypt, its incidence and clinical forms. Acta Un. Int. Cancr. 9, 241–250
    (1953).
[6] DIMMETTE, R. M., H. F. SPROAT, and E. S. SAYEGH: The classification of carcinoma of
    the urinary bladder associated with schistosomiasis and metaplasia. J. Urol. 75,
    680–686 (1956).
[7] DODGE, O. G.: Tumours of the bladder in Uganda Africans. Acta Un. Int. Cancr. 18,
    548–552 (1962).
[8] DOLBEY, R. V., and A. W. MOORO: The incidence of cancer in Egypt. An analysis of
    671 cases. Lancet 1, 587–590 (1924).
[9] EDINGTON, G. M.: Malignant disease in the Gold Coast. Brit. J. Cancer 10, 595–608
    (1956).
[10] FERGUSON, A. R.: Associated bilharziasis and primary malignant disease of the urinary
    bladder with observations on a series of forty cases. J. Path. Bact. 16, 76–94
    (1911/12).
[11] GELFAND, M.: Schistosomiasis in South Central Africa. Capetown and Johannesburg:
    Juta & Co. 1950.
[12] GILLMAN, J., and M. D. PRATES: Histological types of bladder cancer in the Portuguese
    East African with special reference to bilharzial cystitis. Acta Un. Int. Cancr. 18,
    560–574 (1962).

[13] HASHEM, M.: The aetiology and pathogenesis of the bilharzial bladder cancer. J. Egypt. Med. Ass. **44**, 857—966 (1961).

[14] —, and K. BOUTROS: The influence of bilharzial infection on the carcinogenesis of the mouse bladder. An experimental study. J. Egypt. Med. Ass. **44**, 598—606 (1961).

[15] HIGGINSON, J., and A. G. OETTLE: Cancer of the bladder in the South African Bantu. Acta Un. Cancr. **18**, 579—584 (1962).

[16] LE GOLVAN, P. C., K. G. ISHAK, H. K. GRACE, and A. FAM: Carcinoma of the urinary bladder associated with urinary schistosomiasis. Malignant bladder tumors in Egypt — a pathological study of 73 cases. Department of the Navy, U.S. Naval Medical Research Unit-3, Cairo, Egypt, Research Report NM 52 02 03.6.

[17] MAKAR, N.: Urological aspects of bilharziasis in Egypt. Société Orientale de Publicité, Cairo, 1955.

[18] MOHAMED, A. S.: The association of bilharziasis and malignant disease in the urinary bladder. Pathogenesis of bilharzial cancer in the urinary bladder. J. Egypt. Med. Ass. **37**, 1066 (1954).

[19] MOSTOFI, F. K.: Potentialities of bladder epithelium. J. Urol. **71**, 705—714 (1954).

[20] — Pathology of cancer of bladder. Acta Un. Int. Cancr. **18**, 611—615 (1962).

[21] OETTLE, A. G.: Racial differences in cancer in South Africa. S. Afr. Biol. Soc. Pamphlet **17**, 40—49 (1955).

[22] PAYET, M.: Bilharziose et cancer de la vessie au Senegal. Acta Un. Int. Cancr. **18**, 641—642 (1962).

[23] PRATES, M. D.: The rates of cancer of the bladder in the Portuguese East Africans of Lourenço Marques. Acta Un. Int. Cancer. **18**, 643—647 (1962).

[24] SAYEGH, E. S.: Late complications of urinary schistosomiasis. J. Urol. **63**, 353—371 (1950).

[25] SHAMMA, A. H.: Schistosomiasis and cancer in Iraq. Amer. J. Clin. Path. **25**, 1283—1284 (1955).

[26] SOROUR, M. F.: The pathology and morbid histology of bilharzial lesions in various parts of the body. C. R. Congr. Intern. Med. Trop. Hyg. **4**, 321—377 (1928).

[27] TROUT, G. E., J. GILLMAN, and M. D. PRATES: Bilharzial cystitis and the urinary excretion of tryptophan metabolites in the Portuguese East Africans. Acta Un. Int. Cancr. **18**, 575—578 (1962).

The Role of Bilharziasis in the Pathogenesis of Bladder Cancer

M. GAZAYERLI and M. KORAITUM*

Although the general consensus is that cancer of the bladder is related to urinary bilharziasis, the exact relationship still remains unknown. The following theories may be mentioned:

(1) Mechanical irritation theory attributing the process to irritation of the bladder epithelium by the eggs [1, 3].

(2) Chronic irritation theory [2].

(3) Bilharzial toxin theory — toxins produced by the miracidia and worms [6].

(4) Urinary retention theory ascribing the process to destruction of the muscle coat in bilharzial cystitis which could interfere with complete evacuation of the urine. The carcinogen responsible for the development of cancer in any bladder would thus have a chance to act longer on the bladder mucosa in bilharzial bladders resulting in the high incidence of cancer of the bladder in bilharzial countries as compared with that in non-bilharzial countries [4, 5]. The present work gives additional support to this theory.

Material and results

The material consisted of 7 postmortem normal bladders and 61 pathological cases including 38 "operative" cases of bladder neck obstruction, 10 "cystectomy" cases of cancer of the bladder and 13 postmortem bilharzial bladders.

In the 7 normal cases attention was particularly directed to the distribution and arrangement of the muscle in the region of the bladder neck. It was found that the external longitudinal muscle layer of the bladder had its insertion into the middle muscular layer of the bladder neck. This insertion probably helps to pull down the fundus during the process of micturition. Thus fibrosis at this site — a common site involved in bilharziasis of the bladder neck — would interfere with proper evacuation of the urine.

The 61 pathological cases revealed on microscopic examination bilharzial affection of the bladder neck. The bilharzial lesions were both localized and diffuse showing various stages of maturation and involving particularly the submucosa and the inner two-thirds of the muscle coat resulting in marked muscle destruction. In most cases the insertion of the external muscle layer of the bladder into the middle muscular layer of the bladder neck was found replaced by bilharzial inflammatory products. Another common site affected by bilharziasis was found to be the trigone where marked muscular destruction and fibrosis were noticed. The trigonal involvement would interfere with the normal opening of the bladder neck.

* Departments of Pathology and Urology, Alexandria University, Alexandria, Egypt (UAR).

In 70% of the cases the nerves in the various coats of the bladder were also involved in the bilharzial process, most probably interfering with the normal neuromuscular conduction resulting in improper evacuation of the urine.

The bladder neck mucosa of the 10 cancer cases revealed very small bilharzial polypi in 4 cases. The submucous and muscle coats were heavily affected by bilharziasis in the 10 cases.

M. SAFWAT and R. M. FAWZI [8] laid great stress on bilharziasis of the prostate and claimed that it was the major factor in causing bladder neck obstruction. In the present work, 20 prostates were examined and only 5 (25%) cases showed mild bilharzial affection, whereas in the 20 cases the bladder necks were heavily affected by the bilharzial process.

Conclusions

It is postulated that the high incidence of bladder cancer in bilharzial countries may be due to urinary stagnation and consequent prolonged action of carcinogens.

The major factor in the mechanism of this stagnation seems to be marked muscle destruction and fibrosis occurring particularly in the regions of the bladder neck and trigone. Bilharzial polypi and involvement of the intrinsic nerves of the bladder in the bilharzial process may constitute minor factors.

References

[1] DIAMANTIS, A.: Le cancer bilharzien vesical. J. Egypt. Med. Ass. 17, 563—583 (1934).
[2] DOLBEY, R. U., and A. W. MOORO: The incidence of cancer in Egypt. Lancet 1, 587—590 (1924).
[3] FURGUSON, A. R.: Bilharziasis. Cairo Sci. J. 4, 129—134 (1910).
[4] GAZAYERLI, M., and H. A. KHALIL: Bilharziasis and cancer of the urinary tract; some observations. Alexandria Med. J. 5, 31—36 (1959).
[5] GAZAYERLI, M.: The relationship of environment to cancer in Egypt. International Pathology, 4, 37—40 (1963).
[6] MAKAR, N.: Urological aspects of bilharziasis in Egypt. Cairo: S.O.P. Press 1955.
[7] NASR, ABOUL L., M. GAZAYERLI, R. FAWZI, and I. EL SIBAI: Epidemiology and pathology of cancer of the bladder. Symposium on bladder cancer. ACTA. Unio Internationale Contra Cancrum. 18, 528—537 (1962).
[8] SAFWAT, M., and R. E. FAWZI: Pitfalls in the problem of bilharzial bladder neck obstruction. Kasr-El-Aini. J. Surg. 2, 286—292 (1961).

Clinical Patterns in Urinary Schistosomiasis

D. M. Forsyth*

Bilharziasis is of immense antiquity and the clinical signs, symptoms and syndromes attributed to the infection are almost as protean as the papyri, parchments and papers on the subject. The present account is based on personal experience of urinary schistosomiasis in Kuwait and in Tanzania.

Aetiology

Infection is acquired from transmission sites inhabited by a snail intermediate host. The infective larvae, or cercariae, in the water come into contact with and penetrate the skin or mucous membranes, enter the systemic circulation and reach the vessels of the portal system, where development continues. The natural history of bilharzia in the human host is largely determined by the frequency of exposure, by the density of cercariae in the transmission sites and by the numbers of parasites which are able to penetrate and to mature. The adult schistosomes mate and migrate to inhabit the veins and venules related to the bladder, the ureters and other genito-urinary and pelvic organs. By themselves the worms are innocuous; it is their eggs which are responsible for the pathological changes, for the symptoms and signs of infection and the occurrence of irreversible lesions may be directly related to the numbers of ova voided.

Pathology

It has been customary to classify the course of the infection into four phases: invasion, the toxic or anaphylactoid stage and those of early and late established infection [2]. These stages are summarised in Table 1, reproduced from the report to the Director General of the World Health Organisation by the Scientific Group on Research in Bilharziasis (Assessment of Medical and Public Health Importance) [11].

The pathological changes associated with urinary schistosomiasis have been described in the past, notably by MAKAR [9] in Egypt and by HONEY and GELFAND [8] in Rhodesia, but the prevalence was recorded in hospital patients and the importance to the health of the community has remained uncertain. The task of the Bilharzia Research Unit of the Ross Institute was to determine the medical and health importance of the infection in a particular population at Bukumbi, near Mwanza, Tanzania. The observations here described must be taken in this context and are not strictly comparable with those previously reported following the detailed investigation of individual patients.

* Presently: Bilharzia Research Unit, The Ross Institute of Tropical Hygiene, London, W. C. 1, England.

Formerly: Bilharzia Research Unit, The Ross Institute of Tropical Hygiene, Zanzibar, Tanzania.

Table 1. *A classification of the course of bilharziasis — based on parasitological, clinical and pathological aspects*

Stage	Parasitological	Clinical	Pathological
Stage of invasion	Migration and beginning of maturation	Incubation period, including cercarial dermatitis, if present	Slight inflammatory reactions in skin, lungs and liver
Stage of maturation	Completion of maturation and early oviposition	Toxaemic stage of the disease (or acute febrile stage) not always recognised or present	Hyperergic reactions, generalised and local, to products of eggs and/or young schistosomes
Stage of established infection	Intensive oviposition accompanied by a corresponding egg discharge	Stage of early chronic disease, characterised for instance by haematuria, or intestinal and other digestive manifestations possibly with cardio-pulmonary or other complications	Local inflammatory reactions due to ova, resulting mainly in granuloma formation. Fibrosis is not a predominant feature
Stage of irreversible effects	Prolonged infection (usually with reduced or discontinued egg extrusion)	Stage of late chronic disease, due to irreversible effects and/or sequelae or complications	Progressing formation varying with intensity of infection, and possibly other factors of fibrous tissue, with its consequences according to the organs involved

Table 2. *Prevalence of bladder calcification in the Bukumbi survey*

Category	Male			Female			Both		
	Total	No.	%	Total	No.	%	Total	No.	%
Young children	42	6	14.3	11	4	36.4	53	10	18.8
At puberty	15	2	13.3	2	1	50	17	3	17.6
Adolescents	33	5	15.0	1	0	0	34	5	14.7
Total not adult	90	13	14.4	14	5	35.7	104	18	17.3
Young adults, aged 20—29	288	15	5.2	42	8	19.0	330	23	7.0
Middle aged, 30—44 years	160	13	8.1	34	2	5.9	194	15	4.4
Old aged, 45 years and over	74	1	1.4	49	2	4.1	123	3	2.4
Total adult	522	29	5.6	125	12	9.6	647	41	6.3
All	612	42	6.9	139	17	12.2	751	59	7.9

Clinical observations

The stages of invasion and of maturation

In the survey we recognised no case of cercarial dermatitis nor observed any toxaemic or febrile illness which could definitely be attributed to *S. haematobium*. An absolute eosinophilia of more than 800 cells per cmm could be directly related to infection in a proportion of all age and sex groups examined.

The stage of established infection

Past or present haematuria was reported by 64.2% of 976 persons found to be voiding eggs of *S. haematobium* in the urine, and painful micturition in 68.4%. Frequency of urination during the day or by night could not be related to infection. Subacute inflammation of the bladder wall with oedema and congestion, tubercles and papillomata were commonly seen at cystoscopy. These may be resolved by effective treatment [3] and it is probable that some spontaneous re-trogression also occurs.

The stage of irreversible effects

Bilharzia has been indicted as specifically involving the alimentary, genital and urinary tracts; the portal, pulmonary and systemic circulatory systems, and of being responsible for vaguely defined ill-health.

The alimentary tract

Eggs of *S.˙ haematobium* were commonly found in the stools of infected indi-viduals, but no symptoms or signs were observed.

The genital organs

No disease of the genitals attributable to bilharzia was recognised. All women were questioned about their marital status and about the number of children they had borne. It was impossible to establish a relationship between sterility and infection.

The urinary tract

A sample of 824 people, representative of the Bukumbi community, was surveyed radiologically. The films from 44 were technically unsatisfactory or the patient could not be classified according to age and sex group. There were 780 successful examinations, 133 abdominal radiographs and 647 urograms. The plain X-ray of the pelvis was inadequate in 29 of the latter.

Three young adult males and a boy of 12 years had deformity and calcification of both ureters. Ten people, or 1.4% of the total examined had calculi. All were males. Stones were seen in the kidney in 1 young, 1 middleaged and 2 old men; in the ureter of a boy and 2 adults, one old and one middle-aged, and vesical lithiasis was present in 1 young and 2 old men. Pyelography showed that 10 of the 48 people with calcification of the bladder also had more extensive co-existant disease. Unilateral hydronephrosis was seen in a boy of 12 years, in a young woman and in a middle-aged man; another middle-aged man had bilateral hydronephrosis. Two men, one old and the other young, had a non-functioning kidney, and uni-lateral ureteric deformity was present in 1 old man, and 2 old women, and bilateral-ly in a middle-aged man.

The results of intravenous pyelography on 647 men, women and children living in Bukumbi are summarised in Table 3.

Table 3. *Summary of pyelography findings in the Bukumbi survey*

Category	Male			Female			Both		
	Total	No.	%	Total	No.	%	Total	No.	%
Young children	31	10	32	8	2	25	39	12	31
At puberty	13	4	31	4	1	25	17	5	29
Adolescents	31	7	23	1	0	0	32	7	22
Total not adult	75	21	28	13	3	23	88	24	27
Young adults, aged 20—29	251	38	15	42	9	21	293	47	16
Middle aged, 30—44 years	135	23	17	32	2	6	167	25	15
Old aged, over 45 years	59	13	22	40	4	10	99	17	17
Total adult	445	74	17	114	15	13	559	89	16
All	520	95	18	127	18	14	647	113	17

Children attending the primary school at Usagara, the largest settlement in Bukumbi, were excluded from the survey, but were the subject of a separate investigation. Satisfactory urograms were obtained from 405 of the 466 pupils registered and the results are summarised in more detail in Table 4.

Table 4. *Summary of results of radiological survey at Usagara school*

Standard	Number of urograms	Number of abnormals	% abnormal	% with calcified bladder	% with hydro-nephrosis	% with ureteral deformity
1	84	8	10	6	5	1
2	77	19	25	6	10	12
3	70	15	20	9	11	5
4	77	17	22	8	6	13
5	35	11	31	14	3	11
6	33	10	30	9	9	21
7	29	9	31	7	17	14
All	405	89	22	8	8	10

It has been suggested that *S. haematobium* predisposes to secondary bacteriological contamination of the urinary tract. The results of the routine bacteriological examinations of the urines collected from 426 unselected members of the Bukumbi community are shown in Table 5.

No case of carcinoma of the bladder was recognised.

Table 5. *Prevalence of bacterial infection of the urine in those with and without patent S. haematobium infection*

Category	S. haematobium present Bacteriuria			S. haematobium absent Bacteriuria		
	Examined	No. +ve	% +ve	Examined	No. + ve	% + ve
Males	151	13	9	194	14	7
Females	22	5	23	59	12	20
Both sexes	173	18	10	253	26	10

The portal system

The size of the liver and of the spleen of approximately 2,250 men, women and children was recorded systematically. Enlargement of either or both organs was commonplace, but could not be related to bilharzial infection. Thymol flocculation and turbidity tests were performed as a routine and the plasma protein levels of a number of unselected individuals were also estimated. There was no apparent association between abnormal results and the presence of eggs of *S. haematobium* in the urine.

The pulmonary circulation

To detect pulmonary hypertension, standard-lead electrocardiograms were recorded and where these suggested right-ventricular preponderance a postero-anterior skiagram of the chest was taken. To date the electrocardiograms and skiagrams of more than 2,000 people known to be infected with bilharzia have shown no instance of pulmonary hypertension.

The systemic circulation

Blood pressures were recorded routinely and 17 (1.4%) of 1,181 adults apparently free from infection were found to have a diastolic pressure in excess of 100 mms, mercury, compared with 4 (63%) of 635 adults who were voiding eggs of *S. haematobium* in the urine. The differences are not statistically significant. None of the younger people had a diastolic pressure of 100 or more mms of mercury.

Vague non-specific effects

Bilharzia has been said to cause tiredness, apathy and vague ill-health. Absentee rates of infected and uninfected schoolchildren were virtually identical in Usagara and other schools, and it was not possible, even with specially designed tests [1] to demonstrate excessive lassitude in the infected.

The estimation of haemoglobin levels has been routine and after more than 4,500 such examinations we have been unable to relate anaemia with infection with *S. haematobium* in any age or sex group.

We have not found that bilharzia causes impairment of general physique or in the mean height and weight of population groups of any age.

Diagnosis

The diagnosis of active urinary schistosomiasis is made by finding live ova in the centrifuged deposit of a specimen of urine. Cystoscopy or radiography may show the effects of past or present infection; positive skin, agglutination and fluorescent antibody tests indicate that probably the patient has at some time been infected with *S. mansoni, S. haematobium, S. japonica*, or one of the less important schistosomes.

Discussion

It is apparent from the above that haematuria and painful micturition are the only symptoms which consistantly indicate infection with *S. haematobium*. These cause little physical distress and have frequently been considered by doctors, parents and patients alike as phenomena of little significance, to be expected in the normal processes of development and of maturation. They are in reality danger signals giving warning of the possibility of active urological disease. An analogy may be drawn with the symptomatology of rheumatism in childhood where the importance of growing pains, occasional sore throat and minor constitutional upsets may be overlooked by the parents or by the practitioner with disastrous results for the patient. The majority of hydronephroses and almost all calcified bladders and ureteric lesions apparently produced no specific symptoms betraying their presence.

In Kuwait [3, 4], Bukumbi and Zanzibar (unpublished observations) the effects of infection with *S. haematobium* upon the bladder, ureters and kidneys were frequent and severe when compared with those observed in other systems and organs, and it ollows that the pathology of urinary schistosomiasis is essentially that of the associated urological disease.

Little is known of the natural history. Infection was of equal prevalence and intensity in the two sexes, as were calcification of the bladder and ureteric deformity, and the frequency with which these complications were found was directly related to the number of eggs voided in the urine. Hydronephrosis and renal non-function were associated with urinary schistosomiasis but were not dependant upon the intensity of the egg output and were thought to be the sequelea of vesical and ureteral pathology rather than the direct results of infection. Hydronephrosis and non-functioning kidneys were more common in males than in females, and this is due to physiological differences in the mechanisms of urination, which may be demonstrated by micturating cystography [10].

These findings strongly support GELFAND's [7] observations that sequelae were the result of reflux rather than of ureteral stenosis.

The prevalence of urological pathology did not rise in adult males when compared with children, and there was a fall in the rates of bladder calcification and ureteral deformity. There was a slight decrease in the prevalence of hydronephrosis and a rise in the occurrence of non-functioning kidnye with increasing age. These findings indicate a mortality in males with hydronephrosis about the time of adolescence. Bladder calcification and hydronephrosis were often associated, and this mortality was reflected in the observed reduction in the prevalence of calcified bladder and ureteral deformity in adult males. It is thought that these deaths usually occurred in the person's home unobserved and unreported, and that the causes were uraemia and intercurrent disease.

In girls the prevalence of hydronephrosis was lower than in boys, and calcified bladder rates showed no fall with increasing age, which suggested that with the lower hydronephrosis rate significant mortality did not occur.

This indirect evidence will shortly be confirmed or refuted by longitudinal studies.

Summary

The clinical features and natural history of urinary schistosomiasis are briefly described. Haematuria and dysuria are the only consistent symptoms of infection and are inadequate danger signals of possible underlying urological disease. The prevalence of various lesions in the urinary tract is discussed and evidence is given to indicate that S. haematobium is the cause of significant mortality in young adult males. The paper describes the results of community investigations and these are not strictly comparable with studies of hospital patients.

The majority of these data are summarised from the papers of FORSYTH and MACDONALD [6] and FORSYTH and BRADLEY [5] and detailed figures and descriptions of the methods and techniques employed may be found in the originals.

The Bilharzia Research Unit of the Ross Institute of Tropical Hygiene is supported financially by the Rockefeller Foundation, H. M. Treasury and the World Health Organisation.

References

[1] BRADLEY, D. J.: The assessment of lassitude in school children with bilharziasis. Annul report for 1961–1962 of East African Institute for Medical Research, Nairobi, 1962.
[2] FAIRLEY, N. H.: Price's Textbook of the Practice of Medicine, 9th Edition, HUNTER, D. (Ed.) London: Oxford Press 1956.
[3] FORSYTH, D. M.: Post-schistosomal uropathy. Lancet 2, 990–992 (1958).
[4] – Practical difficulties in the treatment of schistomiasis in an Arab community. Trans. Roy. Soc. Trop. Med. Hyg. 55, 168–177 (1961).

[5] Forsyth, D. M., and D. J. Bradley: The consequences of bilharzial infection. Medical and public health importance in North West Tanzania. Bull. World Health Org. (in press).

[6] —, and G. MacDonald: Urologic complications of endemic schistosomiasis in school children. Trans. Roy. Soc. Trop. Med. Hyg. 59, 171—178 (1965).

[7] Gelfand, M.: The diagnosis and prognosis of schistosomiasis. Amer. J. Trop. Med. 29, 945—958 (1949).

[8] Honey, R., and M. Gelfand: The urological aspects of bilharziasis in Rhodesia. Edinburgh: E. & S. Livingstone 1960.

[9] Makar, N.: Urological aspects of Bilharziasis in Egypt, Cairo, Societe Orientale de Publicite 1955.

[10] Middlemiss, J. H.: Personal communication.

[11] World Health Organization: Scientific Group on Research in Bilharziasis (Assessment of medical and public health importance). Report to the Director-General. Geneva 1960.

Egg-Output in Bilharziasis in Relation to Epidemiology, Pathology, Treatment and Control

P. JORDAN*

With 4 figures

Bilharzia must be unique amongst diseases affecting man. It is known to have existed at the time of the Pharaohs in Egypt, and 39 million persons are infected in Africa with *Schistosoma haematobium* [41] to-day, yet, in spite of the antiquity of the disease and all the research that has been done, there is no consistent opinion amongst research workers, clinicians or public health workers as to how important the infection is, and one might add that opinions vary as to how it should be treated — and even whether it should be treated.

In Egypt, the infection is considered important, in Rhodesia also it is thought to be a disease requiring control, but in many other countries in Africa Ministries of Health frequently do not know what priority to give the infection or else it is given a low priority for expenditure of usually limited monies.

Differences in the intensity of infection is said [16] to be the most popular explanation for the apparent differences in severity of the disease which are reported from different parts of Africa. One of the recommendations from the Ciba Symposium on Bilharziasis in 1961 stressed the need for criteria with which to estimate worm load so that it could be related to the clinical and pathological picture.

The determination of worm load is at present impossible and although the egg load may be an inadequate measure of worm load, it is the only measure we have at present of estimating intensity of infection. Certainly, egg output may be affected by many factors, but in the absence of any other method it seems not unreasonable to consider egg output as an indication of worm load. In the older age groups, possible immunological and pathological factors may be operative which might invalidate this relationship, but in the younger age groups where such processes are probably at a minimum it is suggested that egg load might be a useful indication of intensity of infection in groups of people.

Hookworm disease is invariably discussed in relation of egg output. In filariasis studies, where the adult worm load cannot be assessed, therapeutic and clinical studies invariably refer to the number of microfilariae in the blood (varying as it does from hour to hour) or in the skin. In bilharzia, however, little regard has been paid to the quantitative aspect of egg output even though, as BRADLEY [9] has quite rightly pointed out in regard to *S. haematobium* "the parasite (is) kind enough to pour out its eggs suspended in a liquid in pure culture".

Until the middle of the last decade, bilharzia surveys were made in many countries on a qualitative basis. Urines were collected at unspecified times and

* Presently: Research and Control Department, Castries, St. Lucia, West Indies.
Formerly: East African Institute for Medical Research, Mwanza, Tanganyika.

little attention appears to have been paid to the numbers of eggs being excreted. BLAIR [7] considered that egg counts were of little value. BENNIE [6], however, had previously pointed out that more eggs were found in specimens of urine passed in the afternoon than in the early morning and also suggested that exercise increased egg excretion.

GERBER [20] working in Sierra Leone appears to have been the first worker to consider egg output in urines as a measure of intensity of infection. He made rough estimates of intensity by a simple +, ++, or +++ classification of the numbers of eggs in the urinary sediment. DUKE and McCULLOUGH [15] used a similar method in their investigations in the Gambia and found, like GERBER [20], that children showed not only a higher incidence of infection than adults but that also their egg loads were higher.

STIMMEL and SCOTT [40] in a detailed statistical study demonstrated that in Egypt the excretion of eggs of S. haematobium follows a definite pattern and that many more eggs are excreted round about midday than at other times in the 24 hours and SCOTT [39] suggested that egg counts may be used as an indication of the intensity of infection in the study of bilharziasis. The diurnal perodicity of egg output has since been demonstrated in Tanganyika [25], and occurs whether the individual is ambulant or in bed. ONORI [32] also demonstrated the diurnal variation.

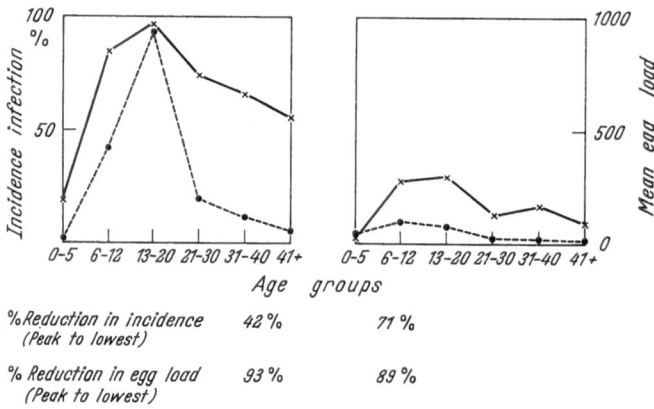

Fig. 1. Showing incidence of infection and egg load (per 10 ml urine) in different age groups in two areas of Zanzibar and Tanganyika

There is, of course, a variation from day to day in egg output at the peak period of egg excretion in individuals, but if one considers a group of people the variation is reduced and it is suggested that egg counts and the calculation of the mean ova load in the group or the median when the urine is collected round the peak of egg excretion is of considerable value in epidemiology.

By collecting urines at about 12 midday from persons of all ages in two different endemic areas, age-incidence graphs and "age-load" graphs were produced (Fig. 1).

As shown in the figure the mean egg load in each age group roughly follows the age incidence curve. The drop in egg load — from the highest mean count to the lowest in each area is similar being 93%, and 89%, in the areas of high and low endemicity respectively.

With the information obtained from such data one can assess with some degree of accuracy which age groups are the greatest public health hazard. It becomes immediately clear that children are potentially responsible for a major part of the contamination of water habitats in Tanganyika. Although there may be a high incidence of egg excretion in the older age groups, the number of eggs passed by them is very much less in proportion than the number passed by the children and teenagers. Added to this is the fact that the younger age groups form nearly 50% of the population and the viability of their eggs is greater than that in the older age groups [20, 21]. Although statistical evidence that children play and urinate in ponds more frequently than adults is lacking it is the general impression in East Africa that this is so and it seems not unreasonable to suppose it is the same throughout Africa.

The above study, by showing a constant pattern, supported the view that if the collection times were standardised, egg counting techniques might give interesting and useful data applicable to survey work.

Surveys were accordingly carried out in different parts of Tanganyika, and urines collected around midday from boys in Standard III and IV at Primary Schools [25, 26]. The incidence was found to vary considerably, and village schools having similar rates of infection have been grouped together to study the distribution of individual high and low egg counts. The results are shown in Fig. 2.

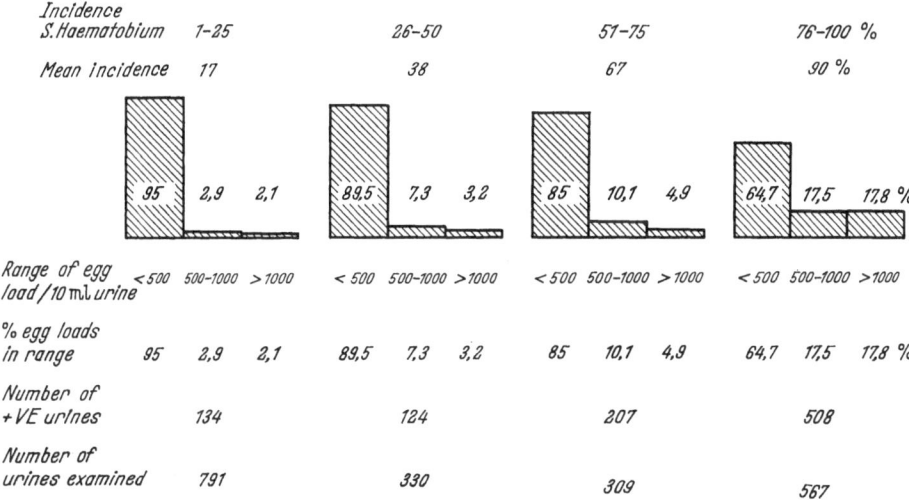

Fig. 2. Percentage frequency distribution of egg load/10 ml urine from boys in standards III and IV at primary schools in Tanganyika. Specimens collected about peak of egg excretion

It is seen that whereas in schoolboys from areas where the incidence of infection was less than 25%, nearly 95% had counts of less than 500 eggs per 10 ml of urine; in the schools where the incidence of infection was between 76 and 100%, 65% had counts in this range and nearly 18% had more than 1,000 eggs per ml of urine compared with only 2.1% in the lower endemic areas — a pattern similar to that found by ONORI [32] in GHANA.

A rough direct correlation was found between incidence of infection and mean egg load in the individual villages but it will be appreciated that when treatment is available the natural incidence/egg load relationship is likely to be upset — the egg load being liable to reduction but the incidence of infection probably being reduced to a lesser degree.

For a given peak incidence of infection, is the intensity the same in other parts of Africa as in Tanganyika? It seems possible that it is and from data given by ONORI [32], the figures from Tanganyika and Ghana appear to be similar.

Of particular interest, however, is the egg load in areas in which every child, or nearly every child, is infected. When incidence is used as the parameter of infection a limit is set at 100%; if intensity of infection is considered, the theoretical upper limit will, presumably, be the egg load just short of that causing death. There might therefore be considerable differences in egg load in different hyper-endemic areas and possibly differences in the incidence of urinary tract complications. Is the egg output in teenagers in such hyperendemic areas of Egypt greater than, similar to, or less than that in hyperendemic areas in East, West and South Africa?

It is suggested that the results of quantitative epidemiological studies in East Africa demonstrate a definite pattern and sufficient differences in egg output in different age groups and different endemic areas to warrant further use of the method to indicate intensity of infection in groups of people.

Eggs may be excreted or retained in the tissues. It is impossible to determine, in humans, the relative proportions, but probably the majority of those remaining, stay in the bladder. Some of course, get swept to the liver and some to the lungs, and some to other organs. It seems reasonable to suppose, however, that the more there are being excreted, the more there will be in the bladder and the greater will be the pathology in that organ.

In the wall of the bladder and ureters, the retained eggs become calcified in their millions — literally millions, the accumulation of years, and will show on X-ray as a calcified bladder and/or ureter. One might expect therefore the incidence of calcified bladder in a community to be related to the incidence (or intensity of infection?) of bilharzia in the area.

HONEY and GELFAND [24] have described the development of the complications of S. haematobium in the urinary tract. The incidence of complications such as hydroureter and hydronephrosis, in persons with calcified bladders is however not known, but it seems possible that persons with calcified bladders are potentially liable to develop later, other severe and possibly fatal changes in the urinary tract and kidney though these may also develop in the absence of a calcified bladder.

HONEY and GELFAND [24] refer to differences in the effect of bilharzia in the African bladder compared with that in the European and consider these differences are due to the African being exposed more often to infection than the European (and thus presumably having a heavier infection). Their cases were all seen in hospital practice and it seems not unlikely that this fact may also be partly responsible for the differences found — Europeans seeking medical attention at an earlier stage than the African. It is noteworthy that they commonly found bilharzial disease, that is, the late complications, in young people, 71% their of African cases with advanced disease being under 30.

Further evidence of the effect of bilharzia in the young has recently come from Egypt where 30% of 132 children between the ages of 4 and 14 suffering with bilharzia were found to have demonstrable changes in the urinary tract on X-ray — including 4% with hydronephrosis [31].

If, as the work reported above suggests, the intensity of infection varies directly with the incidence, the incidence of complications should be greater in those communities where bilharzia is hyperendemic.

In work carried out by the Ross Institute Research Team, working at Mwanza, X-ray examinations both plain and I.V.P. — have been carried out on Primary School children at schools where the incidence — and intensity of infection — were different. It will be seen that in these schools, there was in fact, a difference in incidence of late complications corresponding to incidence and intensity of infection (Table 1).

Table 1. *X-ray examination of primary school children. (Data kindly supplied by Dr.* D. M. FORSYTH*)*

| | I.V.P. | | Plain X-ray abdomen | |
	Usagara	Bukumbi	Bukumbi	Bwiru
Incidence of infection (1962)	88% (Standards I and II)	43% (Standards I and II)	43%	13% (Standards I-IV)
Mean eggs out put / 10 ml urine	517	325	325	88
Nos. X-rayed	406	80	293	146
Standards X-rayed	I—VII	IV and V	I—IV	I—IV
Abnormal (%)	22	15		
Calcified bladder (%)	8	3	6	I + I possible
Hydronephrosis (%)	8	4		
Deformity of ureter (%)	10	10		

All these reports suggest that bilharzia in children and young people in Egypt, East Africa and Rhodesia is not the benign, unimportant infection many authorities consider it to be. In spite of these findings which support the view that serious lesions may be very much more common and that they develop earlier than has been thought, accurate data on their incidence is generally still lacking, and, if they depend on a particularly minimum load of infection, what that load is. It is suggested that further work correlating X-ray findings with incidence and egg load data, from infected populations in areas of differing endemicity might throw light on this aspect of the disease. Large numbers of X-rays would be required from areas of different bilharzial endemicity and it is suggested that the X-ray machines used for mass T.B. surveys might be of value for the detection of calcified bladders the incidence of which might prove to be an index of severe urinary tract disease.

Post-mortem studies are also important in this respect, and a quantitative appraisal of the egg load in the bladder in relation to pathology in the urinary tract might well be rewarding. In a small series of post-mortem examinations at Mwanza [25] a cork borer of 22 mm diameter, was used for removing standard

98   P. JORDAN:

sized pieces of bladder wall. These were removed from different areas of the bladder and digested. In 25 cases the egg load from the site of maximum gross pathology was found to vary up to more than a third of a million eggs. In this, the apparently most heavily infected case, death was due to bilateral hydronephrosis with stones in both hydroureters.

Turning to treatment of bilharzia. — Curative therapy aims at destroying all adult worms which will result in the cessation of the passage of eggs in the urine whatever the method of examination.

Treatment often fails, and eggs are still passed, but in reduced numbers. If a 90% reduction in egg output is obtained in a case excreting, before treatment, few eggs, it is difficult to find the 10% of eggs remaining after treatment — this person is likely therefore to be considered cured. If on the other hand, a 90% reduction in egg output is obtained in a person initially excreting thousands of eggs, the remaining 10% will be comparatively easy to find and the treatment will be considered a failure. Can differences in the egg output of persons with bilharzia account for the different cure rates reported by different workers using the same drug but working in different areas? It might be a possible factor.

Sodium antimony dimercaptosuccinate is being given to children in whom the egg output before treatment is determined. Analysis of "cure" rates after treatment, in relation to pre-treatment egg output suggests — so far — that in the group excreting few eggs cure rates are better than those excreting large numbers of eggs. (Table 2 and Fig. 3). This does not necessarily mean that heavily infected cases are more difficult to cure than lightly infected cases, but merely that

Table 2. *Effect of initial egg out put on results of treatment of S. haematobium (6 months follow-up)*

Egg output range (eggs/10 ml urine)	1—125	126—500	501 +
Mean egg output	62	270	1120
Number in group	68	43	22
Cured	75%	58%	18%
Reduction in egg output	89%	86%	88%

cases finally excreting very few eggs are difficult to prove positive. It may also be that in patients with large numbers of adult worms, there is a greater chance that a few will not be killed by a given dose of drug than in a patient with only a few worms.

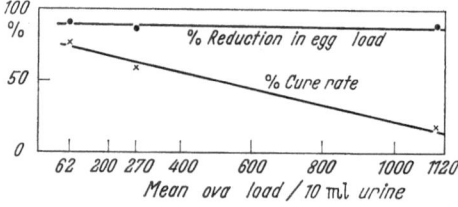

Fig. 3. Figure showing cure rates and percentage reduction in egg load 6 months after treatment in patients with S. *haematobium* grouped according to their egg load before treatment

In the above series of therapeutic trials, which is not yet complete, the percentage reduction in egg load has been calculated for the three different egg load groups. It is seen that percentage reduction in ova load is constant and independant of egg load and supports the view [27] that the percentage reduction in egg output might be a more reliable measure for comparing efficiency of drugs than the cure rate which appears to depend on egg load.

If egg output is to be considered, the question of when to collect urine is an important one in this respect and although the collection of 24 hour specimens might be difficult it seems likely that egg counts based on such collections may be the most satisfactory procedure for accurate assessment of drug efficiency. If this is not possible then the diurnal periodicity of egg excretion makes it imperative that specimens are always taken at the same time, and preferably at the peak of egg excretion.

Control of bilharziasis by therapy is theoretically possible if more satisfactory drugs can be produced or better regimes devised for existing drugs. Even with effective, easily administered drugs it is unlikely that everyone in a population can be treated. Studies of the egg output in different age groups of a population, in relation to the incidence of infection in a community, will show, however, in which group efforts to obtain successful treatment should be concentrated.

Therapeutic control of bilharzia must now include the concept of suppressive therapy — the giving of drugs at — say monthly — intervals in order to reduce egg output for a prolonged period of time and by this means to interfere with transmission of the infection.

Results of this procedure in Tanganyika suggest again that the effectiveness of these regimes depend on the initial egg output of those treated and it was first suggested that the percentage reduction in ova load, rather than the cure rate should be used to assess the effectiveness of suppressive therapy [27]. If results are based only on the proportion of cases becoming negative, results are poor, if based however on percentage reduction of egg loads, they are better. Although the idea of suppressive therapy was initially one of possible control, it is probably of importance to the individuals concerned in that by reducing egg output, a corresponding reduction in the numbers of eggs being retained will presumably be achieved — thus dimishing the risk of late complications if such therapy is repeated annually. Such a view should also be taken of treatment that fails — although the patient may not be cured, the egg load excreted, and the egg load retained will be reduced — perhaps sufficiently to save the patient from gross calcification and other complications in the urinary tract.

The determination of egg output has a further application in assessing the effectiveness of control schemes based on mollusciciding. The mean egg load in infants can be calculated in the area before control measures are commenced. When these have been in operation for a number of years, re-evaluation of the mean egg load in infants of the same age group as were originally examined should show to what extent control has been effective. The children might still be acquiring infection and if the results were based only on qualitative findings, the scheme would be considered a failure, but even under these conditions a substantial lowering of intensity of infection might have been obtained and a degree of control accomplished.

The foregoing remarks apply to infection with *S. haematobium* but any of the points raised are applicable to the study of *Schistosoma mansoni*, a view supported by KLOETZEL [28] who considers that egg output, when studied in groups of

7*

people provides a useful epidemiological tool since SCOTT [37, 38] showed that daily fluctuations in egg output are no greater than in hookworm disease.

In Tanganyika, survey results indicate that egg output is related to the incidence of infection, the mean number of eggs found per direct smear in school children in different areas of the country increasing with the incidence of infection (Table 3).

Table 3. *Mean number of eggs per faecal smear from schools with differing incidence of S. mansoni infection*

Range of incidence	Mean incidence	Mean number of eggs/ positive smear
> 10%	4.8%	2.4
10—20%	13.5%	2.7
21—50%	33.8%	5.9
> 50%	58%	8.5

In circumscribed areas intensity and incidence are probably synonymous and are regarded so by ANNECKE, PITCHFORD and JAKOBS [1]; and FISHER [18] working with *Schistosoma intercalatum*, but a comparable relationship may not apply in other areas where transmission takes place under different conditions and where different intermediate hosts of varying efficiency may be involved. It is interesting in this context, to note that the mean egg output per gramme of faeces of children in Mwanza, and the corresponding incidence of infection show the same relationship one for the other, as do egg load and incidence data from children of the same age group in Almadeira in Brazil [28] (Fig. 4).

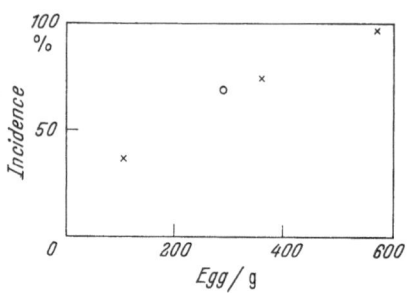

Fig. 4. Showing correlation between incidence and intensity of infection (eggs/gram) in *S. mansoni* infected children (aged 5—9)
× Figure from Brazil; ○ Figure from Mwanza

PESSOA and BARRAS [33] however, consider that incidence is an insufficient index of intensity of infection. This is likely to be the case, particularly, when the incidence of infection is high — a 100% incidence cannot be increased, but the egg load can be.

Support for the view that intensity of infection is responsible for different rates of bilharzial disease is found in the work of PITCHFORD [34] who found that in school children the incidence of enlarged livers in different areas of the Eastern Transvaal was directly correlated with the incidence — (and intensity) — of *S. mansoni*. In Brazil KLOETZEL [28] also showed that the incidence of splenomegaly in different age groups was directly related to the mean egg load. With regard to symptomatology, BELL [4] has shown that the incidence of bilharzial diarrhoea is increased when the egg output is high.

In view of these findings it seems not unreasonable to consider the pathology of *S. mansoni* in relation to egg output — or the number of eggs retained in the tissues.

S. *mansoni* is considered by some [12, 17] to cause fibrosis and cirrhosis of the liver but other workers suggest the parasite might not be responsible for severe diffuse liver disease. GELFAND [19], rightly points out that fibrosis and cirrhosis are caused by other conditions, occur in areas where bilharzia is non-endemic and there is little evidence of more cirrhosis in areas where bilharzia is hyper-endemic than in areas where it is non-endemic. Other workers [13, 30, 42] have also mentioned the complications of the effects of malnutrition in their series of liver biopsy and autopsy investigations.

CARTER and SHALDON [10] have suggested that widespread cellular infiltration of the liver, also reported by DESCHAMPS et al. [11], DIMMETTE [13], and RAGHEB [35] indicates a schistosomal hepatitis. BOGLIOLO [8] from his autopsy series considers the fibrotic and cirrhotic changes brought about by bilharzia to be typical and well defined; and RODRIGUEZ et al. [36] were able to differentiate between bilharzial cirrhosis and cirrhosis due to other conditions.

Although cirrhosis, fibrosis, cellular infiltrations and granulomata are reported by different workers the only lesion apparently of undoubted bilharzial origin appears to be the granuloma or "tubercle". GELFAND [19] refers to the fact that there may be many or few and that the severity of local fibrotic change will depend on the numbers present. This quantitative aspect does not appear to have been investigated in relation to liver damage and it is suggested that such a study might not be inappropriate in view of the differing views of bilharzial liver disease.

In autopsy investigations, it is possible to obtain liver for digest purposes, enabling a quantitative assessment of the egg load in the liver to be correlated with the histological findings as has been done, on a qualitative basis by GELFAND [19] and HIGGINSON and DE MEILLON [23]. The finding of eggs in the digest, however, gives little information as to whether the person is harbouring an active infection or not, since little appears to have been done to determine the longevity of eggs in liver tissues, though GONNERT [22] made some contribution to this problem in mice. The varying capacity amongst peoples in different parts of the world to produce fibrotic reactions [43] may further complicate the picture. Digests of portions of the lower bowel and the examination of faecal material for S. *mansoni* ova may facilitate a conclusion as to whether an active infection is present or not. The finding of adult worms in the portal system, and their numbers, would be useful in this type of investigation, particulary as we have so little information on worm load in human cases of bilharziasis. BECK and GARRETT [2] described a perfusion technique suitable for investigating this in humans but in two bodies in which it was tried at Mwanza, post-mortem clotting of blood appeared to prevent successful results being obtained. Apart from useful data in relation to pathology, the determination of the number of adult adult worms in human cases of bilharziasis is required for other aspects of bilharzial investigations.

Liver biopsy may also be a useful tool with which to investigate bilharzial liver disease, but suffers from the disadvantage that only a small portion of the liver can be removed. If, however, results are considered in relation to the egg load in the excreta, it is likely that more useful information may be obtained.

It is not surprising that bilharzia research is performed in areas where the disease is hyperendemic. This has the disadvantage that those interested in bilharzial liver disease find the vast majority of their subjects infected and there is little opportunity for investigating the non-bilharzial liver for comparison. In view of fibrosis and cirrhosis occurring in non-schistosomal areas it would seem necessary for detailed pathology to be carried out in areas of Africa and S. America known to be free of bilharzia. Apart from an acute lack of pathologists, the problem is complicated in many places by religious objection to autopsy. Could not the viscerotome of yellow fever investigation days — modified to cope with cirrhotic livers — be issued to outlying hospitals and used to obtain large numbers of specimens from a variety of areas for digest and histopathological study at a central laboratory?

In discussing *S. haematobium*, the possible importance of egg output in drug trials was mentioned. BELL [4, 5] has stressed this aspect in relation to *S. mansoni* and has devised a new method for evaluating ova load in faeces.

In conclusion — while the quantitative aspect of bilharzial research has been stressed it is not in the belief that such an approach will solve all the problems. There are many other factors involved but in view of anomalous findings from different endemic areas, a quantitative approach to the problem is considered feasible, worthy of trial, and possibly long overdue.

References

[1] ANNECKE, D. H., J. PITCHFORD, and A. J. JACOBS: Some further observations on bilharziasis in the Transvaal. S. Afr. Med. J. **29**, 314—323 (1955).

[2] BECK, J. W., and F. D. GARRETT: A preliminary report on a perfusion technique for recovering schistosomes at time of autopsy. Amer. J. Trop. Med. Hyg. **6**, 914—919 (1957).

[3] BELL, D. R.: Correlation of daily egg output with symptoms and signs. Ann. Rep. E. Afr. Inst. Med. Res.; Nairobi, 34—35 (1963).

[4] — A new method for counting S. mansoni eggs in faeces with special reference to therapeutic trials. Bull. Wld Hlth Org. **29**, 525 (1963).

[5] — TWSb in Schistosomiasis mansoni: a quantitative evaluation. Ann. Trop. Med. Parasit. **58**, 219—223 (1964).

[6] BENNIE, I.: Urinary schistosomiasis: the best time to obtain specimens: the effect of specific therapy on egg output. S. Afr. Med. J. **23**, 97—100 (1949).

[7] BLAIR, D. M.: Bilharziasis survey in British West and East Africa, Nyasaland and the Rhodesias. Bull. Wld Hlth Org. **15**, 203—273 (1956).

[8] BOGLIOLO, L.: The anatomical picture of the liver in hepato-splenic schistosomiasis mansoni. Ann. Trop. Med. Parasit. **51**, 1—14 (1957).

[9] BRADLEY, D.: A quantitative approach to bilharzia. E. Afr. Med. J. **40**, 240—249 (1963).

[10] CARTER, R. A., and S. SHALDON: The liver in schistosomiasis. Lancet **2**, 1003—1008 (1959).

[11] DESCHAMPS, H. S., J. L. REDMOND, and H. DELEEUW: Hepatic granulomas in schistosomiasis. Gastroenterology **28**, 990—1015 (1955).

[12] DEW, H. R.: Observations on the pathology of schistosomiasis *(S. haematobium and S. mansoni)* in the human subject. J. Path. Bact. **26**, 27—39 (1923).

[13] DIMMETTE, R. M.: Liver biopsy in clinical schistosomiasis. Comparison of wedge and needle types. Gastroenterology **29**, 219—234 (1955).

[14] — Fibrosis of the liver of Egyptian children and adults. Amer. J. Trop. Med. Hyg. **5**, 703—712 (1956).

[15] DUKE, B. O. L., and F. S. McCULLOUGH: Schistosomiasis in the Gambia. II. The epidemiology and distribution of urinary schistosomiasis. Ann. Trop. Med. Parasit. **48**, 287—299 (1954).

[16] ELDSON-DEW, R.: The pathognomy of bilharziasis: an unanswered question. In Ciba Foundation Symposium on Bilharziasis, G. E. W. WOLSTENHOLME, and M. O'CONNOR, (Eds.) pp. 207—214. Boston, Massachusetts, Little Brown and Company 1962.

[17] FAIRLEY, N. H.: Comparative study of experimental bilharziasis in monkeys contrasted with hitherto described lesions in man. J. Path. Bact. 23, 289—314 (1919).
[18] FISHER, A. C.: A study of schistosomiasis of the Stanleyville District of the Belgian Congo. Trans. Roy. Soc. Trop. Med. Hyg. 28, 277—306 (1934).
[19] GELFAND, M.: Schistosomiasis in South Central Africa: a clinico-pathological study. Cape Town and Johannesburg, South Africa. Juta & Co. Ltd. 1950.
[20] GERBER, J. H.: Bilharzia in Boajibu. Part II. The human population. J. Trop. Med. Hyg. 55, 79—93 (1952).
[21] GOATLY, K. D., and P. JORDAN: Schistosomiasis in Zanzibar and Pemba. E. Afr. Med. J. 42, 1—9 (1964).
[22] GONNERT, R.: Studies on schistosomiasis. II Ovulation in S. mansoni and the fate of the egg in the host tissues. Z. Tropenmed. Parasit. 6, 33—52 (1955).
[23] HIGGINSON, J., and B. MEILLON: Schistosoma haematobium infestation and hepatic disease in man. Arch. Path. 60, 341—346 (1955).
[24] HONEY, R. M., and M. GELFAND: The urological aspects of bilharziasis in Rhodesia. Edinburgh and London: E. & S. Livingstone Ltd. 1960.
[25] JORDAN, P.: Annu. Rep. Inst. Med. Res. — E. Afr. Comm. Serv. Org., Nairobi 1961.
[26] — Some quantitative aspects of bilharzia with particular reference to suppressive therapy and mollusciding in control of S. haematobium in Sukumaland, Tanganyika. E. Afr. Med. J. 40, 250—260 (1963).
[27] —, and K. A. E. RANDALL: Schistosomiasis in Tanganyika: Observations on suppressive management of Schistosoma haemtobium with TWSb, with particular reference to reduction in ova load. Trans. Roy. Soc. Trop. Med. Hyg. 56, 523—528 (1962).
[28] KLOETZEL, K.: Splenomegaly in Schistosomiasis mansoni. Amer. J. Trop. Med. Hyg. 11, 472—476 (1962).
[29] — Some quantitative aspects of diagnosis and epidemiology in Schistosomiasis mansoni. Amer. J. Trop. Med. Hyg. 12, 334—337 (1963).
[30] MAGALHAES, A. JR., H. MENEZES, G. M. DA SILVA, and J. DE M. BARBOSA: Incidence of hepatic cirrhosis and schistosomal hepatic fibrosis in autopsies in the department of pathological anatomy in the University of Recife, Brazil. An. Fac. Med. Recife 18, 207—213 (1958); Abstracted in Trop. Dis. Bull. 57, 490 (1958).
[31] NABAWY, M., M. GABR, and M. M. RAGAB: Visceral bilharziasis in children: a clinico-radio-logical study. J. Trop. Med. Hyg. 64, 314—318 (1961).
[32] ONORI, E.: Observations on variations in Schistosoma haematobium egg output of infected persons and the prevalence of infection in a community. Ann. Trop. Med. Parasit. 56, 292—296 (1962).
[33] PESSOA, S. B., L. H. P. DA SILVA, and L. COSTA: Observations on the epidemiology of Schistosoma mansoni infection in the State of Paraiba. Rev. Bras. Malar. 7, 305—310 (1955); abstracted in Trop. Dis. Bull. 53, 1130 (1956).
[34] PITCHFORD, J.: Intestinal bilharziasis in the Eastern Transvaal: A preliminary report. S. Afr. Med. J. 26, 524—528 (1952).
[35] RAGHEB, M.: Schistosomiasis of the liver. Clinical, pathologic and laboratory studies in Egyptian cases. Gastroenterology 30, 631—660 (1956).
[36] RODRIGUEZ, H. F., M. R. GARCIA-PALMIERI, J. V. RIVERA, and R. RODRIGUEZ-MOLINA: A comparative study of portal and bilharzial cirrhosis. Gastroenterology 29, 235—246 (1955).
[37] SCOTT, J. A.: The variability of egg output of infestations of Schistosoma mansoni as compared with hookworm. J. Parasit. 18, 129 (1932).
[38] — Egg counts as estimates of intensity of infection with Schistosoma haematobium. Tex. Rep. Biol. Med. 15, 425—430 (1957).
[39] — The regularity of egg output of helminth infestations with special reference to Schistosoma mansoni. Amer. J. Hyg. 27, 155—175 (1938).
[40] STIMMEL, C. M., and J. A. SCOTT: The regularity of egg output of Schistosoma haematobium. Tex. Rep. Biol. Med. 14, 440—458 (1956).
[41] STOLL, N. R.: This wormy world. J. Parasit. 33, 1—18 (1947).
[42] SYMMERS, D.: Pathogenesis of liver cirrhosis in schistosomiasis. J. Amer. Med. Ass. 147, 304—305 (1951).
[43] WOODRUFF, A. W.: Fibrosing disease of the tropics — some possible causes. E. Afr. Med. J. 36, 527—531 (1959).

Some Remarks on the Clinical and Pathological Aspects of Schistosomiasis in Central Africa

MICHAEL GELFAND*

Much of what I am going to talk about remains conjecture. It is a pity, but this is the situation and if it were otherwise, there would be no reason for a meeting such as this.

When I qualified there were well defined accepted views about the effects of schistosomiasis. Almost all the worthwhile contributions up to that time had come from Egypt, and there were so many that it is difficult to mention them all. The most outstanding, in my opinion, were the description of the clay pipe cirrhosis of the liver recorded in 1904 [15], the association of bladder cancer with urinary bilharziasis and the relationship of ovideposition in the pulmonary arteries to chronic cor pulmonale [14]. Because of the widespread dissemination of ova there was perhaps a tendency to attribute too many complications to schistosomiasis. No doubt these effects occur, but far more rarely than we have been led to believe. For instance I think calculus of the urinary tract is much less frequent in our experience than given in Egyptian literature [12]. Other complications that have been mentioned, such as asthma or diabetes mellitus, are probably not related to the disease at all, although we know ova may be found in the lungs and pancreas. And so in recent years an opposing school of thought came into being and correctly pointed out that because schistosomiasis was so prevalent, it was perfectly feasible for an individual with this disease to have some other disorder at the same time [4]. In Egypt for example we can expect pulmonary hypertension in the population just as in a non-schistosomal country and therefore sooner or later the two diseases are bound to occur in the same person. Of course you will ask why the incidence of pulmonary hypertension in a schistosomal region has not been compared with that in a non endemic one; such a study would be most usefull in determining whether or not pulmonary hypertension is caused by schistosomiasis. Unfortunately, this is a procedure that cannot be contemplated at present in regions where schistosomiasis is endemic.

There are, however, other methods of argument that can be used to strengthen the claim that many of these alleged sequelae are true. Their complications can be grouped into three categories: (1) Highly probable, (2) doubtfully probable, and (3) definitely related.

The *highly probable sequelae of schistosomiasis* include (1) carcinoma of the bladder, (2) clay-pipe stem cirrhosis, and (3) cor pulmonale and pulmonary hypertension. The *doubtfully probable clinical sequelae* are (1) acute appendicitis, cholecystitis, pancreatitis, (2) salpingitis and oophoritis, (3) endometritis, (4) nephrotic syndrome, (5) hypertension and chronic pyelonephritis, and (6) renal osteo-

---

* Department of Medicine, University of Rhodesia, Salisbury, Rhodesia.

dystrophy. Undoubted sequelae: (1) bladder fibrosis, (2) calcification of bladder, (3) stenosis or dilatation of ureter with hydronephrosis, unilateral or bilateral, (4) schistosomal myelitis and cerebral granulomata.

A. Highly probable sequelae

Most authorities hold that schistosomal ovideposition and less often the worms themselves are responsible for this group of complications. There are of course differing schools of thought. For instance we know that in some parts of the Middle East, despite the occurrence of endemic schistosomiasis, bladder cancer is said to be very rare. Yet in Egypt and in Southern Rhodesia we have found the two diseases not uncommonly associated. Further, and perhaps more significant, is that the malignant process is found mostly in relatively young age groups in contradistinction to its incidence in non-schistosomal regions. We also know that carcinoma of the bladder is an apparently uncommon tumour in Leopoldville and Kampala where urinary schistosomiasis is uncommon. Yet I must confess that HONEY [11] over a period of 30 years of urological experience has not met a European in Southern Rhodesia suffering from both diseases. Admittedly schistosomiasis in the European is rarely of such severity as in the African and we have never seen a calcified bladder in the white man [11]. Indeed it would seem that the infestation is comparatively slight in the white man and as the process never reaches the stage of producing a sandy patch in the bladder, this organ is unlikely to develop cancer or may in fact protect the bladder from a future malignant degenerative process. In the African it is most uncommon to find carcinoma of the bladder without being able to discern its calcification on X-ray and usually this calcification is coarser than that ordinarily associated with a chronic inflammatory condition. Is there, therefore, some factor in such a calcified bladder that precipitates malignant degeneration of the tissues?

Liver cirrhosis. This subject has raised much heated debate. In 1904 SYMMERS [15] recorded the special granulomatous fibrotic reaction in the portal tracts of the liver, but with a relatively normal parenchyma. This he described as clay-pipe stem cirrhosis. Workers in Egypt, the Far East and South America [1], have all written extensively on the subject and agree with his findings. However they have usually had to confess that in about a third of their cases they were not able to demonstrate ova in the liver — a rather high percentage. They were at a loss to explain this adequately. Some thought that the fibrosis was caused by a special toxin elaborated by the adult worms, but this has remained merely a hypothesis. Other authorities from these regions seems to mention little about other forms of cirrhosis such as a post-necrotic scarring, which must occur and no doubt some of the so-called schistosomal cirrhosis may in fact be due to causes other than schistosomiasis. As ova are deposited in the liver in about 50% of subjects with schistosomiasis, their presence could be coincidental and thus unrelated to the cirrhosis. This argument has been taken up by workers in the main centres in Africa south of Egypt, especially as cirrhosis is seen so commonly in regions in which schistosomiasis is not encountered or only met very infrequently such as Kampala and Leopoldville. Of course it can be said that the pathological pictures of the schistosomal and non-schistosomal forms of cirrhosis are very different, but it is by no means easy to distinguish between them as fibrosis with leucocytic infiltration is so commonly found in non-schistosomal cirrhosis.

It is worth mentioning my experience at this point. In Mashonaland I encountered many cases of hepatic cirrhosis in Africans and I was puzzled because, despite a fairly high incidence of mansonal disease in the country, there did not seem to be any relationship between it and cirrhosis in the adult. The usual causes seemed to be post hepatitic (viral), nutritional and even siderotic. Rarely have I been able to demonstrate schistosomal lesions in the portal tracts in liver biopsy material. In other words, I supported the view that, at any rate in Central Africa, portal cirrhosis was not usually due to a schistosomal infestation and that our findings must be different to those elsewhere. This fact however worried me greatly. Then I noticed that the coincidence of mansonal disease of the rectum was unusually high in my juveniles with cirrhosis of the liver [5] and after a while I decided to carry out a pericutaneous biopsy on their livers and I was surprised to find that in a significant number of cases schistosomal lesions were found in the portal tract [7]. This finding would suggest that schistosomal portal cirrhosis of the liver manifests itself at this earlier age rather than in the adult. This is very likely as schistosomiasis is usually contracted at a relatively early stage in life so that by the age of 14 to 18 years the granulomatous effect on the liver is established and irreparable damage already done and therefore few of these patients survive as adults. This may be the reason for the difference in findings between the Central and South African workers and those in Egypt and South America.

There also seems to be good evidence that *S. haematobium* does not cause hepatic cirrhosis even though the ova are often deposited in this organ. It is not easy to know why ova of *S. mansoni* and *S. japonicum* are liable to lead to cirrhosis yet those of *S. haematobium* do not appear to have the same effect.

Cor pulmonale. When I read SHAW and GHAREEB's [14] excellent paper written in 1938 on this aspect of the disease I was most impressed, but although I have looked carefully for evidence of this complication, I have seen it only seldom. It certainly does not occur in Mashonaland with the same frequency as in Egypt and South America. In other parts of Africa most workers stress either its infrequency or its entire absence. I believe we shall find more cases once we are able to perform lung biopsies more frequently and better pathological studies can be made. I certainly meet cases of pulmonary hypertension in the African due mostly to lung disease itself, but these occur usually in the more elderly and on X-ray, fibrotic changes are seen in the lungs. Whilst I am certain of the cause of the fibrosis I have not been able to show that it has a schistosomal origin. I have suggested that such fibrosis may indeed be linked with that well known fibroblastic diathesis of the African. I would place greater significance on such a finding if it were in a younger age group similar to that in which we encounter cirrhosis of the liver of schistosomal origin.

I have recorded cases of schistosomal lung disease accompanied by pulmonary hypertension and I believe these cases have a characteristic histological picture in which the most significant feature is the angiomata described by SHAW and GHAREEB [14]. If the angiomata can be demonstrated as well as remants of ova occluding vessels with endarteritis I think we can diagnose schistosomal pulmonary hypertension with justification. However, angiomatosis is not patho-gnomonic of the schistosomal lung as it can occur in other forms of pulmonary hypertension.

B. Doutfully significant clinical group

I think I am safe in stating that an acute superimposed inflammatory reaction on the bilharzial tissue is extremely rare. It has been thought that because of the fibrosis and granulation of the tissues other invading organisms can more readily establish themselves. Thus acute or chronic cystitis, acute appendicitis, acute salpingitis and even, perhaps, cholecystitis and pancreatitis may follow. I must admit that in my experience an acute cystitis developing upon a schistosomal mucosa in extremely rare. On the other hand sometimes a mild chronic infection due to E. coli sets in, but there is no acute inflammatory exudate. The same appears to hold true for the appendix and other conditions just mentioned. There is a large school of thought which believes that a fibrotic appendix due to schisto-somal oviposition is liable to develop acute inflammatory changes. But it must be rembered that in Europeans both diseases are common and therefore the chances of both occurring concurrently are good, especially as ova are deposited in the appendix in over 50% of patients with urinary schistosomiasis. On the other hand despite the fact that ova are found in the appendix, acute appendicitis in the African is about 10 times less common than in the European [4]. Indeed my experience tends to indicate that in schistosomiasis, as in syphilis, an acute inflammation rarely supervenes. The one seems to militate against the other.

Although I have stated that severe chronic urinary schistosomiasis not un-commonly leads to chronic pyelonephritis which in turn is complicated by hyper-tension or a nephrotic syndrome [6], this statement lacks proof and certainly so far there has been no corroborative evidence from other workers. Yet it seems reasonable that this should be the case. Renal biopsy shows that chronic pyelonephritis occurs. On the other hand I must admit that both hypertension and the nephrotic syndrome are common disorders in Africans living in en-demic schistosomal areas. For instance in Kampala and Leopoldville, schisto-somiasis is rarely seen, yet both renal diseases are common and chronic pyelo-nephritis is considered the most important cause of hypertension. Yet since schisto-somiasis leads to chronic pyelonephritis it is difficult to dismiss it as an important factor in any endemic region, especially as hypertension is mostly found in the younger age groups [6].

Undoubted complications of schistosomiasis

In this group we are on more certain ground. We can see the granulomatous and fibrotic tissues in the bladder and ureter both with the naked eye and micro-scopically. When the disease is extensive in the bladder it can be recognized radiologically by the line of calcification due to calcified ova in that organ.

Almost always a vesical carcinoma is found in association with a calcified bladder. It must be exceptional to find bladder cancer in the African living in an endemic bilharzial region without there being some degree of calcification in the organ on X-ray — a further point which tends to show that the severity of infection is all important in leading to the development of carcinoma.

It is quite likely that as a result of fibrosis of the bladder the function of this viscus suffers and in more advanced cases its capacity may be reduced to below 300 ml capacity, the intravesical pressure rises and increased frequency results. The patient has to pass urine more than once during the night. In many cases, however, the bladder capacity is not reduced or in fact altered in any way and in spite of the gross fibrosis it is not easy to discover any change in function. Here then is a line for further study.

It is also possible that some dysuria results from ovideposition and fibrosis in the bladder tissue leading to a bladder wall fibrosis. This condition is well recognized in Egypt, but in Southern Rhodesia there is much argument as to whether it occurs frequently. Some urologists regard it as common, whereas others consider it most unusual. There is no doubt that many ova are deposited in the prostate and seminal vesicles as well but it is difficult to know whether any effects are produced by this. Occasionally a haemospermia occurs, but this appears to be a very unusual complication.

Well over 80% of serious lesions in the ureter are located in its lowest part — usually in its last centimetre and then mostly in its intravesical portion. Thus stenosis and stricture commonly occur here but when the lesions are marked the lower ureter may be dilated instead and admit a catheter with ease. In the European however dilatation alone has not been described [10, 12]. The reason for this is not obvious. In the African a large number — probably over 50% of the lesions in the ureter show dilatation or no narrowing of the ureteric orifice and the segment above. Perhaps the reason lies in the gross disease met with in the African.

The earliest sign of ureteric involvement is persistent filling of the lower segment on intravenous pyelography. The next stage is dilatation of the ureter. The lowest third of the ureter is usually the portion which is dilated. The dilatation may be either slight or gross and may occur in the absence of any stenosis or in conjunction with it. The presence of stenosis cannot be established without a retrograde pyelogram. The dilatation however not infrequently affects the whole ureter with or without the pelvis and calyces. Extensive dilatation is usually associated with either ureteric stenosis or a fibrosed bladder of small capacity or obstruction of the bladder neck. However in 7% of our African series the dilatation of the whole ureter and hydronephrosis occurred without any of the above three causes being present, the sole lesion being an extensive involvement of the ureteric wall, which must have affected its muscle power [3]. When stenosis occurs along the length of the ureter dilatation is almost as great below the stenosis as it is above showing that the dilatation is as much a primary effect of the fibrosis as in the stenosis. Micturating cystograms were done to detect the presence of ureteric reflux. Reflux of dye up the ureter has not been demonstrated by us in the European, but it occurs in a few African cases — less than what we at first found [12].

The majority of stenoses lie at the level of the vesical submucosa. The next most frequent position is the intravesical one up to 1.5 cm from the orifice. These two sites account for 87% of strictures found in European patients and 88% in our Africans. A much lesser number lie in the intravesical portion of the ureter within 5 cm of the orifice in either ureter.

The dilatation may involve only the distal third of the ureter and appears to be due to weakening of this part of the wall which has been replaced by fibrous tissue. Dilatation of the whole ureter is also seen in Africans in whom no stricture can be demonstrated and whose bladders are of normal capacity (7% of our series) [12]. Dilatation involving the whole length of the ureter including the pelvis but associated with a bladder of reduced capacity and increased intravesical pressure was found in 22% of our African series [12].

Frequency of stricture in European and African series [12].

	Number of subjects	Number with stricture (%)
European	300	31
African	100	42

Hydronephrosis which follows a stricture is easy enough to explain. Not so when the lower ureter is dilated [3]. This feature has interested us greatly. We believe that in some cases this might be due to reflux of urine up an incompetent ureter, especially if the intravesical tension rises as a result of bladder fibrosis. But this cannot be the only reason for we meet hydronephrosis in the presence of a bladder of normal capacity and pressure. We should also remember that when there is an incompetent ureteric orifice, there is always a possibility of chronic pyelonephritis supervening and this in turn may produce a pyelectasia when the features are indistinguishable from the appearance attributed to hydronephrosis.

It is impossible almost to list the numerous pathological combinations of ureteric disease in one or both sides and the associated changes which are found in the bladder.

Some degree of hydronephrosis was found in 48% of our Africans admitted with chronic bilharzial disease, but in the European this figure was 14%. In the Africans it was associated with stricture in 26 of the 58 cases, the degree of hydronephrosis being slight to severe. Hydronephrosis was associated with a bladder of reduced capacity and high intravesical pressure in 20 of the 58 cases (20%) and in all of them the ureteric orifices were retracted and distorted.

Incidence of hydronephrosis in the African and European [12].

European	Out of 300 cases there were 42 with hydronephrosis (14%) (only stricture)
African	Out of 100 cases there were 58 cases of hydronephrosis

Bladder of reduced capacity and high intravesical
pressure   26
stricture of ureter   25
Without stricture or small bladder.   7
Total   58

Puzzling pathological points

Now whilst the European may be infested with only a few worms he may suffer more severely from general symptoms and he may be very difficult to cure. Of course it is not easy to judge the severity of symptoms, such as tiredness, and although the African does not complain much of constitutional upset, his tissues show marked fibrotic lesions as already described. As he becomes older his allergy diminishes and he begins to suffer from the effects of a heavier infestation characterised largely by fibrosis and calcification.

I have already referred to our inadequate knowledge of worm load. Are the symptoms proportional to the worm load? I doubt this as Europeans who have only been exposed to infested water once often complain far more bitterly of symptoms than Africans who have been in contact with such waters for years. From egg counts we know many Africans harbour many worms yet their constitutional symptoms are few. These general or constitutional manifestations appear to depend largely on the hypersensitivity of the host at the time the disease is contracted.

The literature constantly refers to the schistosomal pigment so continually seen in the liver. El-Gholmy et al. [2] believe its presence is a sure sign of the disease and as good evidence as finding an egg. However the presence of pigment in the liver has been described in malaria. And as it does not contain iron it should not be confused with that encountered in siderosis. Now how do we distinguish between the malarial and schistosomal pigment? Can there be some confusion as to which of the two diseases produces it? How is this pigment elaborated and at what stage in the disease does it appear in the liver and possibly in other organs. This seems to me a useful line for research.

We are left without a clear idea as to the exact pathological significance of the worm in the production of lesions. There can be little doubt that the Katayama syndrome is produced by the worms as they settle in the liver and portal venous system as at this stage ova are not yet extruded. As mentioned previously temporary allergic lesions are invoked but these disappear some weeks later. When the disease becomes localized haematuria or diarrhoea may follow, but in addition, the patient may suffer from constitutional symptoms, such as tiredness, which may be caused by the living worms rather than by the ova. The lesions in the bladder and appendix can almost be ascribed to the ova as they give rise to the tubercles which can be seen surrounding them. But we have not discovered any definite lesions around the worms themselves. It is doubtful whether living worms produce any but there is some evidence that an endophlebitis with thrombosis develops around dead ones [9, 14]. How significant this is in the total picture of the disease remains unknown and judging from the infrequency of this event I should think these sequelae are relatively unimportant although they may be responsible for lesions of a very localised nature.

The characteristic tubercle with ova or their remnants, giant cells, esoinophils and granulation tissue is not always seen typically in the same organ. Again this may be due to the state of immunity of the particular tissues or viscus. Typical tubercles are generally seen in the appendix, liver and Fallopian tubes, but in the ureter, bladder and lungs, although they are formed at times, we usually only observe eggs lying singly or in groups apparently provoking little reaction around them. The presence of giant cells, often but not invariably, means that eggs are absent from the tubercle or that only remnants or their bare shells are found inside it. But when there are no giant cells, ova are to be expected within the tubercle. It would seem that the giant cells perform the function of absorbing and digesting the ova. When schistosomal granulation tissue is present we can expect no superimposed acute inflammation. The one seems to mitigate against the other. Nevertheless it is held that when schistosomal fibrosis is present in an appendix it may become the seat of an acute superimposed inflammation.

The significance of double schistosomal infestations

When portions of tissue are removed at autopsy and digested in KOH we are able to demonstrate the widespread distribution of ova in both *S. haemtobium* and *S. mansoni* infestation. This has often been recorded by workers in this field, but a point I should like to make is that we observed at autopsy [8] that the ova of *S. haematobium* were not only present much more often than those of *S. mansoni* but they were almost invariably found as well in patients with *S. mansoni*. It was very rare to encounter the eggs of *S. mansoni* alone. This association of both parasites in the same patient is also seen in Europeans although not quite to the same degree. I was able to show that about one quarter of my European cases had a double infestation. Thus when an African patient is admitted with *S. mansoni* infestation we can assume that he is also infected by *S. haematobium* and therefore if he complains of pains in the abdomen and bladder they may in fact be caused by the urinary parasite. More often than not when an I.V.P. was performed on such a case I found lesions in the urinary tract, such as calcification of the bladder, dilatation of the ureter or hydronephrosis.

This autopsy finding has a particular clinical application in those territories in which both parasites are present in association. *S. haematobium* is encountered much more frequently because the snail carrying host of *S. haematobium* (Physopsis) is more frequent and widely distributed than that of *Biomphalaria*.

Immunity (resistance or tolerance to the disease as seen in man).

We possess a certain amount of information on this subject mainly derived from animal experimentation, but it is not always easy to compare these reactions with those we have experienced in man.

It seems obvious that some tolerance must be built up in man. For instance in highly infected regions the disease becomes less common with increasing age and after the age of 50 about 40% of the inhabitants appear to be clear of any active infestation. On the other hand, children from about the toddling age (3 or 4 years onwards) up to 20 practically all harbour the parasite. Between this age and 50 years there is a lowering in the frequency of the disease to about 55%. We assume that after a number of years the host becomes sufficiently capable of throwing off the disease. In the child and young adult the tissue resistance must be poor otherwise it would be impossible to explain the severe lesions with calcification of the bladder and cirrhosis of the liver seen in Africans in this age group — findings practically never seen in the European. We assume that with repeated exposures fresh infections of the body result but not necessarily in proportion. Perhaps the immune processes established in this tissue compare with the state of premunition found in malaria in which the tolerance is not complete. But when I was doing autopsy work I was puzzled because in spite of heavy infestations I recall how difficult it was to find adult worms in the venous plexuses around the bladder and liver area where I fully expected to mett many of them.

The disease is also relatively uncommon before the age of three. It may be argued that a babe in arms is not exposed to infected waters in the same way as a walking child. This is very likely yet I have noticed that very young babies

are bathed in infested water, especially when the mother goes down to the edge
of the river to do her laundry. It seems that the baby has some degree of tolerance
acquired from its mother just as happens with malaria, but this is only a transient
one.

The importance of the sensitivity response

We are still apt to think of schistosomiasis as taking the same course in and
having essentially the same effect on European and African patients. HONEY
and GELFAND [12] suggested that as it clearly produced differences in lesions in
the urinary tract, it should be referred to as Bantu and European schistosomiasis.
Not only were the lesions much more extensive in the African with a much greater
degree of fibrosis in the bladder and ureter, but dilatation without stricture was
not uncommonly met with in the ureter of the African with advanced schistosomiasis whilst in the European, only stricture occurred. This latter finding is borne
out by a recent publication by LANGDALE GREGORY [10] who recorded that he
encountered only stricture. Secondly, calcification of the bladder is almost entirely
limited to the African and we practically never meet with uraemia from bilateral
hydronephrosis in the European, whereas in the African it is a well recognised
complication. Similarly, HONEY and GELFAND [12] pointed out that carcinoma
of the bladder is not uncommonly seen in association with ovideposition in the
African of a relatively young age group, yet in the European of Rhodesia no such
relationship has yet been observed although a careful search has been made.
Thus the picture assumed by the disease in the African is often of greater concern to the urologist than to the physician.

But this does not mean that the European complains of no symptoms when
he develops the disease. At least 60% of my patients suffer from tiredness and
in 30% of European subjects this is quite a striking feature. This complaint is
rarely made by the African who more often mentions pain in one of the loins or
over his loin area. I have already mentioned that, whilst the Katayama syndrome
is occasionally seen in the European, I have never encountered it in the African,
and I attributed this to the fact that the African might not consider these manifestations worth reporting. But this assumption may not be correct as many
Africans seek medical advice for a high fever or urticaria and surely we should
have recognised the syndrome had it been present. In the African too I have not
encountered anything resembling Kabure itch caused by the penetration of
cercariae into the skin. Yet I have occasionally heard of its appearance in Europeans. Perhaps the presence of these early syndromes in the European denotes
that he is hypersensitive to the schistosome and its products in contrast to a normal state of sensitivity in the African who is born as well with some degree of
passive immunity conferred by his mother. Although this protection passes off
in the young African child, who contracts the disease from about the age of three
onwards, he generally then builds up an immunity somewhat similar to that of
the premunition found in malaria. Thus by the time they reach the age of 40 onwards many Africans cease to pass ova in their excreta although they are still
being exposed to the infection [13]

It is therefore suggested that the more severe constitutional symptoms generally complained of by the European are due to his state of sensitivity or allergy

even though the load of infection is much higher in the African who continually infects himself over the years from childhood to adulthood and thus continually adds to his worm load and to the intensity of the ovideposition. In spite of his hypersensitive state with a mild load of schistosomes it is not easy to cure the European of his infestation of either *S. mansoni* or *S. haematobium* although perhaps *S. mansoni* is the more resistant. Indeed it is my impression that the African, despite his heavier load, is as easy to cure as the European. The difference between the two races may be due to a difference in the allergic state of the individual, the degree of antibody formation, or some other similar process. It is on lines such as this that further research might well be directed.

Table showing differences between schistosomiasis as seen in European and African (Central Africa (Central Africa)

Europeans	Africans
Katayama syndrome well recognized.	Not seen
Kabure Itch — seen but rarely	Not seen
Constitutional symptoms, e.g. tiredness, more striking	Not mentioned to same extent
Stricture of ureter common	Common
Dilatation without stricture not encountered	Common
Calcification of bladder and ureter common	Exceptional
Cystoscopy tubercles only	Sandy grain patches usual
Chronic pyelonephritis with hypertension probably common	Very rare
Carcinoma of bladder with bilharziasis not seen	Common in Central Africa
No reflux with micturating cystogram	Reflux occasionally seen
Cure often difficult despite lighter load of schistosomes	Cure probably not more difficult despite a much heavier load

References

[1] BOGLIOLO, L., The anatomical picture of liver in hepatosplenic schistosomiasis mansoni. Ann. Trop. Med. Parasit. **51**, 1—14 (1957).

[2] EL-GHOLMY, A., J. NABAWY, M. GABR, S. AIDAROS, and A. OMAR: Hepatic schistosomiasis in children. J. Trop. Med. Hyg. **58**, 25—33 (1955).

[3] GELFAND, M.: Bilharzial affection of the ureter. A study of 110 consecutive necropsies showing vesical bilharziaris. Brit. Med. J. **2**, 1228—1230 (1948).

[4] — Schistosomiasis in South Central Africa. A Clinicopathological Study. p. 239. Capetown: Juta & Co. 1950.

[5] — A possible relationship between nephrotic syndrome and urinary schistosomiasis. Trans. Roy. Soc. Trop. Med. Hyg. **57**, 191—195 (1963).

[6] — Chronic urinary schistosomiasis and its relationship to hypertension. C. Afr. J. Med. **10**, 1—8 (1964).

[7] — A study of cirrhosis of the liver in (a) adult and (b) juvenile Africans with particular reference to the incidence of schistosomal infestation. Trans. Roy. Soc. Trop. Med. Hyg. **58**, 339—348 (1964).

[8] —, R. H. HUNT and V. DE V. CLARKE: Visceral deposition of schistosome ova in C. Africa. J. Trop. Med. Hyg. **68**, 245—247 (1965).

[9] GILLMAN, T.: Venous obstruction in the pathogenesis of hepatic bilharziasis. A preliminary report of comparative findings in rats, monkeys and man. Ann. Trop. Med. Parasit. **51**, 409—416 (1957).

[10] GREGORY, I. LANGDALE: Bilharzial structure in the terminal ureter. Cent. Afr. J. Med. 10, 119—122 (1964).

[11] HONEY, R. M.: Personal communication.

[12] —, and M. GELFAND: The urological aspects of bilharziasis in Rhodesia. Edinburgh: E. & S. Livingstone 1960.

[13] MORELY-SMITH, F., and M. GELFAND: Bilharziasis in an African infant and child in the Motoko district: Southern Rhodesia. Cent. Afr. J. Med. 4, 287—288 (1958).

[14] SHAW, A. F. B., and A. A. GHAREEB: The pathogenesis of pulmonary schistosomiasis in Egypt with special reference to Ayreza's disease. J. Path. Bact. 46, 401—424 (1938).

[15] SYMMERS, W. ST. C.: Note on a new form of liver cirrhosis due to the presence of the ova of B. haematobia. J. Path. Bact. 9, 237—239 (1904).

The Clinico-Pathological Manifestations of Intestinal Bilharziasis in Durban, South Africa*

S. Brumdutt Bhagwandeen**

With 12 figures

Review of the literature indicates the great variation from country to country of the clinical symptoms and severity of intestinal bilharziasis. While severe clinical symptoms and gross intestinal pathology are experienced in some hyperendemic areas, in places with lower endemicity manifestations may be so light as to pass unnoticed.

Thus the most severe forms of the disease have been reported from Egypt [5, 6, 7, 16]. Less severe forms of the disease are encountered in the Caribbean and South American countries. Koppish [12] from Puerto Rico, Jaffe [10] from Venezuela and Pontes [14] from Brazil are all agreed that in these countries S. mansoni produces less severe intestinal pathology than that reported from Egypt. In the rest of Africa the disease is still milder. Manson-Bahr [13] reported that symptomatology in East Africa due to S. mansoni infection was variable but noted that, in general, the infected indigenous population was symptom-free. Although Wydell [19] demonstrated severe intestinal pathology in the later stages of S. mansoni infection in an isolated African population group on Ukerewe Island in Lake Victoria, and although the incidence of S. mansoni in this group was high, he noted that intestinal symptoms in active infections were uncommon. Further south, Gelfand [8] from S. Rhodesia reported that intestinal bilharziasis is almost asymptomatic and he stressed the benign nature of the intestinal lesions.

Little work has been done on the clinico-pathological aspects of intestinal bilharziasis in South Africa. Turner [18] reported that symptoms due to intestinal bilharziasis were variable and were easily mistaken for chronic diarrhoea or dysentery. Holland [9] considered bilharzial dysentery to be a rare illness. King [11] reported on the similarities in clinical presentation of amoebiasis and bilharzial dysentery. Schneider [11] reported that, when present, symptoms were mild in the Transvaal African.

Present study

The present study was undertaken to assess the intestinal manifestations of bilharziasis in an area where the incidence of S. haematobium and S. mansoni are of the order of 30% and 10% respectively [2].

---

* Extract from Thesis "The Clinico-Pathological Manifestations of Schistosomiasis in the African and Indian in Durban", submitted for the M.D. degree in the department of Pathology, University of Natal.

** Department of Pathology, University of Natal, Durban, South Africa.

8*

Materials and methods

The study was conducted in two parts. The clinical aspects were based on patients attending the Bilharzia Clinic of King Edward VIII Hospital while the pathological aspects were based on autopsies conducted in the same hospital.

In the clinical study three groups of patients were studied:

1. *Clinical group I:* consisting of 225 patients (150 African and 75 Indian) presenting with vesical symptoms. These were questioned specifically to elicit probable latent symptoms of intestinal bilharziasis prior to examination.

2. *Clinical group II:* consisting of 40 patients presenting with vesical bilharziasis. These patients were examined to establish probable intestinal disease due to *S. haematobium.*

3. *Clinical group III:* consisting of 40 patients with known *S. mansoni* infection (proven by rectal biopsy). These patients were examined to determine the clinical presentation of *S. mansoni* infection.

The pathological findings are based on:

1. 900 autopsies constiting of 700 routine hospital and 200 medicolegal autopsies. The age, race and sex of the cases are given in Table 1.

Table 1. *Age, race and sex of autopsy material*

Age	African		Indian		Total
	Male	Female	Male	Female	
2— 9	65	70	6	3	144
10—19	32	31	10	5	78
20—29	72	42	9	4	127
30—39	101	68	10	3	182
40—49	163	79	10	5	257
50 +	60	40	7	5	112
Total	493	330	52	25	900

The bladder and rectum were removed and subjected to digestion, crush and histological examination. Comparison of the three methods has been reported elsewhere [3].

2. Four fatal cases of bilharzial dysentery due to *S. mansoni* infections.

Observations

Clinical study

Clinical group I: Of the 225 patients questioned only 4 had mild symptoms referable to the bowel, and these were all shown to have *S. mansoni* on rectal biopsy. However, rectal, biopsy revealed *S. mansoni* in a further 41 patients and *S. haematobium* in 195, all of whom had no intestinal symptoms. This study revealed that generally intestinal bilharziasis is asymptomatic.

Clinical group II: Of the 40 patients with viable *S. haematobium* in the urine, 8 admitted to bouts of mild diarrhoea with blood-flecked stools, whilst a further 2 complained of hypogastric pain.

Clinical examination failed to reveal any visceromegaly or other abnormality.

The only significant features on proctoscopy were punctate mucosal haemorrhages with focal hyperaemia, which were present in 24/40 (60%). Of the 24 with punctate haemorrhages, rectal biopsy revealed visible *S. mansoni* in 9, and *S. haematobium* in all 24 (9 viable and 15 non-viable). Three showed both viable *S. haematobium* and *S. mansoni*. Of the 6 cases with apparently pure *S. haematobium* 3 had noted blood-flecked stools.

Of the remaining 16 patients with no proctoscopic evidence of rectal involvement, 10 had non-viable, *S. haematobium* ova.

It is therefore apparent that *S. haematobium* may occasionally remain viable in the rectal mucosa and may give rise not only to punctate haemorrhages but also to mild intestinal symptoms.

Clinical group III: The 40 patients in this group all had *S. mansoni* infections (proven by rectal biopsy). In addition, 35 had concomitant *S. haematobium* infections (ova present in urine), while 28 of these also showed *S. haematobium* on rectal biopsy.

The symptomatology of these patients is set out in Table 2.

Table 2. *Presenting symptoms of 40 patients with S. mansoni infections*

Symptoms	No.	%
Diarrhoea with blood and mucus	7	17.5
Diarrhoea only	1	2.5
Diarrhoea and haematuria	1	2.5
Haematuria and blood-flecked stools	3	7.5
Abdominal pain	3	7.5
Haematuria and other symptoms of *S. haematobium* infection	25	62.5

On clinical examination all 40 patients looked well, and were apyrexial. The liver was enlarged in 14 and of these 4 had mild splenomegaly. With one exception the liver was not tender.

On proctoscopy all 40 patients showed punctate haemorrhages, two showed sandy patches, and in only one was a papilloma found (at sigmoidoscopy).

Liver biopsy was performed in 25 of these cases and 22 showed evidence of hepatic bilharziasis with varying degrees of severity. The liver biopsy results will be reported elsewhere [2].

In the one patient with tender hepatomegaly the initial diagnosis was hepatic amoebiasis (a condition common in the area). When antiamoebic therapy failed, liver biopsy was performed and revealed hepatic bilharziasis, and appropriate therapy resulted in some improvement.

A second case, with an initial complaint of diarrhoea with blood and mucus, and abdominal pain had been treated for bacillary dysentery for a month. Subsequent examination revealed *S. mansoni*, which was also found on rectal biopsy. Proctoscopy showed an oedematous mucosa, with clusters of punctate haemorrhage. The liver was enlarged, and biopsy revealed hepatic bilharziasis.

A third case with haematuria, and vague epigastric pain and no history of diarrhoea or of blood and/or mucus, was found to have a 2-finger hepatomegaly. Proctoscopy showed punctate haemorrhages, and "sandy" patches. Rectal biopsy revealed viable ova of *S. mansoni* and *S. haematobium* together with large numbers of calcified *S. haematobium* eggs. Liver biopsy revealed hepatic bilharziasis.

These brief case reports reveal the variety of clinical presentations, and illustrate the point that though the majority (25/40) of patients may have no complaint referable to the bowel, the possibility of a schistosomal origin of such conditions as hepatomegaly should always be considered even in areas of low endemicity of S. mansoni.

Autopsy study

In the 900 autopsies, fresh rectal snip examination revealed 165 cases of rectal bilharziasis.

Of the 165 cases with rectal involvement, including 58 with pure S. mansoni infections, gross intestinal lesions were present in only three. One, who died following perforation of a typhoid ulcer, had a pure S. haematobium infection, "sandy-patch" lesions in the rectum, and typical vesical bilharziasis with bilateral hydroureter and hydronephrosis. The second case, also with a mixed infection, died of Cor-pulmonale due to pulmonary bilharziasis and complicated by bilharzial hepatic fibrosis. The third case, aged 9, with both S. haematobium and S. mansoni died of acute bilharzial dysentery.

Three other cases dying from acute bilharzial dysentery were discovered in departmental records. These were also under the age of ten. In all four cases of fatal bilharzial dysentery the mucosa of the terminal ileum and of the large bowel was intensely congested with myriads of punctate haemorrhagic ulcers. Neither papillomata nor large ulcers were encountered.

Histopathology of the bowel in fatal cases of bilharzial dysentery

Sections from the terminal ileum and colon in all 4 cases revealed large numbers of bilharzial ova, some apparently viable, large numbers calcified and still others as "ghost forms".

Those ova in the mucosa excited no proliferative tissue response (Figs. 1—6) although the mucosa had a "feathery" appearance (Figs. 5 and 9). The apparently viable ova were present in clusters in and around mucosal glands with surrounding areas of moderate eosinophil infiltration (Figs. 2—4). Only the superficial mucosal glands had been shed in these areas and the surface had an exudate of red blood cells, mucoid material and some eosinophils. No true ulceration was evident. The appearance suggested that the ova deposited in the mucosal vessels escaped into the lumen by evoking local necrosis of the mucosa (Figs. 3 and 4) probably by the secretion of toxic metabolites. These focal, microscopic areas are the focal "pin-point" ulcers or punctate haemorrhages seen proctoscopically.

Those ova trapped in the submucosa and muscular layers, however, evoked a typical pseudo-tuberculoid reaction with the ovum, or remnants of the ovum, in the centre attacked by foreign-body giant cells and surrounded by epithelioid cells, eosinophils, fibroblastic reaction and a rim of plasma cells and lymphocytes (Figs. 7 and 8). There were large numbers of these pseudo-tubercles in the sub-mucosa and lesser numbers in the muscle layers.

Histological examination of sections of the bowel in the one case with sandy patches (S. haematobium infection) revealed an atrophic mucosa with large numbers of degenerate ova in the mucosa. The striking feature, however, was a dense plaque of calcified ova in the submucosa without any inflammatory response

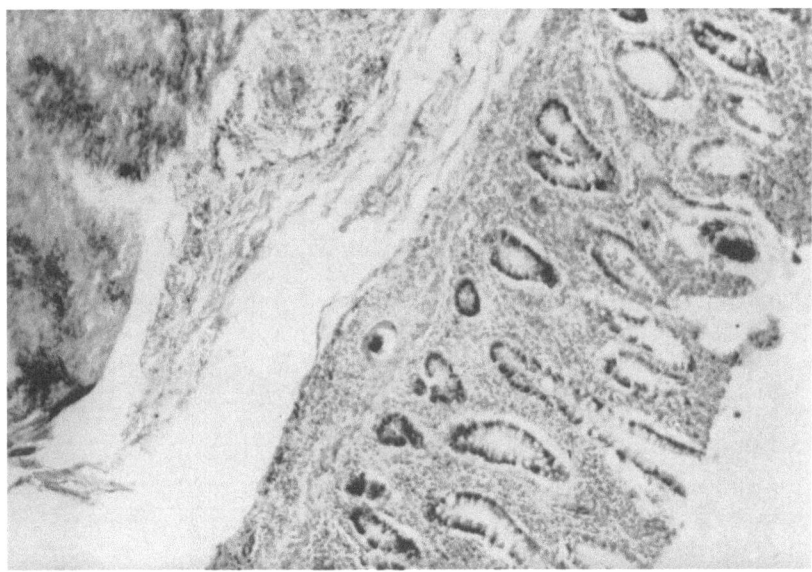

Fig. 1. Section of colon from case with intestinal bilharziasis (S. mansoni) reveals a mature ovum in the mucosal epithelium (left middle) about to enter the bowel lumen. There is minimal inflammatory reaction around it whilst the ovum in the sub-mucosa (right upper) is surrounded by a typical pseudotuberculoid reaction. HE X 50

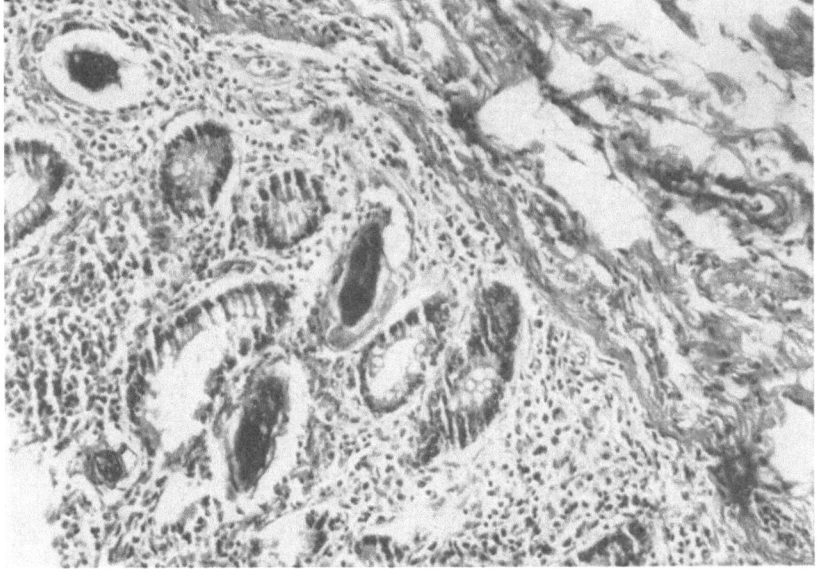

Fig. 2. High power view. 4 mature ova in the mucosa with minimal inflammatory response (chiefly eosinophils). HE X 125

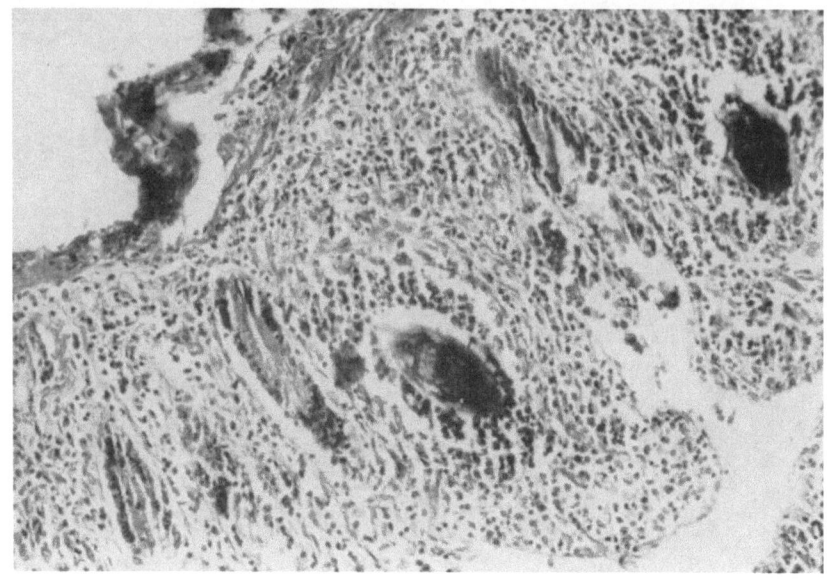

Fig. 3. A mature ovum in a mucosal gland space with eosinophil infiltrate. HE X 125

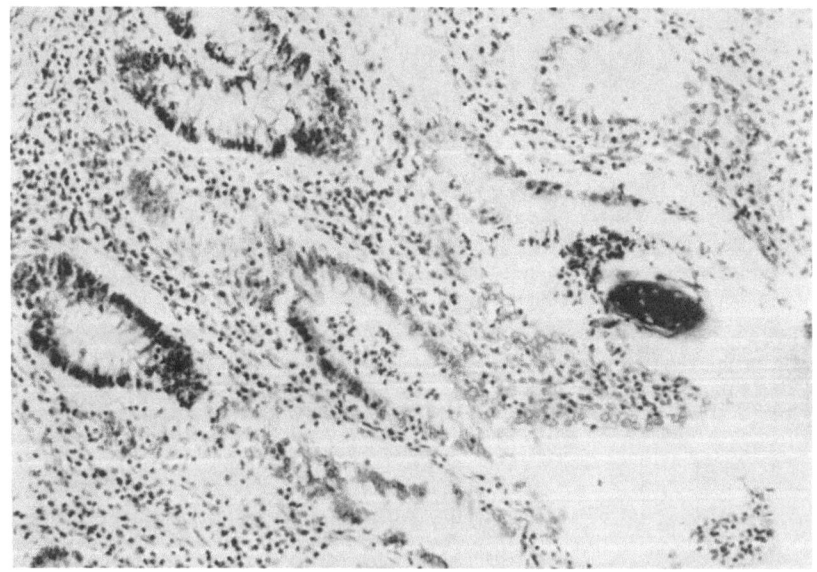

Fig. 4. Mature ovum, with eosinophils tagging it, about to enter the bowel lumen. HE X 125

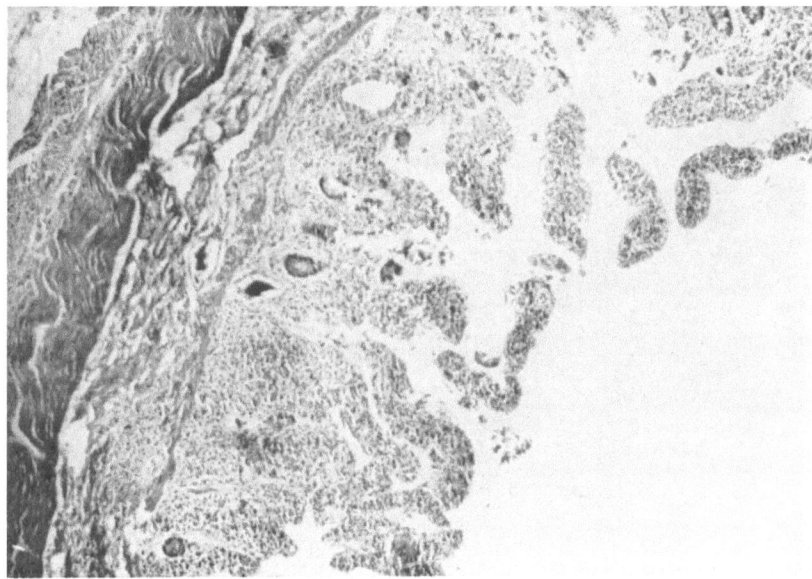

Fig. 5. The "feathery" degeneration of the superficial mucosa is evident. No true ulceration is seen and occasional ova are apparent in the mucosa and submucosa. HE X 20

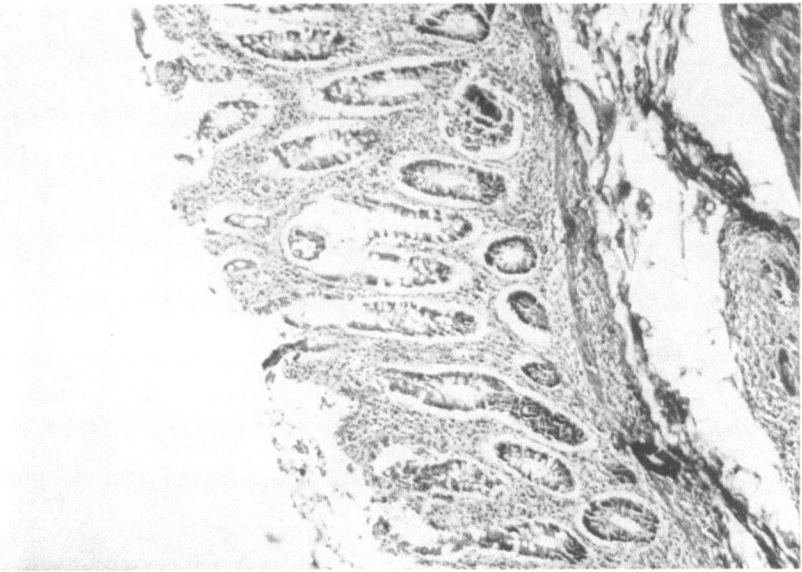

Fig. 6. Another view of the mucosa with a mature ovum in the glandular epithelium surrounded by eosinophils whilst that in the submucosa has evoked the typical pseudotuberculoid reaction. HE X 50

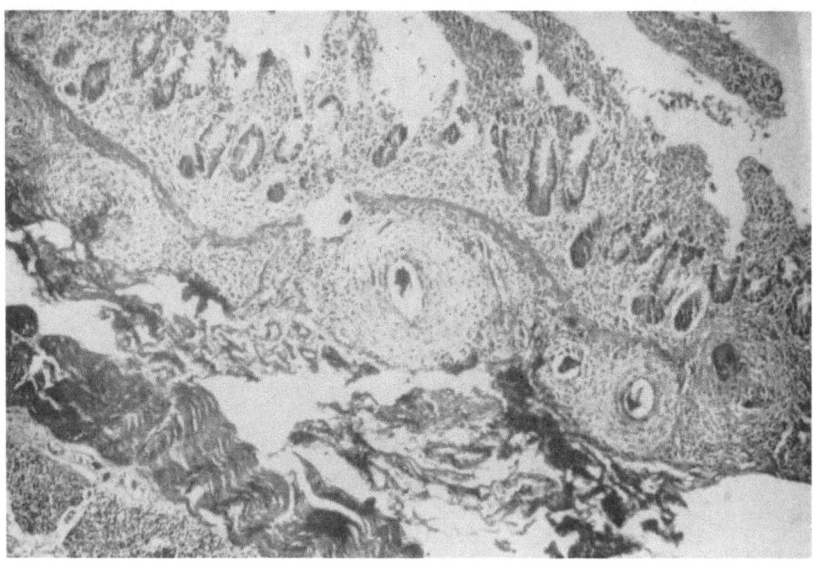

Fig. 7. The prominent, proliferative pseudotuberculoid response evoked by ova in the submucosa is evident. HE X 20

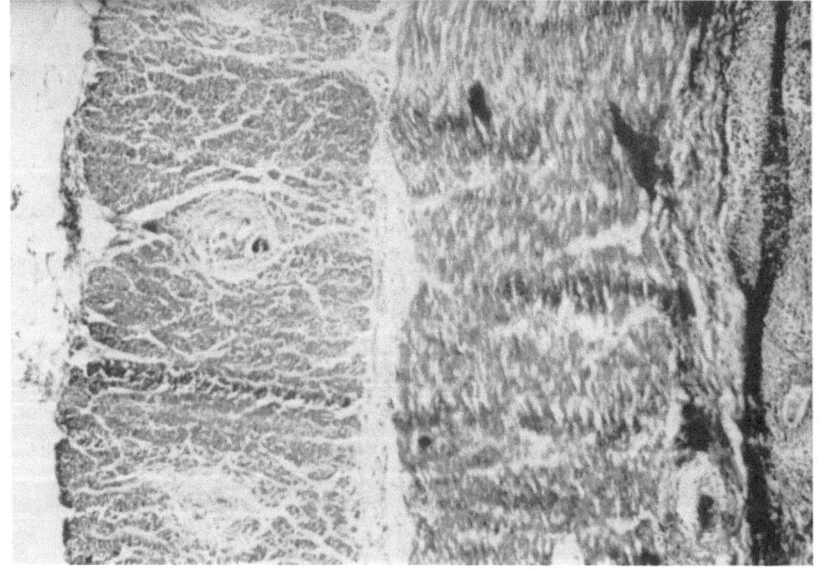

Fig. 8. Typical pseudotubercles in the outer muscule coat. HE X 50

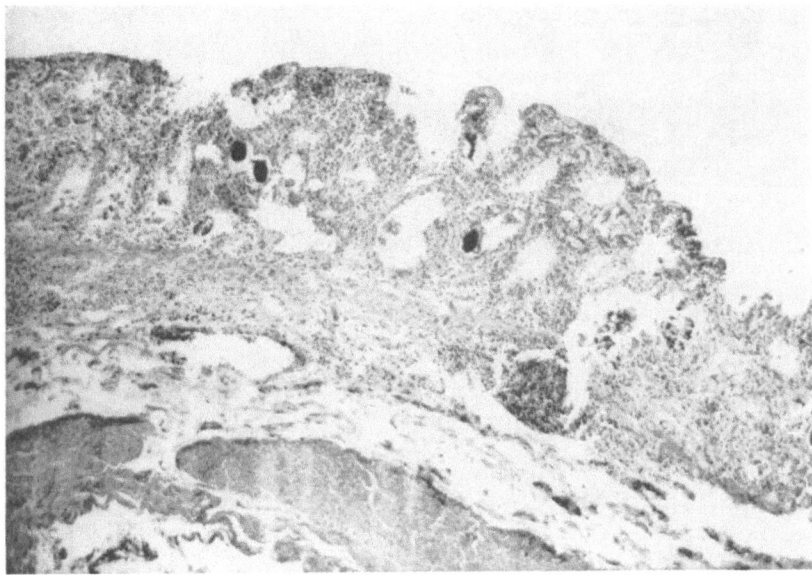

Fig. 9. Mature ova in the mucosa with cellular infiltrate (eosinophils predominating) and pronounced vascularity. HE X 20

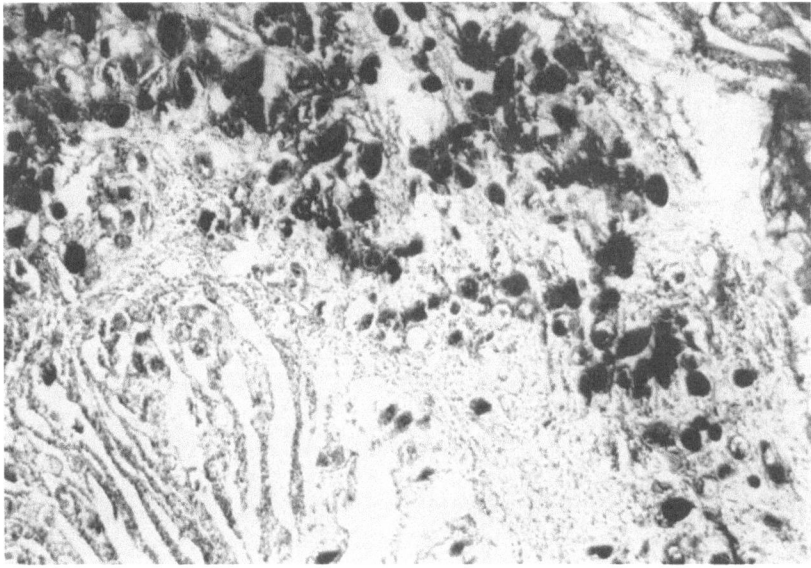

Fig. 10. Histology of a sandy-patch lesion of the bowel with pure *S. Haematobium* infection. Myriads of calcified ova in the submucosa and mucosa with minimal inflammatory reaction. HE X 50

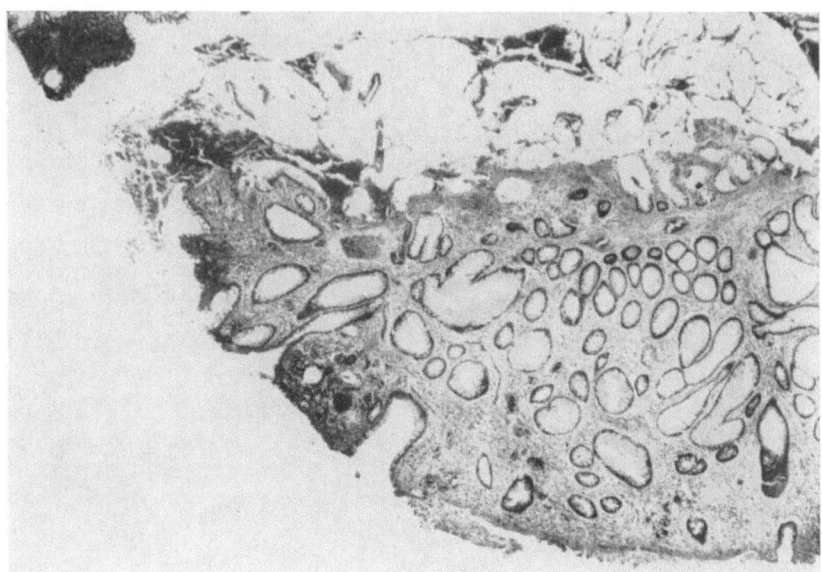

Fig. 11. A bilharzial colonic "polyp". An adenomatous pattern with clusters of ova. HE X 20

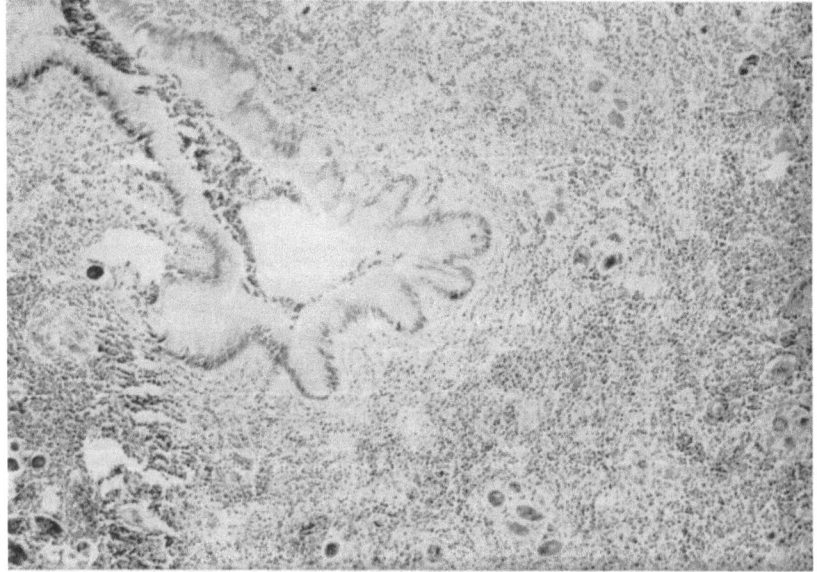

Fig. 12. A higher power view of the same lesion. Intense inflammatory reaction and occasional bilharzial ova.
HE X 50

(Fig. 10). The appearance is identical to that described in late, healed bilharziasis of the bladder.

Moreover, in the clinical cases with "sandy patch" lesions of the rectum, rectal snip revealed, in addition to viable ova, a preponderance of calcified ova. It seems reasonable to conclude then that the "sandy patch" lesions in the rectum, as in the bladder, are the late stage of bilharziasis with myriads of calcified ova layered predominantly in the submucosa with minimal tissue response. The atrophy of the overlaying mucosa contributes to the typical naked-eye appearance.

Histopathology of the rectum in autopsy series

Of the 165 cases of rectal bilharziasis in the autopsy series demonstrated by the snip method, histology was positive in 98 (60%) cases.

The histopathological features are summarised in Table 3.

Table 3. Histopathological features of rectal bilharziasis

Histological features	No.	%
Ova only (mucosa and submucosa)	69	70
Pseudo-tuberculoid reaction (submucosa)	27	28
Acute bilharzial colitis	2	2
Total positive.	98	—

Of the 98 positive cases, histological examination revealed only ova or their remnants in 70%. These were present in the mucosa and submucosa and were accompanied by a little or no inflammatory or fibroblastic response.

In 28% the typical pseudo-tuberculoid type of granulomatous reaction was excited by the ova. All these pseudo-tubercles were confined to the submucosa. In no case were there severe lesions, the large majority showing only a few pseudo-tubercles.

In many cases of pure *S. haematobium* infections, the submucosa harboured, not infrequently, large numbers of calcified ova. The striking feature was, however, the almost total absence of any tissue response.

It would seem that the two species of schistosomes evoke different tissue responses in the rectum. This is probably related to the viability of the eggs. In the clinical cases where biopsies were fresh, eggs of *S. mansoni* were usually viable while those of *S. haematobium* were often more calcified or degenerate.

One may postulate that the proliferative lesions of bilharziasis are provoked by the release of toxic metabolic from viable or recently dead eggs. On the other hand, if the eggs are already non-viable when deposited tissue response will be minimal. PRATES and GILLMAN [15] suggested that bilharzial toxins were responsible for the pronounced tissue response and more recently CAMERON and GANGULEY [4] demonstrated that by comparison with the intact ova of *S. mansoni*, clean eggs shells evoked little or no tissue response.

The rectal mucosa may be considered an ectopic site for *S. haematobium* and may explain the greater numbers of immature, deformed and dead eggs lacking the potential to stimulate proliferative lesions such as are evoked by the mature viable eggs of *S. mansoni*.

Discussion

It is apparent from both the clinical and autopsy observations that intestinal pathology produced by bilharziasis in the Durban population is minimal by comparison with reports from other endemic areas. Two fatal cases were encountered in the present study and search of the records revealed a further two cases who died as a result of acute intestinal bilharziasis.

Contrary to the belief of DEW [5] and DIMMETTE and SPROAT [6] that acute bilharzial dysentery might be a result of secondary bacterial or amoebic invasion, these four cases proved to be pure *S. mansoni* infection confirmed by histopathological studies. Acute bilharzial dysentery is undoubtedly a clinico-pathological entity and almost certainly related to overwhelming infection as revealed by the widespread involvement of the bowel, liver, and to some extent, of the lungs, and mesenteric lymph nodes.

Clinical study of 40 patients with known *S. mansoni* infection demonstrated that 37.5% had symptoms directly related to the infection. Liver biopsy results (to be published) also revealed that the apparent benignity of the intestinal lesions (shown by proctoscopic examination) does not exclude visceral involvement.

Nevertheless, judging by the clinical and autopsy studies, intestinal bilharziasis is, in the majority of Durban patients, a mild, relatively asymptomatic disease, a conclusion supported by the minimal rectal involvement observed both clinically and histopathologically. The punctate haemorrhages revealed by proctoscopy are not true ulcers but focal areas of superficial mucosal necrosis.

Following the classification of RAGHEB [16] all the clinical cases in this study would fall into stage 1 — the earliest manifestations of the disease.

Bilharzial polyps in the large bowel were not encountered in the autopsy series, though, prior to this study, one case had been found with an associated "pipe-stem" cirrhosis of the liver [1]. A solitary bilharzial rectal polyp was discovered in one of the clinical cases (Figs. 11 and 12).

The pathological findings in Durban contrast with those reported by authors from Egypt, East Africa, South America, and the Caribbean countries, where intestinal pathology associated with *S. mansoni* is more severe. Reports suggest that the disease is most virulent in Egypt and less so in the other endemic areas. The picture in Durban is similar to that described by GELFAND [8] in Rhodesia.

Summary

The symptomatology, clinical and pathological findings of intestinal bilharziasis in the Durban, Indian and African populations are presented and compared with those reported by authors from other endemic areas of *S. mansoni*.

Four groups of cases were studied.

(1) Cases of *S. mansoni* infection encountered in the rectal biopsy of 225 cases of known *S. haematobium* infection. Of the 45 cases, only 4 (8.8%) had symptoms related to the intestinal infections.

(2) The role of *S. haematobium* in producing intestinal disease was studied in 40 cases with proven *S. haematobium* infection. Of the 24 cases with proctoscopic evidence of rectal involvement, 15/24 (62.5%) had pure *S. haematobium* infection and in 9/24 (37.5%) viable eggs were shown in rectal biopsies.

Intestinal involvement by this parasite is usually asymptomatic.

(3) The symptomatology, clinical manifestation and rectal and sigmoidoscopic features of *S. mansoni* infection in 40 cases are also presented and discussed. Of these 5 had pure *S. mansoni* infection. Symptoms directly related to *S. mansoni* infection were present in 15/40 (37.5%). The commonest presenting symptom was diarrhoea with blood and mucus with associated abdominal paid.

(4) Of 165 autopsy cases shown by rectal biopsy to have rectal involvement histopathology revealed the condition in 60%.

In addition, 4 fatal cases of acute bilharzial dysentery are reported and the morbid anatomical and histological findings discussed.

The histopathology of intestinal bilharziasis is described and the genesis of punctate haemorrhage is contrasted with that of the sandy patch lesion.

Acknowledgements

I wish to thank Professors R. ELSDON-DEW and J. WAINWRIGHT for their invaluable criticism and guidance; and Dr. R. M. A. NUPEN, acting Medical Superintendent for facilites.

This work was partly financed by a generous grant by Roche Products.

References

[1] BHAGWANDEEN, S. B.: Bilharzial cirrhosis of the liver. Med. Proc. **10**, 199–206 (1964).

[2] — (In preparation).

[3] —, and R. ELSDON-DEW: Comparison of the techniques for the recovery of schistosome eggs in autopsy material. This monograph.

[4] CAMERON, C. R., and N. C. GANGULAY: An experimental study of pathogenesis and reversibility of schistosomal hepatic fibrosis. J. Path. Bact. **87**, 217–237 (1964).

[5] DEW, H. R.: Observations on the pathology of schistosomiasis (S. haematobium and S. mansoni) in the human subjects. J. Path. Bact. **26**, 27–39 (1923).

[6] DIMMETTE, R. M., and H. F. SPROAT: Rectosigmoid polyps in schistosomiasis. 1. General clinical and pathological considerations. Amer. J. Trop. Med. Hyg. **4**, 1057–1067 (1955).

[7] FAIRLEY, N. H.: A comparative study of experimental bilharziasis in monkeys contrasted with hitherto described lesions in man. J. Path. Bact. **23**, 289–314 (1920).

[8] GELFAND, M.: Schistosomiasis in South Central Africa: A clinico-pathological study, p. 239. Capetown: Juta & Co. Ltd. 1950.

[9] HOLLAND, E.: Dysentery. S. Afr. Med. J. **8**, 756–759 (1934).

[10] JAFFE, R.: The anatomical pathology and pathogenesis of bilharziasis mansoni in Venezuela. Trop. Dis. Bull. **46**, 269 (1949) (abstract).

[11] KING, B. A.: Treatment of schistosomiasis with nilodin. Brit. Med. J. **1**, 185–188 (1955).

[12] KOPPISCH, E.: Manson's schistosomiasis. J. Amer. Med. Ass. **121**, 936–942 (1943).

[13] MANSON-BAHR, P. E. C.: The clinical features, diagnosis and host-parasite relationship of schistosomiasis in East Africa. E. Afr. Med. J. **35**, 401–411 (1958).

[14] PONTES, J. T.: Rectosigmoidoscopic aspects of mansonian schistosomiasis in Brazil. Gastroenterology **43**, 244 (1961) (abstract).

[15] PRATES, M. D., and J. GILLMAN: Carcinoma of the urinary bladder in the Portuguese East African with special reference to bilharzial cystitis and preneoplastic reactions. S. Afr. J. Med. Sci. **24**, 13–40 (1959).

[16] RAGHEB, M.: Schistosomiasis of the colon. World Congress of Gastroenterology: Abstract of scientific papers, p. 62–63. Wash. D. C. May 25–31, 1958.

[17] SCHNEIDER, J.: "Intestinal schistosomiasis in Natal and the Northern and Eastern Transvaal". Unpublished Thesis (Witwatersrand University).

[18] TURNER, G. A.: Bilharziasis in South Africa. Parasitology **1**, 195–217 (1908).

[19] WYDELL, S. H.: Some abdominal complications of S. mansoni as seen in Ukerewe Island. E. Afr. Med. J. **35**, 413–426 (1958).

Schistosomiasis in Ibadan, Western Nigeria

G. M. EDINGTON*

The part that schistosomiasis plays in morbidity and mortality rates in West Africa is controversial and has still to be finally assessed. COWPER [3] has recently reviewed the literature on schistosomiasis in Nigeria and considered that Ibadan, the capital city of Western Nigeria with a population of approximately 500,000 was the center of a holoendemic area. The Department of Pathology in the University College Hospital, Ibadan examines 4—5,000 surgical biopsies annually and over 1,000 necropsies are performed — a hospital rate of over 80%. In addition, a three year cancer rate survey in Ibadan has just been completed [6]. It was considered, therefore, that an examination of this material would be of value in assessing the importance of schistosomiasis as a cause of moribidity and mortality in the community.

The incidence of schistosomiasis in surgical biopsy material

In the years 1958—1963, 19,862 surgical biopsies were received, the majority being from the clinical departments in the University College Hospital but about 10% were received from out station hospitals or as referrals from other parts of Nigeria. The incidence of schistosomal lesions in this material is shown in Table 1.

Table 1. *Sites of schistosome lesions seen in 19,862 surgical biopsies 1958—1963*

Site	Number	Age	Site	Number	Age
Appendix	21	12—38	Lymph nodes	2	30
Bladder	16	13—62	Omentum	2	25—41
Bladder carcinoma	15	20—61	Prostate	2	A
Rectum	16	15—60	Testis	1	12
Cervix	6	40—48	Hip joint	1	A
Ureters	5	15—30	Colon	1	25
Vulva and vagina	4	9—63	Lung	1	A
Peritoneum	4	A	Ovary	1	A
Fallopian tube	3	24	Skin	1	?

Total: 102

From this table it will be seen that schistosomiasis was only noted in 102 instances — an incidence of 0.5% and the most common sites affected were the appendix, bladder and rectum. With regard to the appendix, during the period surveyed 304 appendices were received and schistosome ova were noted in 21 whereas in a series of 125 appendices examined post mortem, schistosome ova were only noted in three [9], the incidence in surgically removed specimens being

---

* Department of Pathology, Faculty of Medicine, University of Ibadan, and University College Hospital, Ibadan, Nigeria.

therefore slightly higher than that seen in necropsy material (7 as compared to 3%). The association is not, however, as striking as might have been expected. There was no evidence to suggest that schistosomiasis was associated with carcinoma of the rectum and its association with carcinoma of the bladder is discussed below.

There is no doubt that schistosome ova can initiate a granulomatous reaction in almost any tissue in the body and, on occasion, the lesion so produced requires surgical intervention. From a study of this material no evidence has been produced to suggest that schistosomiasis is a potent cause of morbidity in our hospital patients.

Schistosomiasis in post mortem material

In the years 1958—1962, 3,806 necropsies were performed. 420 being stillbirths, leaving a total of 3,386 to be considered. The pathology of renal disease in this material has already been described and the importance of schistosomiasis as a cause of death briefly discussed [7]. The renal conditions causing death are shown in Table 2.

Table 2. *Renal conditions causing death in 3,386 post mortem examinations, University College Hospital, Ibadan (1958—1962)*

Congenital	16
Glomerulonephritis	
Acute	2
Subacute	18
Chronic	104
Pyelonephritis	
Acute	12
Chronic	51
Others	20
Carcinoma	
Bladder	13
Kidney	10
Prostate	7
Amyloid disease	12
Acute tubular necrosis	10
Schistosomiasis (excluding carcinoma)	7
Total	282

Schistosome ova were found in three patients dying of carcinoma of the bladder. Excluding these cases, it will be seen from Table 2 that schistosomiasis was only considered responsible for death in seven subjects and three of these were children who died from the effects of antimony therapy with mild schistosomal bladder lesions present. Therefore, in over 3,000 necropsies schistosomiasis was only responsible for death in four instances, namely: renal complications of bladder involvement in two instances, cor pulmonale in one and liver abscess following schistosomal appendicitis in the fourth subject (perhaps a doubtful entity).

In a further 51 subjects ova were noted as an incidental finding in bladder lesions at necropsy and the conditions in which these lesions were noted in more than two occasions are shown in Table 3.

Schistosome ova were noted in only one of 65 subjects dying from cirrhosis of the liver and in two dying of primary liver cell carcinoma. When these findings

9 Bilharziasis

are considered in conjunction with Table 3 it would appear that schistosomiasis is unlikely to be the major etiological agent in any of the conditions listed.

Table 3. *Causes of death in which schistosome ova were present as an incidental finding in more than two instances (3,386 necropsies)*

Cause of death	Total	Schistosomiasis
Chronic glomerulonephritis .	104	6
Tetanus	175	5
Chronic pyelonephritis . . .	51	3
Leukaemia	14	3
Sickle-cell hb. C disease . .	48	3

Schistosomiasis and carcinoma of the bladder

During the years 1960—1963, 1,920 tumors were recorded in the Cancer Registry, University College Hospital and of these 43 were carcinomas of the bladder — a relative ratio frequency of 2.3%. This figure is similar to those reported from Ghana and East Africa [2] but much lower than those reported from Egypt and Portuguese East Africa. Approximately 60% of the tumors in the Registry were of the squamous and anaplastic types and schistome ova were noted in 25%. Approximately 46% of the patients were below the age of 50 years with an age range of 18 to 80 and the sex ratio in this material was 3.1 males to females. It is perhaps significant that 70% of the patients with coincident schistosomiasis were below the age of 50 years and the male to female sex ratio was 2 : 1.

A three year cancer rate survey of the population of Ibadan has just been completed and the age specific rates of cancer of the bladder per 100,000 of the population are shown in Table 4 and compared with the rates in Laurenco Marques [8] and in the U.S. White and Non-White [4].

Table 4. *Age specific rates per 100,000 of the population per year for bladder cancer in Ibadan, Laurenco Marques, and in the U.S. White and Non-White population compared in age and sex groups*

Age group	Ibadan		L. M.		U. S. White		U. S. Non-White	
	Male	Female	Male	Female	Male	Female	Male	Female
15—19	—	2.20	—	—	—	—	—	—
20—29	—	—	2.30	4.90	1.00	0.45	—	0.49
30—39	—	—	16.60	7.90	1.30	0.94	1.18	2.07
40—49	7.10	2.00	20.40	29.50	7.54	3.99	4.15	6.23
50—59	4.10	14.30	52.60	44.40	35.29	11.39	15.19	21.53
60++	40.00	—	68.50	67.50	108.78	49.07	36.66	36.68
Crude rate	1.40	0.68	9.2	9.8	17.34	8.06	4.93	5.58

In the Ibadan Rate survey, 648 tumors were considered in the three year period and only 15 were carcinoma of the bladder. The figures are small but when they are compared with those in Table 4, it cannot be claimed that carcinoma of the bladder is common in Ibadan. In contrast in Laurenco Marques [8], the incidence of bladder tumors in the younger age groups is exceedingly high when compared with the White and Non-White population in the United States. Once again this investigation has not suggested that schistosomiasis is a formidable

agent in causing a high incidence of bladder cancer in the population investigated
— although it should be noted that the figures in the 40 to 49 year old age group
do not differ greatly from those recorded in the States and also that schistosome
ova were more commonly found in the younger age groups.

Discussion

The investigations described in this paper would all tend to show that the
morbidity and mortality caused by schistosomiasis in the hospital population
of Ibadan is not high. The mortality figures are in contrast to the writer's findings
in Ghana where, in one year, schistosomiasis was responsible for 2% of deaths in
post mortem material [5] — the inability to incriminate schistosomiasis as a common aetiological agent in cirrhosis of the liver, however, agrees with the findings
in Ibadan. In Ibadan in the absence of digest studies in the post mortem material and accurate epidemiological data it is considered that the findings should
be accepted with reserve. Although high infestation rates have been described in
Ibadan school children recent figures would suggest that the incidence is falling
[1] and the incidence of *S. haematobium* ova in the urines of 8,662 in patients in
the University College Hospital was only 3.1% [3]. It would appear, therefore,
that although the incidence of schistosomiasis is high in surrounding areas, the
material studies in this investigation has most probably come from a population
in which the intensity, if not the incidence, of infection has been low. In this
connection the writer has been fortunate in obtaining preliminary figures from a
group of workers in Ibadan who are studying the clinical effects of *S. haematobium*
infection in selected populations in which the intensity of infection is high [2].
Table 5 shows the results of intravenous pyelography in 12 adults working in a
boat yard in a holoendemic area and 19 pupils in an Ibadan school — all of whom
were passing ova of *S. haematobium* in the urine at the time of examination.

Table 5. *Results of I VP in 12 egg positive adults (Epe boat yard) and 19 pupils 9—15 years old
(Ibadan)*

Group	Number	Bladder		Ureters	
		Normal	Calc.	Normal	Dilated
Adults	12	6	6	7	5
Pupils	19	11	8	16	3

Thus almost 50% of those examined exhibited calcification of the bladder and
a high proportion of these showed dilatation of the ureters — in one child the
calyceal system was also dilated. These figures suggest, in contrast to the findings
in hospital patients, that the urological effects of schistosomiasis in the Ibadan
area may be considerable in selected populations in which the intensity of infection is high. The final assessment of the pathological importance of schistosomiasis
in Nigeria, therefore, must await the outcome of investigations performed on
these selected communities following accurate epidemiological studies. The writer,
however, feels strongly that the lack of accurate morbidity and mortality figures
should not be allowed to distract workers from the most important aspect of
schistosomiasis — namely prevention.

9*

Summary

A study of material in the Department of Pathology, University College Hospital, Ibadan, Nigeria has revealed a relatively low incidence of pathological lesions due to schistosomiasis.

The findings should be accepted with reserve and further investigations on selected populations performed.

References

[1] AKINKUGBE, O., O.: Urinary schistosomiasis in Ibadan school children. W. Afr. Med. J. **11**, 124—127 (1962).

[2] ANNAND, S. V., I. BRABANT, H. M. GILLES, R. LINDER, and S. PI-SUNYER: Personal communication.

[3] COWPER, S. G.: Schistosomiasis in Nigeria. Ann. Trop. Med. Parasit. **57**, 307—322 (1963).

[4] CUTLER, S. J., and H. F. DORN: Morbidity from Cancer in the United States. Public Health Monograph No. 29, U.S. Govt. Printing Office, Washington 1955.

[5] EDINGTON, G. M.: Schistosomiasis in Ghana with special reference to its pathology. W. Afr. Med. J. **6**, 45—57 (1957).

[6] —, and G. M. U. MACLEAN: A cancer rate survey in Ibadan, Western Nigeria. Brit. J. Cancer. (In Press).

[7] —, and A. R. MAINWARING: Pathology of renal disease in West Africa. In: Kidney. F. K. MOSTOFI, (Ed.). Baltimore: Williams and Wilkins 1966.

[8] PRATES, M. D.: The rates of cancer of the bladder in the Portuguese East Africans of Laurenco Marques. Symposium on cancer of the urinary bladder. Acta Un. Int. Cancer **18**, 643—647 (1962).

[9] SOLANKE, T. F.: Personal communication.

Bilharziasis in French Speaking West Africa

M. Payet and R. Camain*

Endemic bilharziasis was described 50 years ago in French speaking West Africa and now the main foci of bilharziasis are well localized. S. mansoni and S. haematobium)[1] are the chief pathogens.

Information on the pathology of the disease has been obtained from two different sources [1—42].

A. Routine microscopic examination of biopsy and necropsy material.

B. Systematic and associated epidemiological, parasitological and pathological surveys in endemic zones.

A. Pathological examination

Except when the eggs are detected in the excreta of the patients or when the symptomatology is in favour of bilharziasis (dysentery, hematuria), the diagnosis of the disease is difficult.

Schistosomiasis is in fact pleomorphic. However, it may be suspected when interstitial nephritis or hepatic fibrosis occur, associated with splenomegaly, as well as in some cases of epididymitis, salpingitis and cervitis. A positive diagnosis may be also presumed from radiological investigations (calcifications of urinary bladder and ureters).

Table 1

Organ	Schistosoma haematobium	Schistosoma mansoni	Questionable species
Urinary bladder	65		
Ureter	2		
Testicle	2		
Epididymis	10		
Spermatic cord	6		
Prostate	1		
Ovary	10		
Fallopian tube	10		
Uterus	44		
Vagina	6		
Vulva	4		
Appendix	30		
Omemtum	7		
Intestine	5		
Mesenteric glands	1	1	1
Spleen	2		
Liver	29	34	55
Lung	1		3
Skin	2		
Bilharzian sepsis	3		

* Faculté de Médecine et de Pharmacie, University of Dakar, Dakar, Senegal.

[1] Some parasitologists (Gretillat) consider that S. curassoni is locally responsible of urinary bilharziasis in Senegal. S. curassoni has nearly a similar morphology as S. haematobium, but some of its biological characteristics are different.

In most cases the diagnosis of bilharziasis is a pathological one, but as the eggs of parasites are often altered, the diagnosis of species is not always obtained.

The results of our own investigations in "Institut Pasteur" of Dakar (1950 to 1964) are reported (Table 1) and will be shortly commented upon.

1. Lesions of urogenital tract (S. haematobium)

Urinary bladder. – Various types of lesions may be recognized (erosio simplex, sclerosis, nodules, tubercles, polyps, papilloma, carcinoma). Correlation between bilharziasis and carcinoma of the bladder was not evident, though 26 epidermoid carcinomas were detected among 65 bilharzial bladders. But during the same period (1950—1964) 95 carcinoma of the bladder without bilharziasis were observed (a total of 119 bladder carcinomas among 5000 malignant tumors).

Pathological examination allows assessment of ureteral lesions when stenosed ureters are reimplanted in the bladder.

In 14 years' experience we never detected bilharzial eggs in the kidneys, though ascending interstitial nephritis is frequently observed and represents about 50% of all nephritis. The relationship between bilharziasis and interstitial nephritis is nevertheless a positive fact, for stasis or atrophy of the bladder, ureteric and pelvic dilatation are often complicated by bacterial infection due to repeated destructions of the surface of the epithelium. These lesions of the urinary tract may be absent and nephritis may, in such cases, be related to bilharziasis by the early occurrence of hematuria and other related symptoms.

Nephritis is one of the most severe complications of schistosomiasis, and must be systematically investigated (by renal needle biopsy) when a patient suffering from bilharziasis has to undergo a bladder or ureteral operation. When recognized, kidney alterations may change the attitude of the surgeon and give a better approximation of the prognosis.

Acute infection may complicate urinary bilharziasis. Such a case occurred in an 18 months old African girl who rapidly died from a perivesical phlegmon in relation to severe bilharziasis, complicated by acute pyelonephritis.

The testes are rare sites of localisation. The epididymis, spermatic cord, seminal vesicles and prostate are more frequently involved. In epididymis, the differential diagnosis is between bilharziasis and tuberculosis since the bilharzial tubercles which are observed during an operation are similar to those seen in tuberculosis. A bilharzial vesiculitis may constrict the terminal ureter and a bilharzial prostatitis may be associated with painful erection, impotence and dysuria.

Bilharzial oophoritis with reactive sclerosis of the cortex, as well as chronic or subacute salpingitis with sclerosis and stenosis of the tube may lead to sterility. The Corpus uteri is less frequently invaded by the parasites than the cervix, where all grades of lesions may be seen. In many cases clinical confusion is possible between bilharzial outgrowths of the cervix and carcinoma. In 4 of 38 cases carcinoma of cervix was associated with bilharziasis but it was impossible to determine the specific relationship.

In one case many eggs of *S. haematobium* were found in a disrupted uterine scar of a former cesarean operation.

Schistosomiasis may cause papillomatous or tumour-like changes of vagina and vulva. We have observed bilharzial inflammatory tumours as large as an orange, even a foetus head.

Eggs of parasites were occasionally seen in ectopic testicles. (Feminizing testicles).

Bilharzial appendicitis is frequent and the anastomosis between pelvic and appendicular veins explains the invasion of the organ by S. *haematobium*. This invasion, if mild, leads to sclerosis and chronic appendicitis; if severe, acute appendicitis, secondary to destruction of the mucosa.

2. Lesions of digestive tract

Excluding the rectal lesions but including the well-described hepatic injuries, we may report that all gradings were observed (plain presence of eggs, follicles, interstitial fibrosis, severe Symmers fibrosis, cirrhosis). S. *mansoni* was more frequently observed than S. *haematobium* but in many cases the discrimination was impossible, due to great alterations of the eggs.

Whether bilharziasis is the cause of African cirrhosis remains controversial. When eggs coexist with cirrhosis the probability exists but when they have disappeared, as in the so-called bilharzial Banti syndrome, the relationship is much more hypothetical.

The association of bilharziasis-primary carcinoma of the liver is regarded, in West Africa, as fortuitous (10/1000 of the cases of primary carcinoma of the liver.

3. Bilharzial splenomegaly

Splenomegaly is frequent in West Africa, but in many hundreds of cases of enlarged spleens examined after necropsy and more than one hundred after splenectomy eggs were detected only twice (one case of Banti syndrome, one case of reticulosarcoma of the spleen). Perhaps potassic digestion of these samples would have given us more accurate results, but, notwithstanding, the association of splenomegaly and eggs is rare. In order to explain the frequency of splenomegaly in bilharziasis and especially in urinary schistosomiasis, possibly a rapid destruction of eggs in spleen may explain their rarity. But would it not be more probable that spleen enlargement is due to a reaction of the splenic R.E.S. to the waste-products of the worm?

The problem of large spleens seems to us more and more difficult to resolve. A recent study showed the impossibility of determining a reliable etiological basis in more than 1/4 of the cases (Table 2).

Table 2

Etiology	No. of cases
Malaria	2
Bilharziasis	3
Hemopathies, tumors	10
Sepsis	1
Typhoid fever	2
Tuberculosis	6
Icterus	1
Trypanosiomasis	2
Unknown	74

4. Pulmonary localization and secondary cardiac effects

Eggs were observed in lung parenchyma in seven cases. Three of them were associated with a real bilharzial sepsis. In two the eggs were free in the capillaries, in four they were embedded in numerous follicles, and in one there was a huge embolism of eggs in the capillary net with about 15 eggs in each microscopic field. Twice there was a close relationship between lung involvement and cardiac failure; the last case above mentioned was associated with a glioblastoma of the brain and, though a pulmonary edema with cardiac failure was present, it was not possible to relate its existence to massive bilharziasis.

B. Systematic surveys based on cooperation

Cooperation between parasitologists, internists and pathologists.

In 1954 we attempted to clarify the importance of malarial and bilharzial parasitism in hepatic and splenic pathology in children. Interstitial or portal fibrosis were related to these infestations, more severely when they were coexisted. During this investigation the type of schistosomiasis was not considered.

A second investigation (1962—1964) was more satisfactory. In a first step, the parasitologists detected in Senegal, at about 100 km from Dakar, two foci of bilharziasis, the one with pure infestation by *S. haematobium* (Kirène), the other with pure infestation by *S. mansoni* (Fandène). These two foci, separated no more than twenty kilometers, presented similar environmental conditions. The tribal and religion (Catholic) were also the same.

Sixteen Africans from Kirène, aged 6—23, and presenting eggs of *S. haematobium* in the urine, as well as 28 Africans from Fandène, aged 6—23, with eggs of *S. mansoni* in feces, were admitted during a fortnight into Infections Diseases Hospital of Dakar (Prof. ARMENGAUD).

In addition to the clinical and biological tests each patient was subjected to a liver biopsy (needle). All were apparently healthy in spite of their parasitism and had normal activity.

In the liver biopsy, a substantial difference was observed between the livers infested by *S. haematobium* and those by *S. mansoni*. The latter showed a higher frequency of eggs and of fibrosis (Table 3).

Table 3

Species	No. of cases	Normal liver	Lymphocytic infiltration Portal Fibrosis +	Portal Fibrosis + +	Cirrhosis	Presence of eggs
S. H.	16	8	7		1	1
S. M.	28	5	6	17		21

It must be noted that biological liver tests were not in accordance with pathological findings and that the splenic enlargement occurred in 6 of 16, with vesical schistosomiasis, and 8 of 28 with MANSON's schistosomiasis.

Such results indicate the higher frequency of splenomegaly in urinary bilharziasis, and the gravity of liver damage in MANSON's schistosomiasis. The presence of eggs in 21/28 of the livers is remarkable when one considers the small size of a biopsy sample (a 15 mm × 2 mm cylinder).

During these investigations rectal biopsies were obtained from Africans suffering from rectal bilharziasis. These biopsies were examined in two different ways: (1) clearing by potash and direct microscopic examination and (2) histological routine examination. The first of the of the two technics is considered as the most suitable.

The 16 Africans from Kirène and the 28 from Fandène were treated with combined amphotalide -anthiolidine and most of them came back to the hospital one year later to be investigated. Unfortunately, those from Kirène *(S. haematobium)* had recurrent parasitic infections and a reliable estimation of the treatment was impossible. On the contrary no superimposed infections occurred in Fandène *(S. mansoni)* because the infective pond remained dry during the year.

The results of the 17 investigations before and after treatment are reported in Table 4.

Table 4

Survey Fandène			Stools		Eggs or follicles		Liver			
							Fibrosis		Lymphocytic infiltration	
No.	Age	Sex	A*	B**	A*	B**	A*	B**	A*	B**
1	10	M	+	+ (1)	+	0	+	+	+	0
2	9	F	+	0	0	0	+	0	+ +	±
3	12	F	+	0	0	0	0	0	+	0
4	11	F	+	0	0	0	+ +	0	+ +	+
5	9	F	+	0	+	0	+	+	+	±
6	10	F	+	0	+	0	+ +	+	+	±
7	7	F	+	0	+	0	+ +	+	+	0
8	10	F	+	+ (2)	+	+	+ +	+	+	±
9	9	F	+	+ (1)	+	+	+ +	+	+ +	±
10	9	F	+	0	+	0	+ +	+	+	±
11	11	M	+	0	+	0	+	+	+	±
12	7	F	+	0	+	0	+ +	+	+ +	0
13	15	F	+	0	0	0	+	0	+	±
14	10	F	+	+ (4)	+	0	+ +	+	+	±
15	7	M	+	0	+	0	+	+	+	±
16	11	M	+	0	+	0	+	+ +	+	+
17	12	F	+	0	0	0	+	+	+	±

* A = before treatment. ** B = one year after treatment

There was a spectacular fall in fecal excretion of eggs corresponding to decrease of eggs and follicles in the liver biopsy. In the same way, hepatic fibrosis regressed in most cases with the loss of its inflammatory and evolutive process after the antiparasitic therapy.

The value of this form of inquiry should be confirmed in other countries and we suggest it to epidemiologists and pathologists. For example, gynecologists here follow with repeated biopsies of the cervix, the bilharzial lesions of women cured by the combined amphotalide-anthiomaline; where eggs were shown to have disappeared from the cervical mucosa. Such studies would help in making allowance for bilharziasis illness and bilharziasis sequela.

In bilharzial endemic areas, pathological research should be accompanied by immunological studies. As the used antigens are actually of inequal quality, it is difficult to interpret skin reaction and complement fixation reaction. But if we follow some authors to whom these reactions have a very large sensitivity and a good specificity, it would be possible to determine quantitatively the bilharzial endemicity. However, we have to consider the opinion of other authors who only retain the sensitiviness of these reactions and deny the specificity.

In conclusion, pathological study of bilharziasis is important in different ways: to resolve a medical or a surgical problem, to investigate the unsettled pathogenesis, to provide useful controls for epidemiological, parasitological and therapeutic studies. It would be most valuable to determine the etiology of bilharzial splenomegaly and the relationship between bilharziasis and urinary bladder cancer.

In French speaking West Africa, pathological study of bilharziasis confirms
the numerous diversity of schistosomiasis aspects. Systematically used during
polyvalent survey, it helps to define the pathology of bilharziasis in African
rural areas.

References

[1] Armengaud, M., M. Lariviere, P. Hocquet et R. Camain: A propos de deux foyers de
Bilharziose au Sénégal — Considérations cliniques et anatomiques. Méd. Afr. Noire
(Numéro spécial) juillet, 177 (1963).

[2] Boiron, H., et R. Koerber: Contribution a l'étude de la bilharziose urinaire en Afrique
Occidentale Française. Bull. Soc. Path. Exot. 40, 118—124 (1947).

[3] Bouet, G., et E. Roubaud: Bilharziose au Dahomey et en Haute-Casamance. Bull.
Soc. Path. Exot. 5, 837—842 (1912).

[4] Bouffard, et Neveux: Bilharziose dans le Haut-Sénégal et le Haut-Niger. Bull. Soc.
Path. Exot. 1, 420—432 (1908).

[5] Camain, R.: Sur quelques tumeurs bilharziennes de l'appareil gential masculin observées
en Afrique Occidentale Français. Bull. Méd. A. O. F. 9, 265—269 (1952).

[6] — Aspects histopathologiques des schistosomiases en A. O/F. — Bull. Ec. Nat. Méd.
Pharm. Dakar 1, 167—174 (1952/53).

[7] — Schistosomiases genitales féminines et masculines à S. haematobium observées en
A.O.F. Bull. Soc. Path. Exot. 46, 412—434 (1953).

[8] —, J. Vernier, P. Navarranne, et E. Ayite: Schistosomiase cervico-vaginald à S. haematobium. Bull. Méd. A. O. F. 9, 81—84 (1952).

[9] —, et M. Armengaud: Aspects anatomo-cliniques des splénomégalies. Méd. Afr. Noire.
(Numéro spécial) juillet, 31—35 (1963).

[10] —, P. Navaranne et E. Ayite: Deux cas d'annexite à S. haematobium observés à
Dakar. Bull. Soc. Path. Exot. 44, 202—208 (1951).

[11] Daget, J.: Le Parc National du Niokolo-Koba, II. Mollusques d'eau douce. Mém. IFAN
62, 13—29 (1961).

[12] Dejou, L., et. P. Navaranne: Aspects chirurgicaux de quelques localisations abdo-
minales des bilharzioses. Méd. Trop. 14, 513—541 (1954).

[13] Deschiens, R.: Le problème sanitaire des bilharzioses dans les territoires de l'Union
Française. Généralités et reparatition géographique. Bull. Soc. Path. Exot. 44, 350—
377 (1951).

[14] Gaud, J.: Les bilharzioses en Afrique Occidentale et en Afrique Centrale. Bull. O.M.S.
13, 209—259 (1955).

[15] Gretillat, S.: Epidémiologie de la bilharziose vésicale au Sénégal Oriental. Observations sur l'écologie de Bulinus guernei et de Bulinus senegalensis. Bull. O. M. S.
25, 459—466 (1961).

[16] — Recherches sur le cycle évolutif du Schistosome des Ruminants domestiques de l'Ouest
Africain (Schistosoma curassoni Brumpt, 1931) C. R. Acad. Sci. 255, 1657—1659
(1962).

[17] — Une nouvelle zoonose, la »Bilharziose Ouest-Africaine« à Schistosoma currasoni, com-
mune à l'homme et aux Ruminants domestiques. C. R. Acad. Sci. 255, 1805—1807
(1962).

[18] Larivière, M., et M. Charnier: Contribution à l'étude des bilharzioses au Sénégal. Re-
cherche des mollusques sur la Presqui'lle du Cap-Vert. Bull Ec. Nat. Méd. Pharm.
Dakar 5, 336—339 (1957).

[19] —, P. Correa et J. Lauroy: A propos de 2 cas de cervicité bilharzienne. Bull. Méd.
A. O. F. 4, 313 (1959).

[20] —, R. Aretas, A. Raba et M. Charnier: Index d'infestation bilharzienne au Sénégal
(Cercles de Thies et de Kaolack). Bull. Méd A. O. F. 3, 239—243 (1958).

[21] —, J. Lapierre, P. Hocquet et P. Camerlynck: Etude d'un foyer de bilharziose à
S. mansini dans un village du cercle de Thies (Sénégal). Bull. Soc. Méd. Afr. Noire
Langue Franç. 5, 88 (1960).

[22] LARIVIÈRE, M., P. HOCQUET et P. CAMERLYNCK: Enquète parasitaire chez les enfants de Basse-Casamance (République du Sénégal). Bull. Soc. Méd. Afr. Noire Langue Franç. 6, 717 (1961).

[23] —, S. GRETILLAT et P. HOCCQUET: Considérations et recherches sur l'épidémiologie des bilharzioses au Sénégal. Méd. Afr. Noire (Numéro spécial) juillet, 61 (1963).

[24] LEGER, M.: Les bilharzioses urinaire et intestinale au Sénégal. Bull. Soc. Path. Exot. 16, 141−144 (1923).

[25] —, et E. BEDIER: Index bilharzien (S. haematobium) chez les enfants de Dakar. Bull. Soc. Path. Exot. 16, 276−278 (1923).

[26] LEFROU, G.: Présence de Bulinus dybowski au Sénégal. La diagnose des Bulinidae Africains. Bull. Soc. Path. Exot. 26, 1099−1105 (1933).

[27] NAVARANNE, P., P. PARIS et R. CAMAIN: Note sur l'appendicité en milieu Africain. Bull. Méd. A. O. F. 11, 309 (1952).

[28] NEVEU-LEMAIRE, M., et A. ROTON: Trois cas de bilharziose vésicale observés à Dakar. Arch. Parasitol. 15, 474−477 (1911).

[29] NOSNY, D., R. CAMAIN et L. J. COURBIL: Aspects cliniques et anatomo-pathologiques des bilharzioses génito-urinaires. Méd. Afr. Noire (Numéro spécial) juillet, 69 (1963).

[30] — La bilharziose génito-urinaire (Etude anatomo-pathologique). Bull. Soc. Path. Exot. 56, 999 (1963).

[31] PAYET, M., et R. CAMAIN: Pneumopathie aigue à S. haematobium. Bull. Soc. Path. Exot. 45, 680−687 (1952).

[32] —, E. BERTHE, R. CAMAIN et P. PENE: Accidents cardiaques aigus de la bilharziose à S. haematobium; à propos de deux observations. Bull. Soc. Path. Exot. 46, 688−692 (1953).

[33] — P. PENE, R. CAMAIN et C. ARDOUIN: Bilharziose viscérale à S. haematobium. Gaz. Méd. Fr. 61, 813−819 (1954).

[34] — — — Considérations sur la bilharziose à S. haematobium dans la région de Dakar. Bull. Mém. Ecole Prépar. Méd. Pharm. Dakar 11, 23−35 (1954).

[35] — — — Les néphrites bilharziennes. Bull. Méd. A. O. F. 11, 141−143 (1954).

[36] PELLEGRINO, A., et P. GIUDICELLI: Confrontations radio-cliniques dans 85 cas de bilharziose urinaire. Méd. Trop. 17, 7−27 (1957).

[37] — L'urographie intra-veineuse dans la bilharziose urinaire. J. Radiol. Electrol. 39, 599−609 (1958).

[38] — Le radiodiagnostic dans la bilharziose urinaire. Gaz. Méd. Fr. 68, 2155−2162 (1961).

[39] REY, M., R. CAMAIN, P. HOCQUET et A. BOURGEADE: Modifiications des lésions hépatiques de la bilharziose intestinale après traitement par Amphotalide et Anthiolimine associés. Bull. Soc. Méd. Afr. Noire Langue Franc. 9, 204−208 (1964).

[40] SERAFINO, X., X. TOSSOU et B. DIOUF: Aspects chirurgicaux des bilharzioses. Bull. Soc. Méd. Afr. Noire (Numéro spécial) juillet, 85 (1963).

[41] — — — A propos d'une urétero colocystoplastie pour bilharziose urétero-vésicale. Bull. Soc. Méd. Afr. Noire Langue Franç. 2, 232 (1963).

[42] — B. DIOUF, CL. RICHIR et PH. BRETON: Sur un nouveau cas de faux-cancer du col. utérin d'origine bilharzienne. Bull. Soc. Méd. Afr. Noire Langue Franç. No. 5, p. 690 (1963).

The Pathology of Schistosomiasis in Japan

Historical Review of the Research in Japan and its Relation to the Liver Cirrhosis

MASAHI MIYAKE*

With 15 figures

1. Distribution of schistosomiasis japonicum

The main endemic areas of Japanese schistosomiasis are Japan, mainland China, Formosa, the Philippine Islands, and the Celebes Islands. In mainland China, it occurs along the Yangtze River, and in Fkien, Kwangtung and Yunnan. In the Philippine Islands, it covers Mindoro, Leyte, Mindanao and Samar Islands. In Formosa, there are no cases of human schistosomiasis, although a specific form of Japanese schistosomiasis has been reported (Fig. 1).

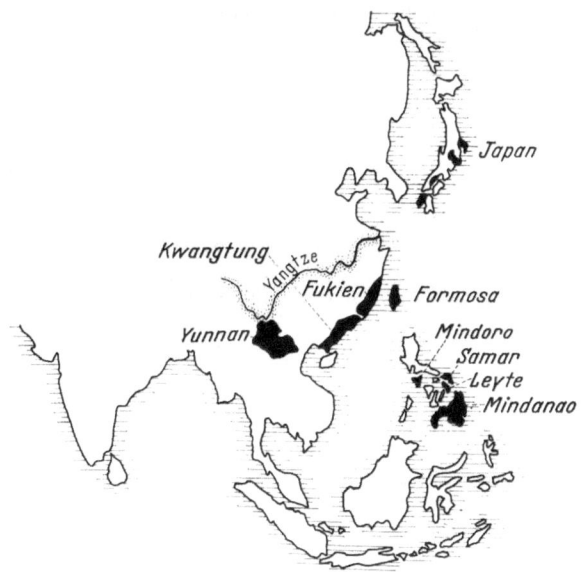

Fig. 1. Distribution of schistosomiasis japonicum in Asia

In Japan, the main endemic areas are the Kohfu Valleys in Yamanashi Prefecture; Numazu, Shizuoka Prefecture; the Katayama (Fukuyama) area, which extends from Okayama Prefecture to the Hiroshima Prefecture; the Kurume area, covering Fukuoka and Saga Prefectures, and the Tone River area, covering Chiba and Ibaragi Prefectures. Recently the presence of Oncomelania nosophora, intermediate host of this disease, has been reported in Fujikawacho, Shizuoka Prefecture and in Nakagawa area, Saitama Prefecture. In the past

* Department of Pathology, Faculty of Medicine. The University of Tokyo, Hongo, Tokyo, Japan.

Oncomelania nosophora has been found along Edogawa River and Arakawa River in the Tokyo Metropolitan area.

The location of the endemic areas of schistosomiasis in Japan depends upon the distribution of Oncomelania nosophora (Fig. 2).

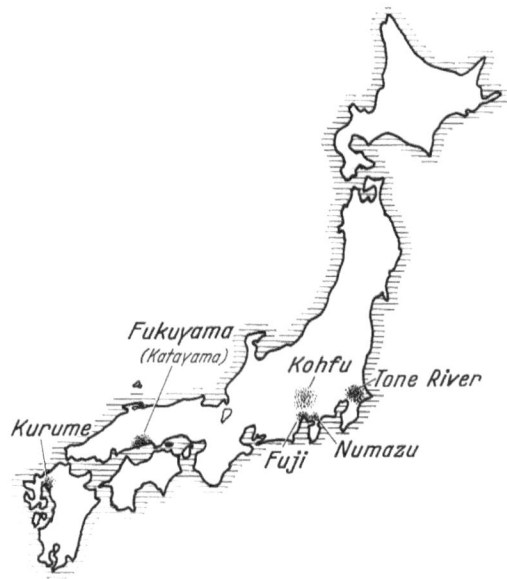

Fig. 2. Distribution of schistosomiasis japonicum in Japan

2. History of Japanese schistosomiasis

Schistosomiasis in Japan was first reported by FUJII [6] in 1847 in his book "Katayama-ki", in which he described a specific endemic focus in Katayama area, near Fukuyama City, Hiroshima Prefecture.

The history of discovery of the worm as a pathogen of Japanese schistosomiasis began in 1888 when MASHIMA [18] found the eggs in the liver at autopsy. In 1904, KAWANISHI [14] found the eggs in feces of the patients and the same year, FUJINAMI [7] discovered the eggs in the visceral organs at autopsy of patients with schistosomiasis (Table 1).

Table 1. *History of researches on Japanese schistosomiasis*

1847	FUJI [6]	First description			
1888	MASHIMA [18]	Autopsy	Human	Liver	Eggs
1904	KAWANISHI [14]	Patient	Human	Feces	Eggs
1904	FUJINAMI [7]	Autopsy	Human	Organs	Eggs
1904	KATSURADA [12]	Autopsy	Dog and cat	Portal vein	Worms
1905	STILES [33]	Schistosoma japonicum			
1913—1914	MIYAIRI and SUZUKI [20]	Oncomelania nosophora			

Furthermore in the same year, KATSURADA [12] first found many male and female adult worms and named them as schistosomum japonicum. In the following year (1905), STILES [33] renamed this worm as schistosoma japonicum.

In 1913—1914, MIYAIRI and SUZUKI [20] found the intermediate host of Japanese schistosomiasis and named it as KATAYAMA nosophora or Miyairi nosophora (Oncomelania nosophora) (Fig. 3).

Although the eggs were found in 1888 [18], 26 years were needed to complete thediscoveries of the adult worms in 1904 [11, 12], and the intermediate host in 1913 and 1914 [20]. These observations led the researchers of Egyptian and Mansonian schistosomiasis to focus attention on the shellfish in their respective areas.

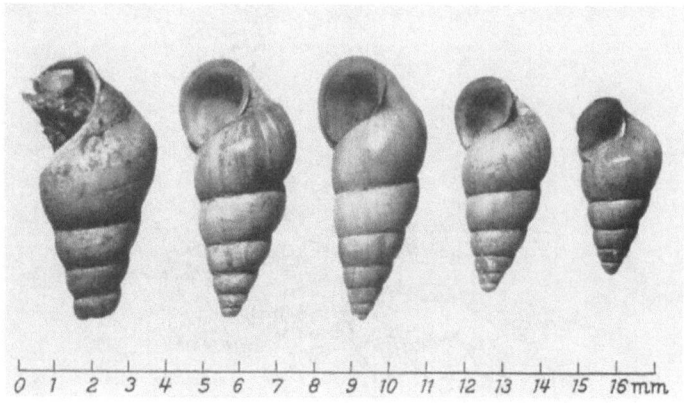

Fig. 3. Katayama nosophora or Miyairi nosophora

It is evident from this brief historical review that studies of Japanese schistosomiasis have been one of the main concerns of Japanese scientists for over 75 years.

It is of interest to note that schistosomiasis including the pathological, clinical and parasitological aspects was the subject of the main lecture [13] at the first annual meeting of the Japanese Pathological Society held in 1911 in Tokyo. At the present time, although the incidence of the disease has sharply decreased in the Tokyo Metropolitan area where it is rarely encountered at autopsy, a fairly large number of cases is still being reported from Kurume area and Yamanashi Prefecture and research on this disease is continuing.

3. Statistical study of parasitic hepatic diseases

Statistical survey has been made of the parasitic diseases of the liver in autopsy material seen at the Department of Pathology, Faculty of Medicine, University of Tokyo from 1901 to 1954. This is summarized from HIKI's [9] report for 30 years from 1901 to 1930 and the report of MIYAKE and OKUDAIRA [21] for the 24 years from 1931 to 1954. The two parasites solely responsible for liver disease are schistosoma japonicum and clonorchis sinensis (Distoma sinensis). In Japan the parasitic diseases of the liver, especially cirrhosis, have been considered important because of the relatively high frequency (Fig. 4).

According to HIKI [9] from 1901 to 1930, parasitic cirrhosis of the liver was encountered in 1.31% of all the autopsy cases. Cirrhosis due to schistosoma japonicum constituted 0.31% and that due to clonorchis sinensis 1.0%. In contrast

MIYAKE and OKUDAIRA [21] found, from 1931 to 1954, only 20 cases of parasitic cirrhosis of the liver among the total autopsies of 5774 cases (0.35%). During this period schistosoma japonicum accounted for 0.30% and clonorchis sinensis for 0.05%, indicating remarkable decrease of cases in cirrhosis of the liver due to clonorchiasis. In addition to the 20 cases of cirrhosis during the period between

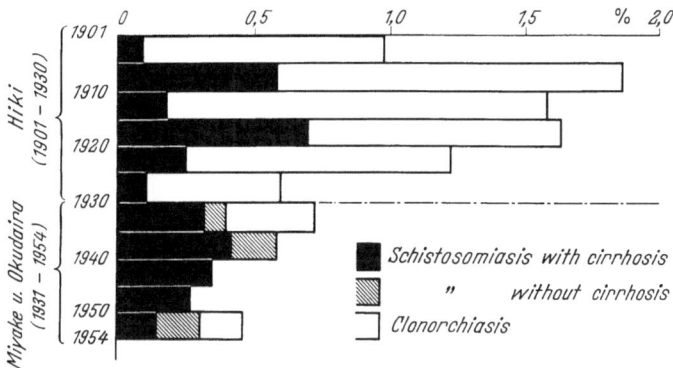

Fig. 4. Diagram of hepatic disease due to parasites in the University of Tokyo (1931—1954)

1931 and 1954, 11 cases of parasitic diseases of the liver without cirrhosis were found. These 31 cases constituted 0.52%, of all autopsies. Twenty-two of these (0.38%) were Japanese schistosomiasis while 9 (0.14%) were clonorchiasis (Table 2).

Table 2. *Statistical survey of hepatic disease due to parasites in the University of Tokyo*

Group	HIKI (1901—1930) in % [9]	MIYAKE and OKUDAIRA (1931—1954) in % [21]
Schistosomiasis with cirrhosis	0.31	0.30
Schistosomiasis without cirrhosis		0.08
		0.38
Clonorchiasis with cirrhosis	1.00	0.05
Clonorchiasis without cirrhosis		0.09
		0.14
Total	1.31	0.52

No cases occurred below 30 years of age. The peak incidence was between 45 and 65 years of age, indicating that the disease occurs almost exclusively after middle age. Of the 22 cases of Japanese schistosomiasis (1931—1954), there were 19 males and 3 females showing male preponderance of 6 to 1 (Fig. 5). During the same period, 17 (77.2%) of 22 cases of Japanese schistosomiasis were complicated by cirrhosis of the liver, whereas only 3 (33.3%) of the 9 cases of clonorchiasis were observed with cirrhosis (Table 3).

In these 31 cases found at autopsy only 7 (22.6%) were diagnosed clinically (4 of Japanese schistosomiasis and 3 of clonorchiasis). The other 24 cases (77.4%) were discovered at the time of autopsy. This is due to lack of specific clinical characteristics. Three of the 18 cases of cirrhosis due to schistosomiasis were diagnosed clinically as BANTI's disease (Table 4). Marked clinical jaundice, ascites, decreased weight of the liver and increased weight of the spleen were seen in the cases with cirrhosis of the liver, whereas no remarkable changes in the weight of the liver and spleen occurred in cases without cirrhosis (Table 5). There were 2 cases of hepatocellular carcinoma complicating cirrhosis due to schistosomiasis (Table 6).

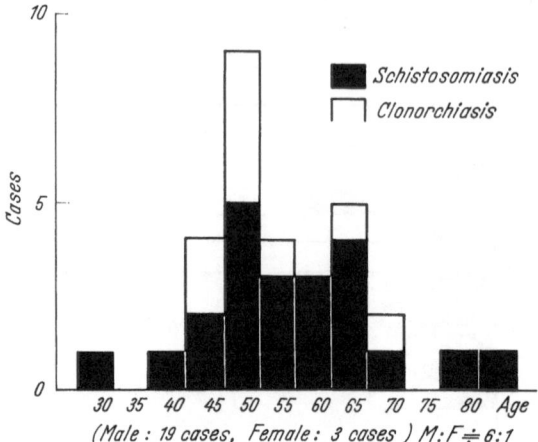

Fig. 5. Age distribution of hepatic disease due to parasites (University of Tokyo 1931—1954)

Table 3. *Hepatic disease due to parasites in relation to liver cirrhosis* *

		Schistosomiasis	Clonorchiasis	Total
Cirrhosis	+	17 (77.2%)	3 (33.3%)	20
	—	5	6	11
Total		22	9	31

* (Univ. of Tokyo, 1931—1954).

Table 4. *Discrepancies between pathological and clinical diagnoses* *

Clinical diagnosis	Pathological diagnosis	Cases	Total
Schistosomiasis	Schistosomiasis	4	7
Clonorchiasis	Clonorchiasis	3	
Other diagnosis	Schistosomiasis	15	24
	Clonorchiasis	6	
Banti's disease	Schistosomiasis	3	

* (Univ. of Tokyo, 1931—1954).

Table 5. *Clinical symptoms and weight of liver and spleen in hepatic diseases due to parasites in relation to cirrhosis* *

Parasite	Cirrhosis	Cases	Icterus ++	+	—	?	Ascites ++	+	—	?	Liver weight (average)	Spleen weight (average)
Schistosomiasis	+	15	2	2	10	1	4	5	5	1	901	376
Clonorchiasis	+	3	2	1			3				907	170
Schistosomiasis	—	5		2	1	2		1	1	3	1390	113
Clonorchiasis	—	6		1	4	1	2	2	2		1245	126

* (Univ. of Tokyo, 1931—1954).

Table 6. *Hepatoma and cirrhosis* *

Type of cirrhosis	Icterus				Ascites				Total
	++	+	—	?	++	+	—	?	
Hepatoma with cirrhosis									
Annular cirrhosis	29	26	5	10	45	7	2	6	60
A type cirrhosis	2				1			1	2
B type cirrhosis	3	2	1		4	1	1		6
Schistosomal			1	1	1			1	2
Biliary cirrhosis	1				1				1
Congest. cirrhosis	1	1				1	1		2
Pigment cirrhosis		1			1				1
Hepatoma without cirrhosis	5	8	7	3	11	8	2	2	23

* Univ. of Tokyo (1931 — 1954)

The statistics of other endemic areas are different from the foregoing statistics of the Tokyo Metropolitan area, which was one of the lighter endemic areas. For instance, NAKAJIMA'S [24] statistics at the Department of Pathology, School of Medicine, Kurume University, during the period between 1956 and 1960 show that 53 (12.0%) of 442 cases of liver biopsies showed eggs. In Kurume area, YOSHIZUMI

Table 7. *Schistosomiasis in Kurume area*

	Reporter		No. of cases	Schistoso-miasis	%
1956—1960	NAKAJIMA [24]	Liver biopsy	442	53	12
1961	YOSHIZUMI [41]	Liver biopsy	470	317	67
1962	KUWANO [15]	Appendices	235	25	10.6
1942	AONUMA [1]	Autopsy	180	25	13.9
1955—1962	NAKAJIMA [25]	Autopsy	180	38	4.6

[41] reported that 317 (67%) of 470 patients had eggs of schistosoma japonicum in liver biospies. KUWANO [15] also reported in the same area that 25 (10.6%) of 235 surgically removed appendices contained ova. Although the incidence of this disease in the endemic area appears to be decreasing, it is still relatively high.

According to AONUMA [1], in 1942, there were 25 cases (13.9%) of Japanese schistosomiasis in 180 consecutive autopsies in Kurume area, whereas NAKAJIMA [25] has reported only 38 such cases (4.6%) in 828 autopsies during 1955 to 1962. This is still a much higher incidence compared with the observations in the Department of Pathology, Faculty of Medicine, University of Tokyo [9, 21] where it was only 0.3%.

4. Gross observations of livers in schistosomiasis

NAKAJIMA [25] has reviewed 38 autopsies from the Department of Pathology, School of Medicine, Kurume University, since 1955 and also 8 autopsies from the Department of Pathology, School of Medicine, Kyushu University. In both series eggs of schistosoma japonicum were found. Based on the degree of gross fibrosis of the liver, the livers were classified as follows (Fig. 6—10) (Table 8):

Table 8. *Incidence in each grade of fibrosis in Nakajima's series*

Fibrosis	cases
Grade I	16
Grade II	17
Grade III	13

1. Grade I: smooth surface   16 cases
2. Grade II: recognizably uneven surface   17 cases
3. Grade III: remarkably uneven surface   13 cases

The majority of the patients were from agricultural profession and those who had more chances to be reinfected had the more severe fibrosis.

Seven (53.7%) of 13 cases of Grade III were clinically diagnosed as cirrhosis of the liver. NAKAJIMA, TSUTUMI and WATANABE [25] further classified Grade III fibrosis of the liver into 3 subgroups:

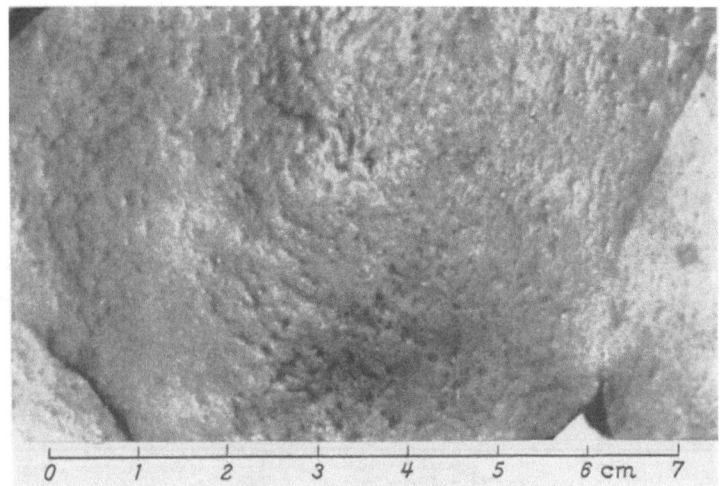

Fig. 6. Grade I fibrosis (with the courtesy of Dr. TSUTUMI H. [25])

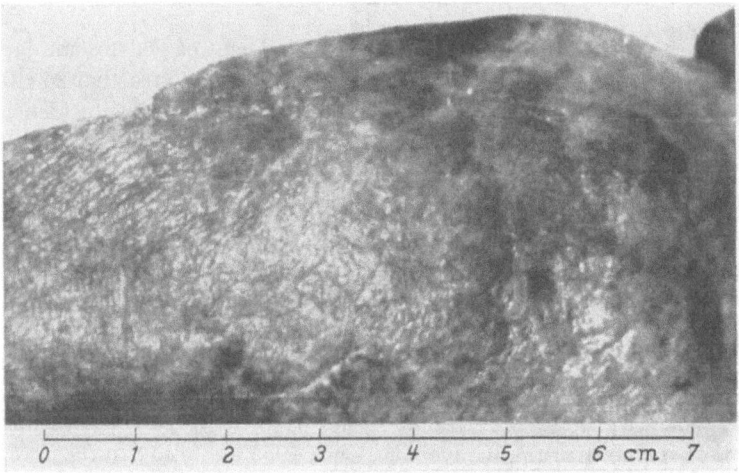

Fig. 7. Grade II fibrosis (with the courtesy of Dr. TSUTUMI H. [25])

1. The lobular type resembling congenital syphilitic cirrhosis of the liver (Hepar lobatum) and showing coarsely indented liver surface (Fig. 7).

2. The granular type with irregular small nodular or granular liver surface which is similar to atrophic cirrhosis of the liver (Fig. 8).

3. Mixed type showing both the fine nodular or granular surface and larger nodules (Fig. 10).

According to this classification 5 were of the lobular type, 4 granular and 4 mixed (Table 9).

The degree of the fibrosis usually, but not necessarily, paralled the number of eggs in the liver. Livers from cases having the larger numbers of eggs in the gastrointestinal tract usually showed the granular type

Table 9. *Incidence in subtypes of grade III fibrosis in Nakajima's series* [25]

Grade III	cases
Lobular type	5
Granular type	4
Mixed type	4
	13

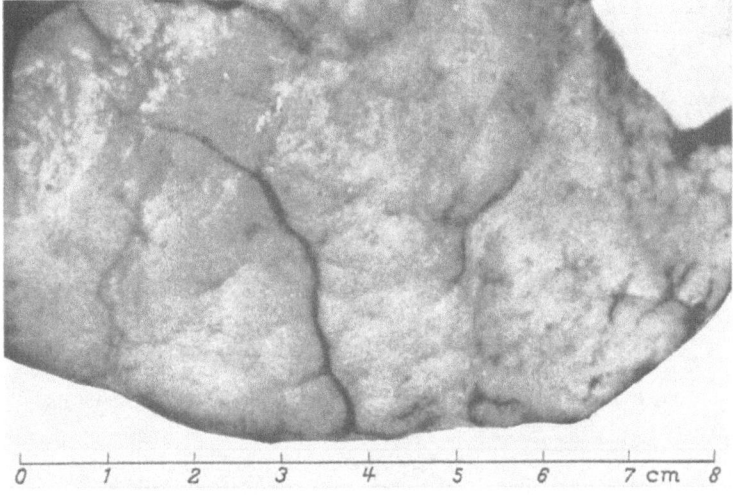

Fig. 8. Lobular type of grade III fibrosis (with the courtesy of Dr. TSUTUMI H. [25])

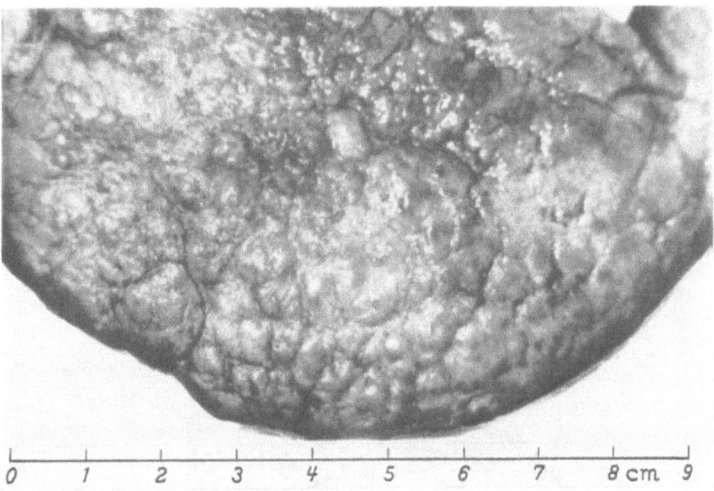

Fig. 9. Granular type of Grade III fibrosis (with the courtesy of Dr. TSUTUMI H. [25])

of Grade III fibrosis, while in patients with fewer eggs in the gastrointestinal tract the hepatic fibrosis is of lesser degree. It should be noted that YAMAGIWA [40] (at the University of Tokyo) in 1904 had already described the gross characteristics of cirrhosis of the liver due to Japanese schistosomiasis as being an intermediate form between the syphilitic hepar lobatum and the fine granular atrophic cirrhosis of the liver of Laennec type, and that NAKAJIMA'S [25] granular type of Grade III fibrosis had already been reported by FUJINAMI in 1916 [8].

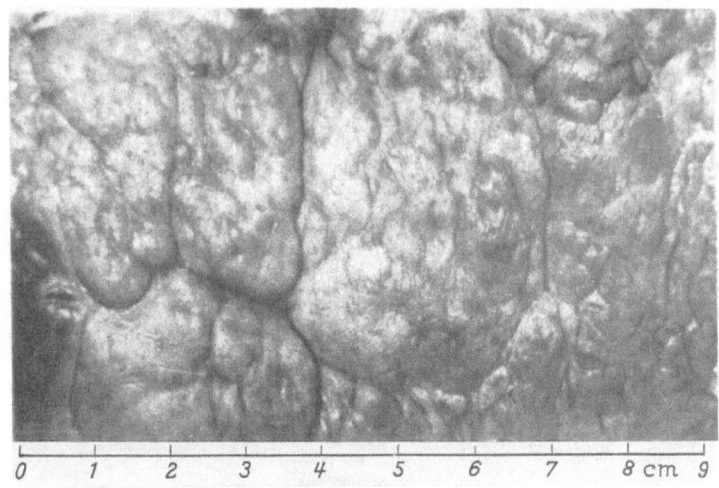

Fig. 10. Mixed type of grade III fibrosis (with the courtesy of Dr. H. TSUTUMI [25])

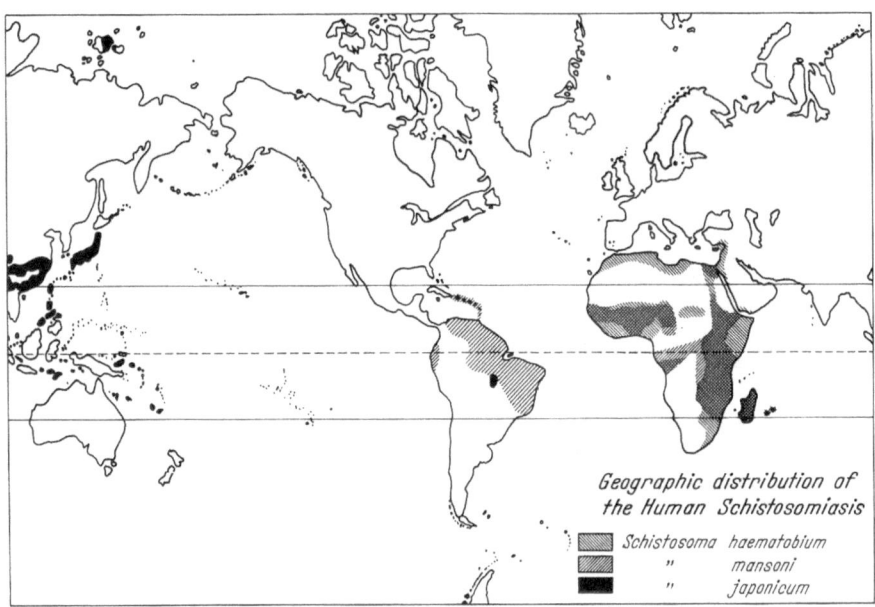

Fig. 11. World distribution of human schistosomiasis. (Cited in MARTINEZ BAEZ, [17])

The hepatic changes in Mansonian schistosomiasis (Fig. 11) reported from other countries are similar to that of Japanese schistosomiasis. For example, the white, clay-pipe stem cirrhosis of SYMMERS [34] corresponds to the lobular type of Grade III fibrosis of NAKAJIMA [25]. The gross characteristics of cirrhosis of the liver due to Mansonian schistosomiasis are said to be the white clay-pipe stem cirrhosis, but cases similar to NAKAJIMA's granular type have also been reported [3], so that both changes can be said to be almost alike.

5. Clinical features of schistosomiasis

Patients who have been suffering from Japanese schistosomiasis for a long time will often proceed into more severe cirrhosis. According to MORITA [23], who studied patients with cirrhosis due to Japanese schistosomiasis in the Kohfu Valley before 1905, cirrhosis developed where treatment was inadequate or where infestation of minor degree persisted for a long period. The liver generally decreases in size and becomes firmer. The anterior edge of the liver becomes sharper and its surface is finely granular. The spleen becomes large, elastic and firm and has a smooth surface.

With portal hypertension, there may be dilatation of the veins of the abdominal wall and gastrointestinal bleedings. Hemorrhagic diathesis due to thrombocytopenia will often cause slight anemia. MORITA [23] has summarized the findings in the peripheral blood and bone marrow and stated that signs of hypersplenism increase gradually with the progression of the disease. Changes in leucocytes also occur, particularly eosinophilia due to the presence of worms.

6. Avian schistosomes in Japan

CORT [5] first reported that cercaria of the avian schistosomes could cause exanthemic dermatitis upon penetration of the human skin by the worms. In this case, he reported infestation of the fresh water shellfish in Douglas Lake, Michigan, U.S.A., by the cercaria Trichobilharzia ocellata. In 1950, PENNER [30] reported a dermatitis due to cercaria littorinalinae from another species of shellfish on a California beach. In Japan a specific form of exanthemic dermatitis with itch known as KABURE has frequently appeared among workers in rice fields of endemic areas. The disease was first mentioned in 1847 by FUJII [6] in "Katayamaki" as one of the symptoms of Katayama disease, a severe endemic dermatitis in Katayama area, near Fukuyama city, Hiroshima Prefecture.

The discussion of the pathogenesis of the disease focused on whether or not the cercaria would actually cause "Kabure" at the time of penetration.

In 1948, TANABE [36] found a new species of avian schistosome, the cercaria of gigantobilharzia sturniae or gray starling's schistosome, to be the pathogen of rice-field dermatitis (Lakeside disease: Kogan-byo) on Shinji lake side, Tottori Prefecture (Fig. 12).

In the same year, ODA [27, 28] clarified the cause of "Kabure" in Katayama disease. He found cercaria of grey starling's schistosome in the rice fields of that area. The intermediate host was HIRAMAKIMODOKI (Polypylis hemisphaerula, BENSON 1842 [2]; Segmentia nitidella v, MARTENS 1877 [16]). This cercaria was confirmed to be the causative factor of Katayama dermatitis by an infestation experiment in human subjects including Oda himself (Fig. 13). He also studied grey starlings in Hiroshima and Yamanashi Prefectures which are endemic areas

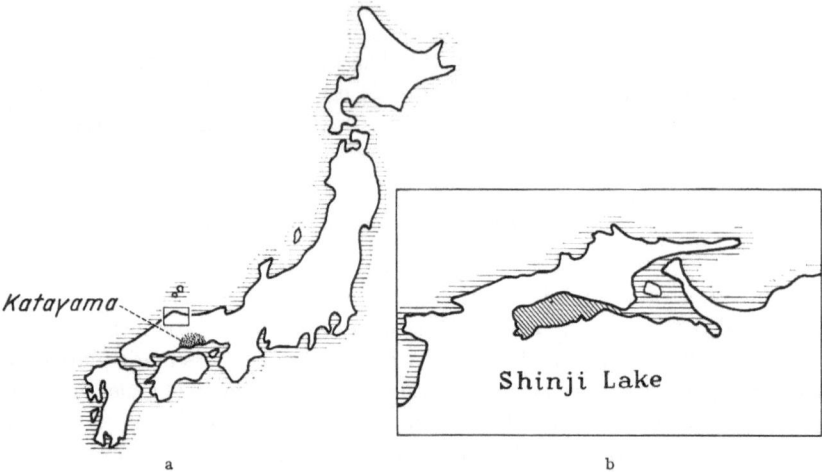

Fig. 12. a. Area of Lake-side disease or Kogan-byo, in relation to Japan. b. Enlargement of the area shown in a.

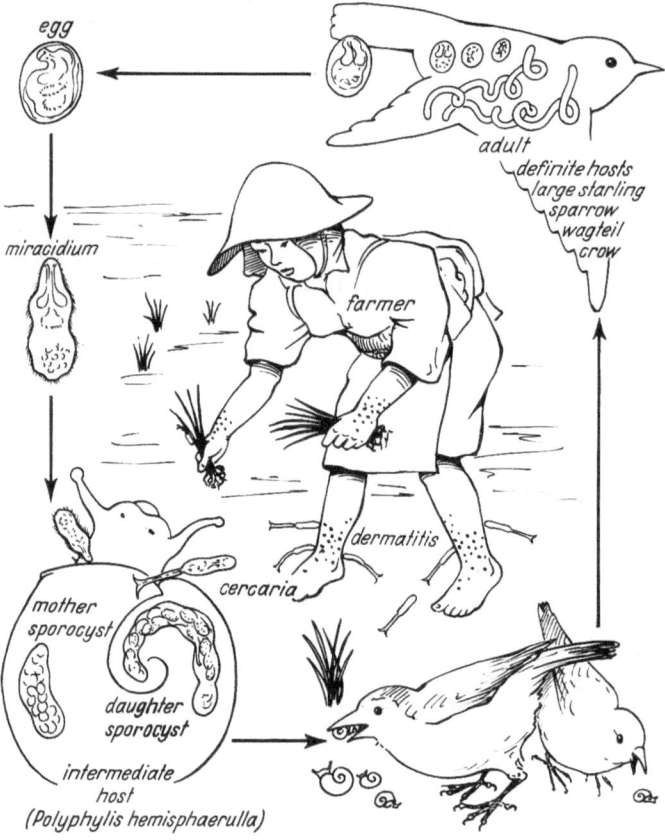

Fig. 13. Diagram of life history of Gigantobilharzia sturuniae and mode of infection by its cercaria into the human skin.
(With the courtesy of Dr. T. ODA, [27, 28])

of Japanese schistosomiasis. Adult worms of this species were found mainly in the portal system of the intestinal wall, particularly in the venous plexus of the submucosa and small vessels in the subserosa. ODA [28] obtained adult worms, by experimental infestation of domestic ducks with the cercaria and confirmed these as identical with Gigantobilharzia sturinae, discovered by TANABE [36] in Shinji Lake, Tottori Prefecture. The distribution of the Miyairi nosophora (Oncomelania nosophora), the intermediate host of schistosoma japonicum, is limited particularly to the irrigating drains of the rice fields, rather than the rice-fields proper. On the other hand Polypylis hemisphaerula (HIRAMAKIMODOKI), the intermediate host of grey starling's schistosome is more wide spread and it is found in irrigating drains and in the rice-fields as well. Thus irrespective of the distribution of Miyairi nosophora there are many areas where Polypylis hemisphaerula nosophora (HIRAMAKOMODOKI) are found and account for the endemic dermatitis.

Dermatitis as one of the main symptoms of so-called Katayama disease is therefore caused at least in part by the cercaria of the grey starling's schistosome. This was confirmed by the examination of 34 cases of dermatitis in patients with Katayama in Hiroshima Prefecture. Seven were positive (6 due to cercaria of grey starling's schistosome and one due to that of schistosoma japonicum).

The histological changes in the skin of patients with dermatitis of grey starlings' schistosome are more severe than those of Japanese schistosomiasis. Two types of reaction are found often coexisting: (a) the traumatic changes in skin secondary to the cercaria, and (b) the reactive changes to the cercaria itself. The latter may be further divided into the reaction to toxic substances from cercarial glands and those due to the decomposition products of dead cercaria. The reaction to the toxic substance of cercarial glands may be either monocytic, in the case of normergic reaction, or neutrophilic and eosinophilic in the case of allergic reaction (Arthus type). The reaction to the decomposition products of dead cercaria may be either monocytic (normergy), or eosinophilic (allergy). Cases of repeated infestation show marked eosinophilia in the dermis, which is interpreted to represent an allergic reaction and considered to have some functional significance in preventing possible tissue damage (Table 10).

Table 10. *Histopathological changes of dermatitis in grey starling's schistosomiasis*

Reactive change	against substance of poisonous gland of cercaria	monocyte	eosinophil
	against decomposed products of Dead cercaria	(Normergy)	(Allergy)

In 1958, ODA [29] studied rice-field dermatitis in the Oki Islands (Fig. 14) and found cercaria of a species of schistosome in Monoaragai (Lymnaea japonica), which was thought to be similar to that of cercaria physellae [35]. His attention was drawn to the fact that the incidence of dermatititis is higher in rice-fields, where there are more wild ducks than in fields with fewer ducks. This led him to investigate the wild ducks in those areas and resulted in the discovery of two kinds of eggs and adult male and female worms of the Trichobilharzia group (Fig. 15) which inhabited the veins of the intestinal wall and the mesentery and the hepatic portal system. One of those Trichobilharzia is very similar to Trichobilharzia ocellata [4, 39].

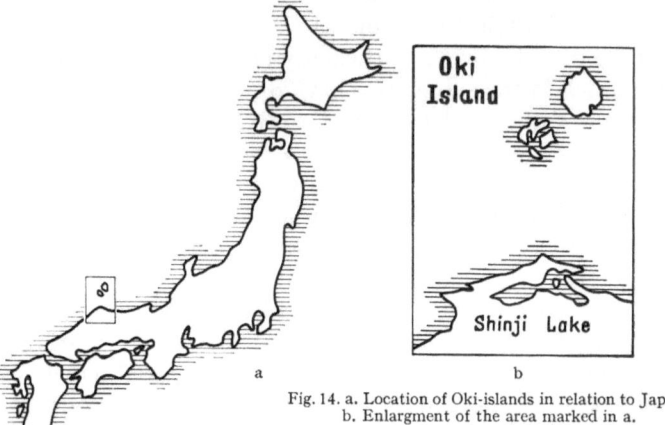

Fig. 14. a. Location of Oki-islands in relation to Japan.
b. Enlargment of the area marked in a.

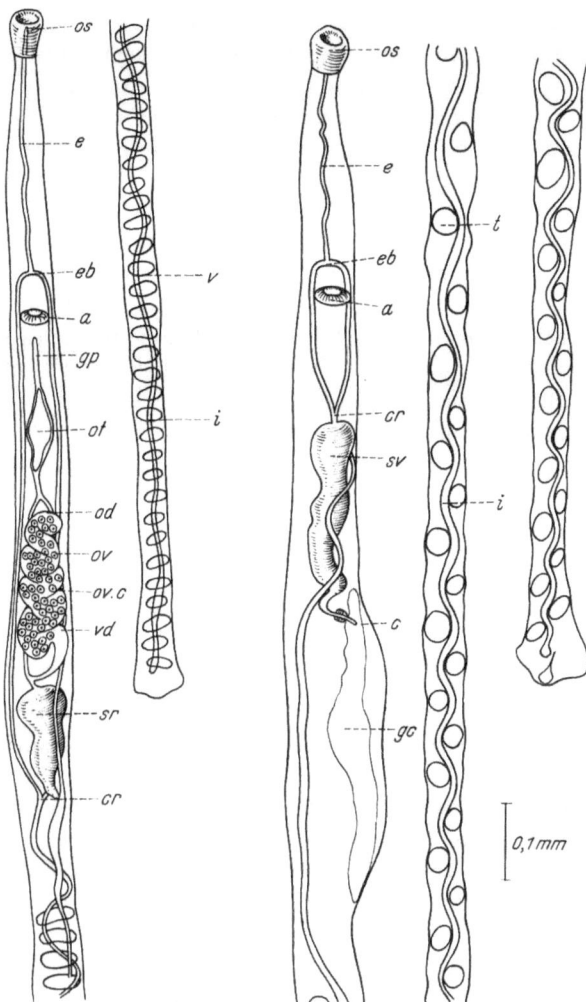

Fig. 15. Schema of Trichobilharzia
os-oral sucker; e-esophagus; eb-eso-
phageal bifurcation; a-acetabulum;
gp-genital pore; ot-ootype; od-ovi-
duct; ov-ovum; ov. c-ovarian con-
volutions; vd-vitelline duct; sr-
seminal receptacle; v-vittelaria;
i-intestine; cr-cecal reunion; sv-
seminal vesicle; c-cirrus; gc-gyneco-
phoric canal; t-testis (With the
courtesy of Dr. M. Tanaka [37])

0,1mm

7. Skin test of schistosomiasis

Allergic skin reaction in Japanese schistosomiasis has been studied by INOUE et al. [10]. During the period between 1949 and 1951 MORITA [23] succeeded in extracting an excellent antigen from the worm body by a simple method for use in diagnostic skin reaction in man.

Cercaria obtained from Miyairi nosophora were inoculated into rabbits and sheep. These were sacrficed when the cercaria reached adulthood. Adult worms were harvested from the blood vessels of portal system and stored in physiological saline with 0.5% phenol. The solution was filtered again by Seitz' apparatus, and diluted with the same solution (Table 11). The antigen was tested on 2 groups. In the infested

Table 11. *Morita's method: extraction of antigen from schistosomiasis japonica*

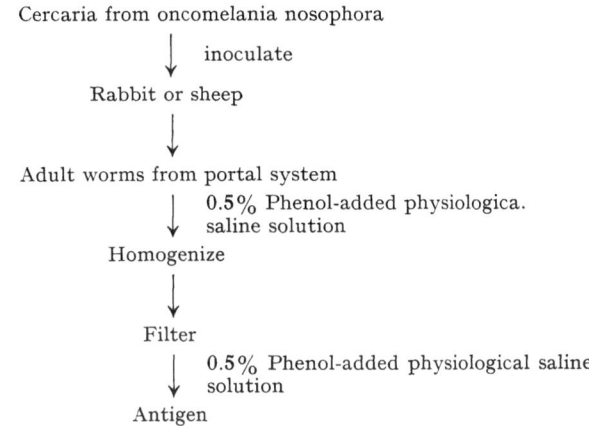

group with positive egg excretion it gave a 94% positive result; while in another group considered to be absolutely non-infested there was a 4% weakly positive result. The interval between the initial infestation and the development of a positive skin reaction was about 30 days after the onset of signs and symptoms in human patients, i. e., about 2 months after cercarial penetration.

A new endemic area developed after 1945 in the town of Fujikawa along the Fuji River which flows through the large endemic area of Kohfu Valley. NOGUCHI and others [26] surveyed, by means of an intradermal reaction and examination of feces, the junior high school children in the area of Ukishima-numa and the Fujikawa area. Antigen for intradermal reactions obtained from the 406th Medical General Laboratory of the United States Army was SM-antigen [38] (acid soluble proteid fraction) (Table 12). 0.01 ml of this antigen was injected intradermally in the forearm and the results were read by measuring the papular area 15 minutes after injection. Positive intradermal reaction was seen in 137 out of 1903 children examined (6.6%) but examination of the feces was negative in all cases. These positive results were considered non-specific.

8. Therapy and prophylaxis

Among numerous chemotherapeutic agents used in treatment of this disease, the most effective at present time are the antimonyl derivatives. In contrast to

Table 12. *Method of extraction of SM-antigen for skin test of schistosomiasis*

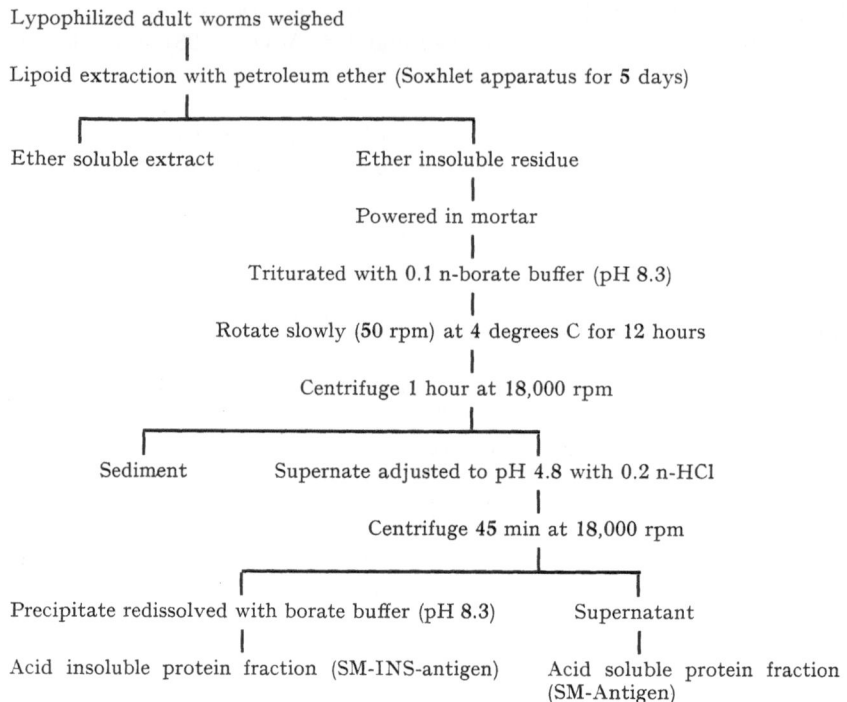

Lypophilized adult worms weighed
|
Lipoid extraction with petroleum ether (Soxhlet apparatus for 5 days)
|
Ether soluble extract   Ether insoluble residue
|
Powered in mortar
|
Triturated with 0.1 n-borate buffer (pH 8.3)
|
Rotate slowly (50 rpm) at 4 degrees C for 12 hours
|
Centrifuge 1 hour at 18,000 rpm
|
Sediment   Supernate adjusted to pH 4.8 with 0.2 n-HCl
|
Centrifuge 45 min at 18,000 rpm
|
Precipitate redissolved with borate buffer (pH 8.3)   Supernatant
| |
Acid insoluble protein fraction (SM-INS-antigen)   Acid soluble protein fraction
                                                     (SM-Antigen)

the potassium salts of antimonyltartrate in Europe and America, in Japan sodium antimonyltartrate marketed as Stibnal is widely used. In adult patients, 20 cc are administered intravenously every other day for 20 to 30 doses.

The site of action of antimonyl derivatives is said to be in the ovaries of the worm and to consist of inhibition of ovulation. Eggs disappear from the feces of patients in a relatively short time and the symptoms disappear but if treatment is stopped at an early stage, the worms again ovulate actively and the symptoms reappear. It is, therefore, recommended that the treatment begin early and continue long after symptoms disappear. According to MORITA [22] there has been a remarkable decrease recently in the high incidence of cirrhosis of the liver due to schistosomiasis in the Kohfu Valleys due to wide use of antimonyl derivatives.

A personal prophylactic measure consists of rubbing the exposed parts with benzyl benzoate to prevent penetration of cercaria whenever visiting an endemic area. Since the main source of infestation is egg-contaminated human and bovine feces, mixing quick lime or lime nitrogen with feces would kill the eggs and cercaria. The cercaria are very sensitive to lime and will be dead in 30 minutes by a 0.001% solution. For the intermediate host, Miyairi nosophora, lime (quick lime, lime nitrogen and superphosphate of lime) should be sprayed over the areas constantly, a measure which is not only effective for the control of Miyairi nosophora, but also increases the fertilizer quality.

After World War II, a large scale research on this disease has been performed by American workers in the Kohfu Valleys. They found drugs effective against

Miyairi nosophora, but since these are also harmful to agricultural products, they are not used. Although certain drugs such as Benzene hexachloride (B.H.C.) are highly effective against shellfish, and this has considerably reduced the number of new patients, it has also caused a shortage of shellfish (Table 13).

Table 13. *Prophylaxis of Schistosomiasis*

Personal prevention	Skin	Benzyl benzonate
Source of infestation	Feces	Quick lime. Lime nitrogen
Intermediate host	Oncomelania nosophora	Lime (Quick lime. Lime nitrogen. Superphosphate of lime.) B. H. C.

References

[1] AONUMA, T.: Histopathological studies on schistosomiasis in Kurume area. Nippon Igaku Kenkohoken **3283**, 1099 (1942).

[2] BENSON, W. S.: Mollusca: In: T. CANTOR: General features of Chusan with remarks on the flora and fauna of that island. Ann. Mag. Natural History **9**, 486—490 (1855).

[3] BOGLIOLO, L.: The anatomical picture of the liver in hepatosplenic schistosomiasis Mansonii. Ann. Trop. Méd. Parasit. **51**, 1 (1959).

[4] BRUMPT, E.: Cercaria ocellata, determinant la dermatite des nagers, provient d'une bilharzie des canards. C. R. Acad. Sci. **193**, 612—614 (1931).

[5] CORT, W. W.: Schistosome dermatitis in the United States. J. Amer. Med. Ass. **90**, 1027—1029 (1928).

[6] FUJII, Y.: As quoted in [11].

[7] FUJINAMI, K.: Study on eggs of bilharzia as cause of Katayama disease. Kyoto Med. J. **2**, 106 (1904).

[8] — Pathological anatomy of schistosomiasis japonicum. Jap.J.Med.Prog. **6**,101—182 (1916).

[9] HIKI, Y., T. BAN, Y. MIYAZAKI, E. TAKIZAWA, and K. AKAZAKI: Statistical analysis of liver cirrhosis out of autopsy cases for 30 years from 1901 to 1930. Nippon Iji Shimpo **468**, 2024—2026 (1931).

[10] INOUE, T., K. MATSUBARA, Y. KAKU, K. HIRAKAWA, and Y. WATANABE: Screening test of schistosomiasis for primary school children in an endemic area. Kurume Med. J. **6**, 145—154 (1941).

[11] KATSURADA, F.: Causes of parasitic diseases. Iji Shinbun **669**, 1325—1332 (1904).

[12] — Schistosomum Japonicum, ein neuer menschlicher Parasit, durch welchen eine endemische Krankheit in verschiedenen Gegenden Japans verursacht wird. Ann. Zool. Jap. **5**, 147—160 (1904).

[13] — Schistosomiasis japonica. Transactiones Societatis. Path. Jap. **1**, 1 (1911).

[14] KAWANISHI, K.: Reports on investigation of Katayama disease in Bingo area. Tokyo J. Med. Sci. **18**, 165—182 (1904). Continued Tokyo J. Med. Sci. **18**, 183—213 (1904).

[15] KUWANO, M.: Schistosoma ova observed in appendices from operation materials. Kurume Med. J. **25**, 1130 (1962).

[16] MARTENS, VON, F. HILGENDORF, and W. DONITZ: Im Japan gesammelten dinnen Mollusken in Sitzungsbericht der Gesell. Naturforsch. Freund zu Berlin **17**, 96—123 (1877).

[17] MARTINEZ-BAEZ, M.: Manual de Parasitologia Medica. Mexico, Prensa: Medica Mexicana 1953.

[18] MASHIMA, E.: Über Wurmeier in der cirrhotischen Leber. Z. Tokio med. Gesellsch. **2**, 821—826 (1888).

[19] — Fortsetzung. Z. Tokio Med. Ges. **2**, 898—901 (1888).

[20] MIYAIRI, K., and M. SUZUKI: Der Zwischenwirt des Shistosomum japonicum Katsurada. Mitt. Med. Fak. Univ. Kyushu **1**, 187—197 (1914).

[21] MIYAKE, M., and M. OKUDAIRA: Statistical analysis of liver cirrhosis out of autopsy cases for 24 years from 1931 to 1954. Saishin Igaku **12**, 1421—1433 (1957).

[22] MORITA, H.: Personal communication.

[23] — H. YOSHIMURA, A. HINO, T. SAITO, K. MIYAZAWA, and Y. AOYAGI: Japanese schistosomiasis. Diagn. and Therapy. Shindan to Chiryo **50**, 1567—1576 (1962).

[24] Nakajima, T.: Personal letter.

[25] —, H. Tsutumi, and A. Watanabe: Studies on liver fibrosis (cirrhosis) due to schistosomiasis japonicum. Morphology of liver: Part 1, The Kurume Med. J. 10, 51—61 (1963).

[26] Noguchi, N., G. Itoh, and H. Mochizuki: Studies on the schistosomiasis japonicum in
Shizuoka Prefecture. Survey on the Fujikawa River Basin and the Ukishimanuma
district. Parasitol. J. 12, 437—439 (1963).

[27] Oda, T.: Studies on Katayama disease dermatitis. Okayama Med. J. 65, 839—878 (1958).

[28] — Studies on the life cycle of grey starling schistosoma. Okayama Med. J. 65, 879—888
(1958).

[29] — Studies on pathogenic schistosomes in the Oki-islands. Ann. Hyg. Lab. Okayama
Prefecture 8, 50—62 (1958).

[30] Penner, L. R.: Cercariae littorinalinae sp. nov., dermatitis-producing schistosome larva
from marine snail, Littorina planaxis Philippi. J. Parasitol. 36, 466—472 (1950).

[31] Saito, T.: Skin reaction in schistosomiasis. Sohgoh Igaku 19, 917—921 (1962).

[32] Shinpo, S.: Studies on the histopathology of Gigantobilharziosis. Ann. Hyg. Lab.
Okayma Prefecture 10, 77—90 (1960).

[33] Stiles, C. W.: The new Asiatic blood fluke (Schistosoma japonicum, 1904, Schistosoma.
Cattol, 1905) of man and cats. Amer. Med. 9, 821—823 (1905).

[34] Symmers, W.: Note on new form of liver cirrhosis due to the presence of the ova of
bilharzia haematobia. J. Path. Bact. 4, 237—239 (1904).

[35] Talbot, S. B.: Studies on schistosome dermatitis; morphological and life history studies
on 3 dermatitis-producing schistosome cercariae, C. elvae Miller, 1923, C. stagnicolae
n. sp., and C. physellae n. sp. Amer. J. Hyg. 23, 372—384 (1936).

[36] Tanabe, H.: Cause of "Lake-side disease" (Kogan-byo) (Special speech). Yonago Med. J.
1, 2—3 (1948).

[37] Tanaka, M.: Studies on trichobilharzie physellae in Oki Island. Kiseichugaku Zasshi
9, 604—609 (1960).

[38] U.S. Army Medical General Laboratory 406, Professional report, 106 Tokyo (1959).

[39] Valette, La, St. George, von H. J. H.: Symbolae ad Trematodum evolutionis historium,
Berolina, Westphalia, 1855.

[40] Yamagiwa, K.: Views on the work by Fujinami and Kon. On the pathological anatomy
of the so-called Katayama-disease, an endemic in the Province of Bingo. J. Kyoto
Med. Ass. 1, 181—184 (1904).

[41] Yoshizumi, Y.: On diagnosis of schistosomiasis japonicum by fresh liver side method.
Acta Hepat. Jap. 2 (4), 373—380 (1961).

Clinical and Pathological Aspects of Schistosomiasis in Brazil*

Zilton A. Andrade,** and Allen W. Cheever***

With 8 figures

Schistosoma mansoni was first identified in Brazil by Pirajá da Silva [25] in 1908. The disease was introduced into this country from Africa, and today Brazil constitutes one of the most important endemic areas of schistosomiasis in the world. The area of highest endemicity is in the northeastern states, and there are about 3 million infected people in this zone alone. The disease also exists in isolated foci in several other states in north, south and central Brazil, and it seems that schistosomiasis will pose even greater problems with its increasing geographic spread [24].

Several snail species are known to act as intermediate hosts for Brazilian strains of *S. mansoni*. Different geographic strains of Brazilian *S. mansoni* have been shown biologically distinct in terms of their varying abilities to infect different snail species and strains [23, 6]. The response of man or experimental animals to infection is not known to be influenced by the parasite strain, although this field of investigation is virtually unexplored.

Numerous animal species have been found naturally infected with *S. mansoni* in Brazil, but they are probably of little consequence in maintaining the life cycle of the parasite, since in the majority of these hosts maturation of eggs does not take place and eggs are not excreted in the feces [7].

The clinical and pathological picture of the disease as seen in Brazil can be considered under the following headings:

A. The acute or toxemic form

This term refers to the period of toxic manifestations occuring during larval migration and the period of early oviposition. This form of the disease appears to be caused by a heavy initial exposure and is almost never seen in persons living in an endemic area.

Itching may or may not be noted at the time of exposure. The explosive onset of fever, diarrhea, abdominal pains etc. 3–5 weeks after exposure has been well described by Díaz-Rivera et al. in Puerto Rican cases [15]. The clinical picture in Brazil [8, 18] resembles that in Puerto Rico and in *S. japonicum* infections in China [13].

* Suported by Grant No. AI-D 6209 from USPHS National Institute of Allergy and Infections Disases. Bethesda, Maryland, U.S.A.

** Department, of Pathology. Hospital Prof. Edgard Santos, University of Bahia School of Medicine, Salvador, Bahia, Brazil.

*** Laboratory of Parasitic Diseases. National Institute of Allergy and Infectious Diseases. National Institutes of Health, Public Health Service, U.S. Department of Health Education and Welfare, Bethesda, Maryland, U.S.A. — Department of Pathology. Hospital Prof. Edgard Santos. University of Bahia School of Medicine Salvador, Bahia, Brazil.

Few cases having the acute form of the disease have been necropsied. In these cases the gross findings were limited to the presence of small white granulomas, most conspicuous on the intestinal serosa, in the liver and sometimes in the lungs, toxic splenomegaly and numerous shallow ulcerations in the small intestine or colon [8, 15]. Microscopically all periovular granulomas were noted to be in the same evolutionary phase and frequently showed central necrosis and numerous eosinophiles. Besides miliary granulomas, diffuse, non-specific portal inflammation was present in the liver.Kupffer cell mobilization and focal cloudy swelling or fatty degeneration were also noted. In some cases focal areas of parenchymal necrosis were seen, but it is not known if these were caused by antimony treatment or by the infection itself [1, 8]. The spleen showed marked reticuloendothelial hyperplasia, congestion, infiltration by plasma cells and eosinophiles and hyperplasia of the germinal centers.

Many manifestations of the acute form are probably caused by hypersensitivity reactions. Thus patients frequently present urticaria,asthmatic attacks, blood and tissue eosinophilia, central necrosis in granulomas, and acute infectious splenitis.

The symptoms of the acute phase usually subside spontaneously or after treatment [15, 18], but in rare cases rapid progression to the hepatosplenic or cardio-pulmonary forms of the disease has been reported [22, 30].

B. The chronic form

1. Mild or asymptomatic schistosomiasis

This represents the largest group of infected persons. Although these individuals have viable eggs in the stools and strong skin sensitivity to injected schistosomal antigens, they show no evidence of disease attributable to schistosomiasis. Sometimes vague complaints such as abdominal pains, diarrhea or constipation, anorexia and dizziness are present, but without controlled studies it is difficult to attribute these symptoms to schistosomiasis. Physical examination may disclose a palpable liver, sometimes with a hard and prominent left lobe, and pain may be provoked by palpation of the colon.

At necropsy gross changes are usually not seen and microscopically granulomas are noted in various organs, particularly the liver and intestines. In the liver there are also mild lympho-plasmocytic portal infiltrates and slight fibrosis of small portal tracts. In the intestines eggs and granulomas are found mainly in the mucosa and submucosa, but in heavier infections they may be found in the muscular layers and serosa.

2. Symptomatic intestinal schistosomiasis

Infected patients with abdominal complaints are usually considered to have intestinal schistosomiasis. Although symptoms may improve with treatment, no published controlled studies are known to us. Mucosal congestion, edema and petechiae may be seen at proctoscopy.

Schistosomal polyps are not commonly seen in Brazil by clinicians [21] or pathologists [9], in contrast to their apparently high incidence in Egypt [16]. In the few cases seen by us, eggs were particularly numerous in the mucosa of the polyps.

Ulcerative colitis attributed to schistosomiasis is also uncommon. In rare cases with massive infections a carcinoma of the colon has been simulated by schistosomal lesions. At operation extensive segmental fibrosis of the intestinal submucosa was seen and microscopically numerous granulomas around schistosome eggs were found [3].

3. Hepatosplenic schistosomiasis

In this form of 'the disease extensive periportal fibrosis is accompanied by portal hypertension, splenomegaly and esophageal varices. Usually the patients

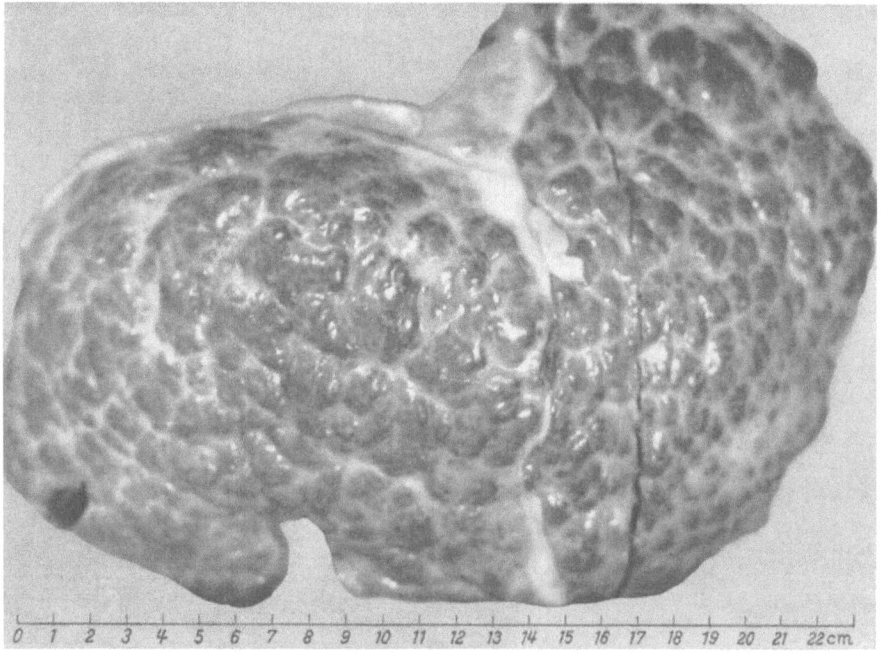

Fig. 1. External appearance of the liver, resembling postnecrotic cirrhosis, in a case of advanced schistosomiasis

present manifestations of portal hypertension with little evidence of hepatic dysfunction [28, 33]. These patients are usually well nourished and have good muscular mass. Other patients may present a picture difficult to differentiate from true cirrhosis and may die in hepatic coma. In our necropsy material, 20% of patients with hepatosplenic schistosomiasis died in hepatic coma as compared to 68% of cirrhotic patients.

The gross appearance of the liver is characteristic (Fig. 1, 2, 3). The left lobe is disproportionately enlarged. The external surface is macronodular and may resemble the liver of postnecrotic cirrhosis, but the cut surface reveals pathognomonic dense periportal fibrosis (Symmers' clay pipestem fibrosis) [31]. The liver parenchyma maintains its lobular structure, but focal areas of nodular regeneration can be seen, particularly in the subcapsular zone. Occasionally Symmers' fibrosis is seen in the absence of splenomegaly [27].

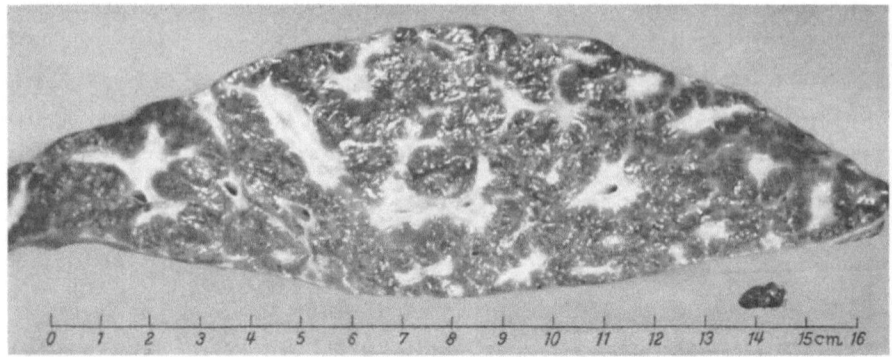
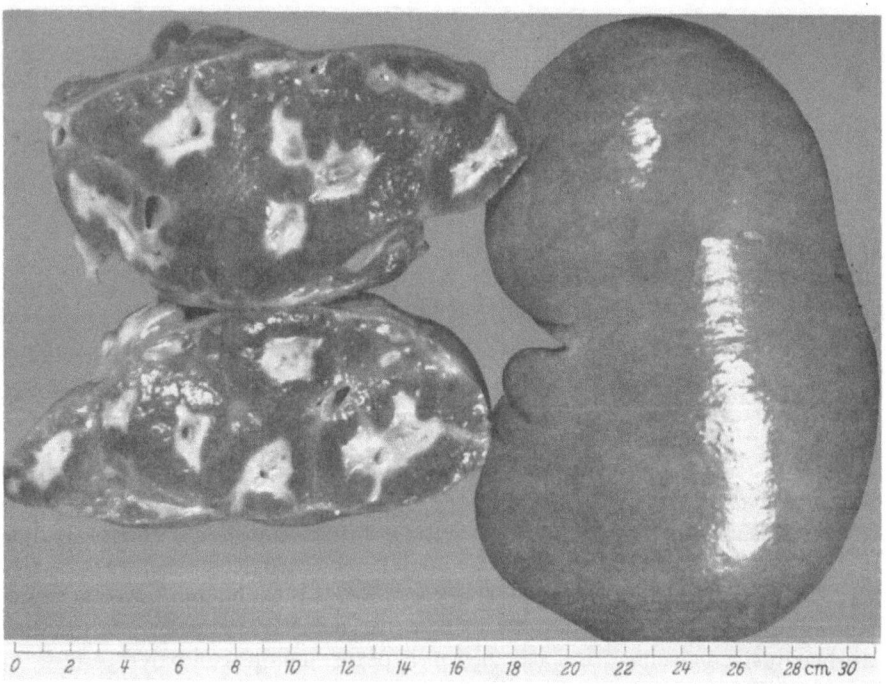

All of approximately 100 cases of hepatosplenic schistosomiasis autopsied in this hospital showed Symmers' fibrosis of the liver. In all infected patients with portal hypertension, Symmers' fibrosis or cirrhosis was present. We have not seen

Fig. 2. Cut surface of the liver shown in Fig. 1, presenting the characteristic "pipestem" fibrosis in the portal areas

Fig. 3. Hepato-splenic schistosomiasis. Enlarged spleen associated with dense peri-portal fibrosis of the liver. The liver parenchyma is normal in appearance despite the portal changes

cases of Hashem's fine periportal fibrosis [19], and this lesion is rarely seen in Brazil [9, 10].

Microscopically the fibrosed portal spaces are infiltrated by lymphocytes and plasma cells and present telangectasia. Schistosome eggs are most often abundant but may be scarce or absent. Vascular lesions are frequent [20]. These include

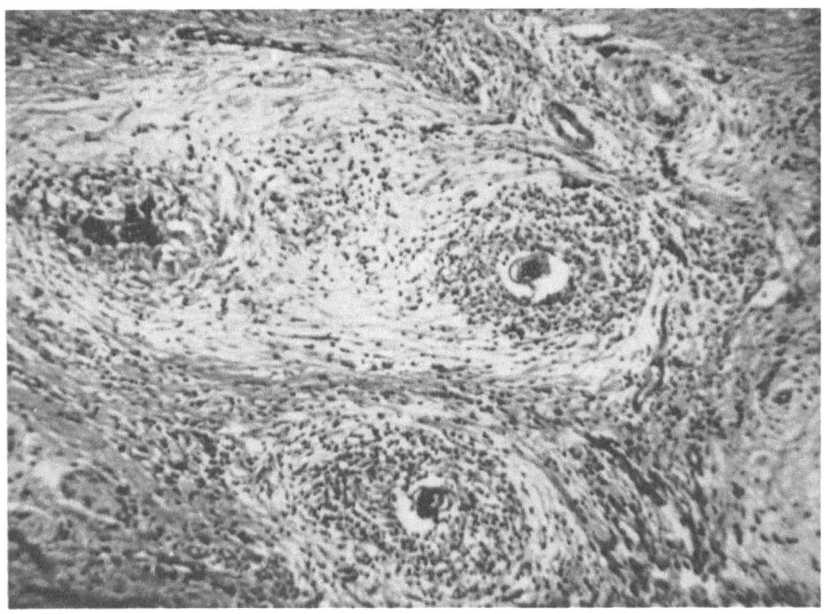

Fig. 4. Portal fibrosis and granulomas around eggs of *S. mansoni*, a common finding in hepatic schistosomiasis. Hematoxylin and eosin. 200 ×

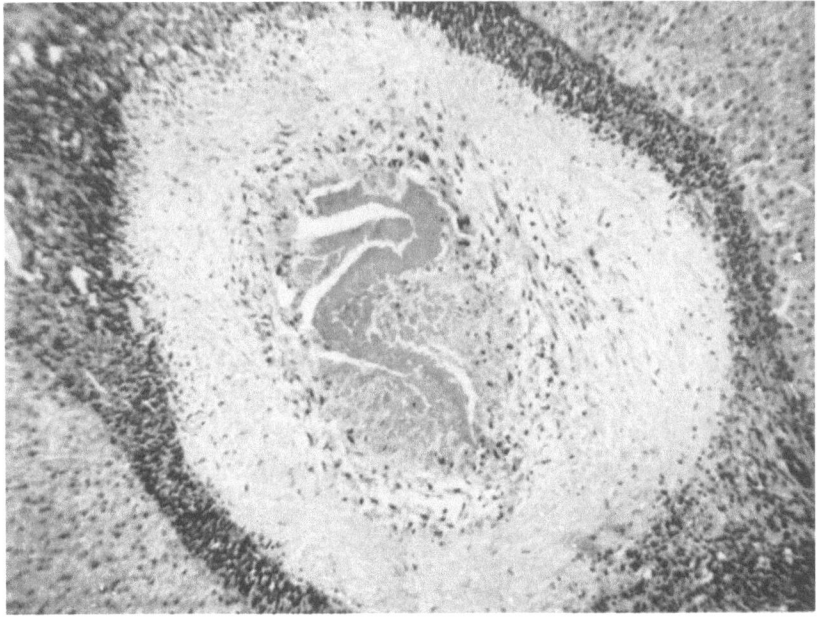

Fig. 5. Lesion caused by a dead worm in the liver of a patient with advanced schistosomiasis. There are central necrosis, presence of dense fibrous tissue and peripheral infiltration of lymphocytes. Hematoxylin and eosin. 100 ×

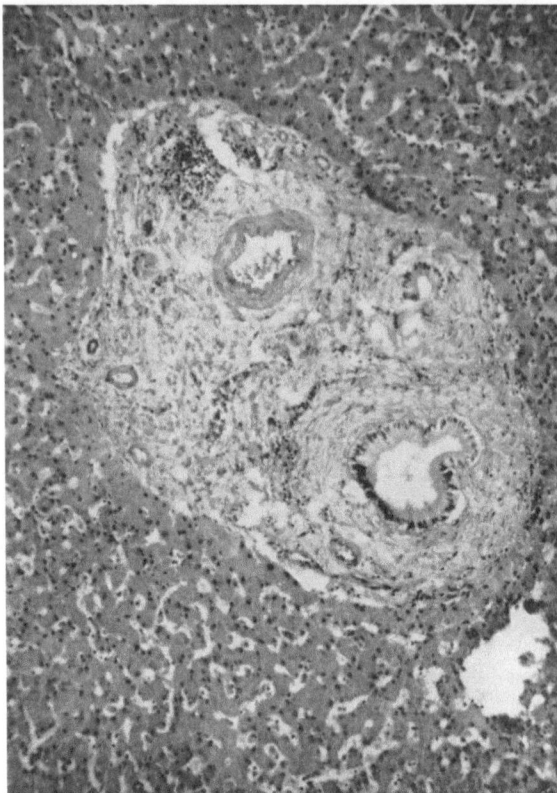

Fig. 6. A characteristic finding of schistosomiasis frequently seen in wedge biopsies of the liver. An enlarged and fibrosed portal space with preservation of the bile duct and hepatic artery, but with destruction of the portal vein branch. The hepatic parenchyma appears normal. Hematoxylin and eosin. 150 ×

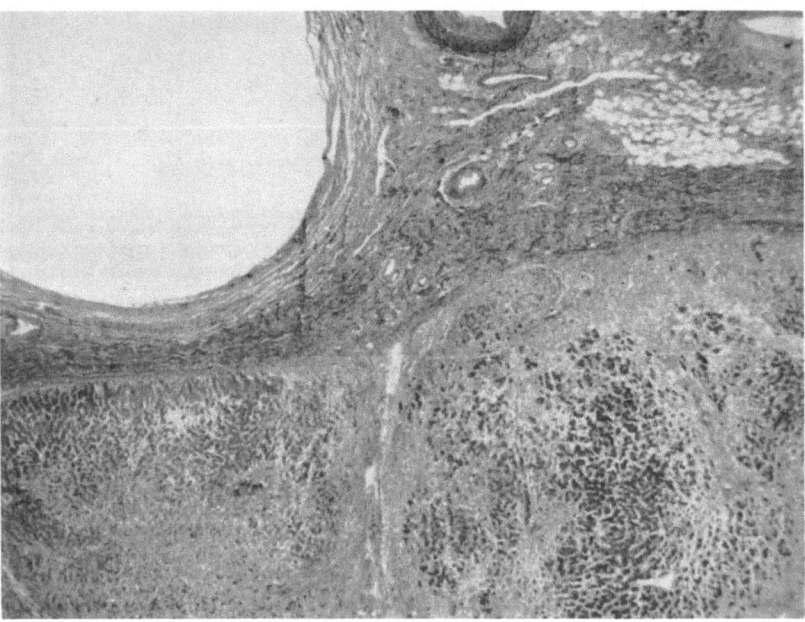

Fig. 7. Hepato-splenic schistosomiasis. The liver shows portal fibrosis and dilatation of the portal vein. The parenchyma is nodular and presents evidences of ischemic destruction. Mallory's line blue. 20 ×

occlusion of small vessels by granulomas, by dead worms, (Fig. 5) thrombophlebitis of larger portal branches, narrowing of portal venules by phlebosclerosis
and intimal thickening of arterioles. Thrombophlebitic lesions are usually seen
in the stage of recanalization and are most frequent near the periphery of the liver
(Fig. 6). The portal obstruction has been shown, by comparison of wedged hepatic

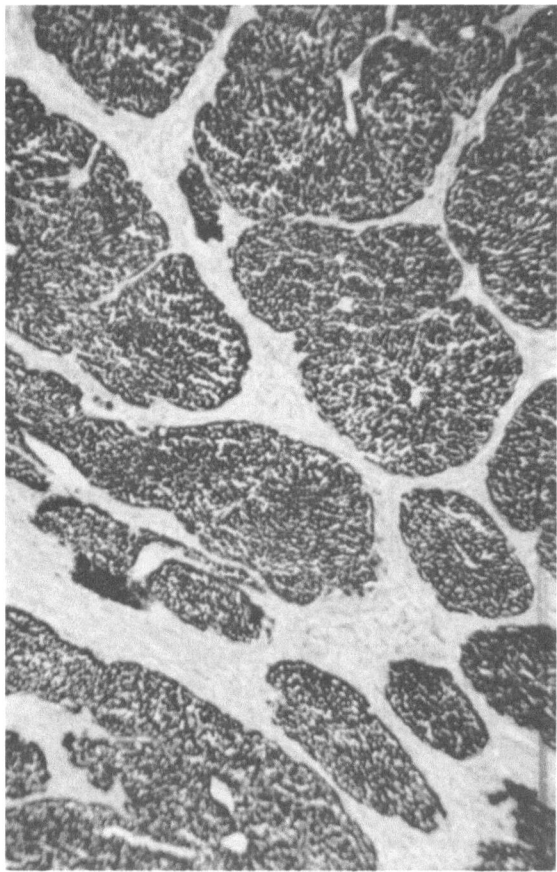

Fig. 8. Post-necrotic cicatrization in the subcapsular area of the liver in a case of hepato-splenic schistosomiasis. Davies'
method for non-specific esterase. Incubation time 5 min. 50 ×

vein pressures with portal vein or splenic pulp pressures, to be functionally presinusoidal [5, 14, 28]. The obstructive vascular lesions may also cause parenchymal changes, particularly during episodes of gastrointestinal hemorrhage and
shock, when extensive areas of necrosis may be seen (Fig. 7). Since bleeding from
varices occurs repeatedly, focal postnecrotic changes may be superimposed upon
the basic pattern of Symmers' pipestem fibrosis [4] (Fig. 8).

In wedge biopsies, focal postnecrotic cicatrization may lead to an erroneous
diagnosis of postnecrotic cirrhosis. True cirrhosis has not been considered to be
related to schistosomiasis in most Brazilian studies [4, 9]. In our autopsy material
the incidence of schistosome infection in patients with cirrhosis was equal to that

11*

in non-cirrhotic patients of comparable age. In 20 cases of hepatoma studied in this hospital, no relation with schistosome infection was found [29].

The spleen is greatly enlarged, averaging 1000 grams in weight in surgical material [2] and only slightly less in our autopsy cases. The usual changes of so-called congestive splenomegaly are seen, and special techniques show marked reticuloendothelial hyperplasia and infiltration by gamma globulin-producing plasma cells. The venous sinuses are dilated and may function as venules permitting rapid blood flow and perhaps the transmission of pressure from the arterial to the venous sector [2]. Manifestations of hypersplenism are frequent.

Macroscopically intestinal lesions are generally not seen, although occasional cases show isolated polyps or areas of marked serosal or peri-intestinal fibrosis. In cases with Symmers' fibrosis of the liver, large numbers of eggs are found in the proximal colon and small intestine, while the rectal mucosa contains few eggs. In cases without Symmers' fibrosis, eggs are most numerous in the rectal mucosa and distal colon [32]. The reason for this shift in the site of oviposition is not known. Rectal fibrosis is uncommon.

4. Cardiopulmonary schistosomiasis

Pulmonary hypertension with cor pulmonale appears in some patients with hepato-splenic schistosomiasis. Collateral portal-systemic veins facilitate the passage of adult schistosomes and their eggs from the portal into the pulmonary circulation, where they provoke arteritis and vascular occlusion. Atherosclerosis of the pulmonary arteries, arteriolar medial hypertrophy and fibrous or fibro-elastic intimal thickening and plexiform (angiomatoid) lesions are seen later as a result of the pulmonary hypertension itself [12, 17]. Patients with schistosomal cor pulmonale have a grave prognosis and are very poor surgical risks.

It has been claimed that schistosomal cor pulmonale may be seen rarely in the absence of hepato-splenic schistomiasis and portal hypertension [11]. If really caused by schistosomiasis, hypersensitive vascular damage caused by a few eggs or by periodic migration of schistosomulae through the lungs may be important pathogenetic pathways in such cases [12, 17].

Cyanosis and clubbing of the fingers are rarely associated with schistosomal cor pulmonale. However a new syndrome has recently been described in which marked cyanosis is noted in patients with hepatosplenic schistosomiasis, but in the absence of pulmonary hypertension. In these cases cyanosis is probably related to numerous minute pulmonary arterio-venous fistulae or to anastomoses between portal-systemic collateral veins and the pulmonary veins [11], as sometimes occurs in cirrhosis.

In the necropsies performed in this hospital, pulmonary arteritis and cor pulmonale have been noted in 15% of patients with Symmers' fibrosis, while only 2 questionable cases have been seen in 397 infected persons without Symmers' fibrosis.

5. Ectopic lesions

Isolated granulomas have been found in practically every organ, but generally no clinical manifestations are noted. Ectopic granulomas are most frequently noted in cases with massive infections or with portal-systemic collateral circulation, when worms and eggs can more easily bypass the liver. Numerous eggs may be seen in ectopic foci when the worms themselves are present in the ectopic site. In our material one patient with transverse myelitis [26] and one with a nodule in the epididymis are the only cases in which the ectopic lesions were clinically evident. In both cases numerous granulomas were present.

Summary

Clinical and pathological features of *Schistosoma mansoni* infections in Brazil are briefly presented. The great majority of patients with severe illness caused by schistosomiasis have the hepato-splenic form of the disease. In these patients liver function is usually well preserved, and the clinical picture is dominated by portal hypertension and its consequences. Bleeding from esophago-gastric varices is the most common cause of death. The hepatic lesion of Symmers' clay pipestem fibrosis is a characteristic and constant feature in these cases. True cirrhosis is not related to schistosome infection, nor is hepatoma. Intestinal complaints are frequently attributed to schistosome infection, but severe intestinal lesions are uncommon. Schistosomal pulmonary arteritis and cor pulmonale are seen principally in patients with hepato-splenic schistosomiasis. Ectopic lesions are frequent but seldom of clinical importance.

References

[1] ALVARIZ, F. G., O. N. FREITAS e P. DACORSO FILHO: Hepatite tóxica no decurso do tratamento anti-esquistossomótico por antimoniais. Hospital (Rio de J.) **67**, 451—466 (1965).

[2] ANDRADE, Z. A., e S. G. ANDRADE: Patologia do baço na esquistossomose hepatoesplenica. Rev. Inst. Med. Trop. S. Paulo **7**, 218—227 (1965).

[3] —, e G. R. SILVA: Manifestações pseudo-neoplásicas na esquistossomose intestinal. Arch. Bras. Med. **44**, 437—444 (1954).

[4] — S. SANTANA, and E. RUBIN: Hepatic changes in advanced schistosomiasis. Gastroenterology **42**, 393—400 (1962).

[5] AUFSES, A. H., F. SCHAFFNER, W. S. ROSENTHAL, and B. E. HERMAN: Portal venous pressure in "pipestem" fibrosis of the liver due to schistosomiasis. Amer. J. Med. **27**, 807—810 (1959).

[6] BARBOSA, F. S., and A. C. BARRETO: Differences in susceptibility of Brazilian strains of Australorbis glabratus to Schistosoma mansoni. Exp. Parasit. **9**, 137—140 (1960).

[7] BARRETO, A. C.: Reservoir hosts in schistosomiasis. Proceedings Seventh Internat. Cong. Trop. Med. Mal. **2**, 25—26, Rio de Janeiro 1963.

[8] BOGLIOLO, L.: Subsídios para o estudo da anatomia patológica da forma aguda toxêmica da esquistossomose mansoni. Organ Official de la Socieded Venezolana de Gastroenterologia, Endocrinologia y Nutricin. (G. E.N). **19**, 157—236 (1964).

[9] — Pathological changes in Mansonic Bilharziasis. Riv. Anat. Pat. **23**, 269—297 (1963).

[10] — Anatomical picture of the liver in hepato-splenic schistosomiasis mansoni. Ann. trop. Med. Parasit. **51**, 1—14 (1957).

[11] CAVALCANTI, I., e G. THOMPSON: Cianose, cirrose hepática e esquistossomose. An. Fac. Med. (Racife) **22**, 93—121 (1962).

[12] CHAVES, E.: Cor pulmonale crônico esquistossomótico. I. Estudo das lesões vasculares associadas á hipertensão pulmonar. Rev. Inst. Med. Trop. S. Paulo **2**, 78—89 (1960).

[13] CHING, WEI-HSIN: Acute schistosomiasis. Clinical manifestations of 96 cases. Chin. Med. J. **76**, 1—10 (1958).

[14] Coutinho, A., I. Cavalcanti, e G. Thompson: Cateterização de uma veia hepática na Síndrome hepato-esplênica esquistossomótica. Pressão da veia hepática ocluida. An. Fac. Med. (Racife) **19**, 157—159 (1959).
[15] Díaz-Rivera, R. S., F. Ramos-Morales, E. Koppish, M. R. Garcia Palmieri, A. A. Cintrón-Rivera, E. J. Marchand, O. Gonzáles, and M. V. Torregrosa: Acute Manson's schistosomiasis. Amer. J. Med. **21**, 918—943 (1962).
[16] Dimmette, R. M., and H. F. Sproat: Recto-signmoid polyps in schistosomiasis. Amer. J. Trop. Med. Hyg. **4**, 1057—1067 (1955).
[17] Faria, J. L.: Pulmonary vascular changes in schistosomal cor pulmonale. J. Path. Bact. **68**, 589—602 (1954).
[18] Ferreira, L. F., J. B. Naveira, i. J. R. Silva: Fase toxêmica da esquistossomose mansoni. Considerações a propósito de alguns casos coletivamente contaminados em uma piscina. Rev. Inst. Med. Trop. S. Paulo **2**, 112—120 (1960).
[19] Hashem, M.: The etiology and pathogenesis of the endemic form of splenomegaly: Egyptian splenomegaly. J. Egypt. Med. Ass. **30**, 48—79 (1947).
[20] Lichtenberg, F.: Lesions of the intrahepatic portal radicles in Manson's schistosomiasis. Amer. J. Path. **31**, 757—771 (1955).
[21] Meira, J. A.: Quadro clínico da esquistossomose mansônica. Rev. Bras. Malar. **11**, 247—357 (1959).
[22] Meves, J., e. P. Raso: Estudo anátomo-clínico de um caso de forma toxêmica da esquistossomose mansoni que evoluiu para a forma hepatesplenica em 130 dias (fibrose hepática tipo Symmers). Rev. Inst. Med. Trop. S. Paulo **7**, 256—266 (1965).
[23] Paraense, W. L., and L. R. Corrèa: Susceptibility of Australorbis tenagophilus to infection with Schistosoma mansoni. Rev. Inst. Med. Trop. S. Paulo **5**, 23—29 (1963).
[24] Pellon, B., e I. Teixeira: Distribuição da esquistossomose mansônica no Brasil. Divisão de Organização Sanitária. Publication of the Public Health Department of Brazil (1950).
[25] Pirajá da Silva, M. A.: La schistosomose à Bahia. Arch. Parasit. **13**, 415 (1908).
[26] Pondé, E., E. Chaves, e P. G. Sena: Esquistossomiase medular. Arch. Neuro-psiquiat. **18**, 166—175 (1960).
[27] Prata, A., e Z. A. Andrade: Fibrose hepatica da Symmers sem esplenomegalia. Hospital (Rio de J.) **63**, 617—623 (1963).
[28] Ramos, O., F. Saad, and W. P. Leser: Portal hemodynamics and liver cell function in hepatic schistosomiasis. Gastroenterology **47**, 241—247 (1964).
[29] Santana Filho, S.: Carcinoma primário do fígado (Estudo de 20 casos autopsiados). Thesis, University of Bahia, Brazil (1964).
[30] Santiago, J. M., J. Neves e J. L. A. Ratton: Evolução da forma toxêmica da esquistossomose mansoni para o cor pulmonale. Rev. Inst. Med. Trop. S. Paulo **7**, 295—304 (1965).
[31] Symmers, W. St. C.: Note on a new form of liver cirrhosis due to the presence of the ova of Bilharzia haematobia. J. Path. Bact. **9**, 237—239 (1904).
[32] Valladares, C. P.: Determinações intestinais na doença de Manson-Pirajá da Silva. Thesis, University of Bahia, Brazil (1953).
[33] Warren, K. S. G. Reboucas, and A. G. Batista: Ammonia metabolism and hepatic coma in hepatosplenic schistosomiasis. Ann. Intern. Med. **62**, 1113—1133 (1965).

Studies on Schistosomiasis mansoni[1]
Correlation between Clinical Finding, Liver Pathology and Portal Circulation Hemodynamics

E. A. Saad[2], S. G. Coutinho[3], J. Barbosa Filho[4]
and J. Rodrigues da Silva[5]

Catheterization of hepatic veins was performed for the first time by Warren and Brannon [20] for biochemical study purposes. Later on this technic was used to measure hepatic and splanchnic blood flow through Fick principle or through bromosulphalein clearance studies [2, 3, 20].

Studies in experimental animals [15] and man [21] have shown that if a catheter is wedged in a hepatic venule (hepatic "capillary") a pressure could be measured which reflects portal vein pressure as the pulmonary wedge pressure represents left strium pressure [10, 11].

Normal values for wedged (WHVP) and free hepatic vein pressure (FHVP) so determined are 3–12 mm Hg and 1–6 mm Hg respectively. A pressure gradient up to 5 mm Hg exists normally between wedged and free hepatic vein positions. Hepatic vein catheterization has therefore been used for studies on portal hypertension.

Paton et al. [16] were able to distinguish two different hemodynamic patterns in portal hypertension.

1. Post sinusoidal portal hypertension in which wedge hepatic vein pressure (WHVP) is very high, usually between 15–25 mm Hg. This group includes nutritional and post necrotic cirrhosis.

2. Pre-sinusoidal portal hypertension as found in prehepatic causes of portal hypertension in which WHVP is within normal limits.

In schistosomiasis mansoni Coutinho et al. [8] found normal WHVP in around 70% of the cases and slightly elevated pressures in 30% of the cases.

This was the first demonstration that an intrahepatic portal hypertension could exist with nearly normal portal vein wedge pressure (WHVP) and these findings were confirmed by other authors [1, 6, 12, 13, 17, 18].

Simultaneous measurements of WHVP and intrasplenic pressure by Coutinho [6, 7] and Becker et al. [2] discovered another important feature of hepato-

---

[1] From the Department of Tropical Medicine and Infectious Diseases, University of Brazil (Prof. J. Rodrigues da Silva) and Department of Cardiology, Guanabara State University Hospital "Pedro Ernesto" (Prof. A. B. Benchimal). This study was supported by research grant No. AI—05188 —01 from the National Institute of Allergy and Infectious Diseases, National Institutes of Health, United States Public Health Service.

[2] Department of Tropical Medicine and Cardiology.

[3] Departments of Tropical Medicine.

[4] Heart Laboratory, University Hospital "Pedro Ernesto".

[5] Department of Tropical Medicine and Infectious Diseases.

splenic schistosomiasis mansoni. Splenic pressure is almost always very high so that a pressure gradient exists between the splenic pulp and WHVP.

It was concluded that in hepatosplenic schistosomiasis mansoni WHVP does not exactly measure portal vein pressure.

A comprehensive review of hepatic vein catheterization was recently published by COUTINHO [6].

Our study correlates hepatic vein catheterization data with clinical and histopathological findings. It aims at having more conclusive data than that published by other workers since in a previous communication by one of us [9] it was found that some cases of hepato-splenic schistosomiasis could exhibit a hemodynamic pattern similar to that of portal cirrhosis.

Material and methods

Thirty three cases were studied (Table 1). In every case the diagnosis of schistosomiasis and portal hypertension were confirmed by finding the ova in faeces and/or rectal biopsy, roentgen and endoscopic study of esophagus and stomach, splenoportography and needle liver biopsy. Five cases were submitted to shunt operations for portal hypertension and had surgical biopsy of the liver performed.

Table 1. *Clinical cases submitted to hepatic vein catheterization*

1. Intestinal form of Schistosomiasis Mansoni .	8 cases
2. Hepatosplenic form of Schistosomiasis Mansoni	22 cases
3. Laennec cirrhosis	2 cases
4. Cavernous malformation of portal vein . . .	1 case
Total	33 cases

Our pathological data is based only on these five cases because of obvious limitations of needle biopsy.

Splenic pressure was measured through a common pressure device.

With the patient in fasting state and without sedatives a Cournand No 7 or 8 catheter was introduced under local anesthesia in an arm vein and advanced up to the right atrium where the tip near the column was rotated backward and so advanced into the inferior vena cava.

Once in the inferior vena cava, the catheter tip below the diaphragm is rotated on-ward and so advanced into the hepatic vein until the wedge position.

Holding the breath in deep inspiration makes procedure easier.

Wedge position is obtained ordinarily with catheter tip very near the ribs; only twice did we succeed wedging in a medial position.

Records were made with the Statham P 23D pressure transducer coupled with Strain-gage manometer or with a Sanborn 267 B-FE pressure transducer and carrier preamplifier; both systems were in use with a Sanborn Twin-Viso Electrocardiograph.

Zero reference line was arbitrarily chosen at 10 cm above the catheterization table.

Results

Analyses of 8 cases of intestinal form and of 22 cases of hepatosplenic form of schistosomiasis are shown in Tables 2 and 3.

Results in both these schistosomiasis forms are shown in Tables 4, 5 and 6. Intrasplenic-suprahepatic gradient is analysed in Table 7.

Correlation between liver pathology and portal hemodynamics

Five cases of hepatosplenic schistosomiasis were studied by liver catheterization and wedge biopsy (Table 8).

Table 2. *Hepatic vein catheterization in intestinal form of Schistosomiasis mansoni*

Identification data	WHVP mm Hg	FHVP mm Hg	WHVP-FHVP Gradient mm Hg
1. PCC*/5593 25 female, white	8.5	5.1	3.4
2. PCC/5593 22 white female	6.0	2.6	3.4
3. Pcc/6321 29 white, female	8.8	7.9	0.9
4. PCC/5559 14 black, male	9.6	5.8	3.8
5. PCC/6319 25 white, male	11.0	6.0	5.0
6. PCC/7358 23 white, female	5.0	1.0	4.0
7. PCC/6331 23 white, male	9.0	4.0	5.0
8. HCPE**/101.930 26 white, male	7.5	5.0	2.5

* PCC-Tropical and Infections diseases clinic, University of Brasil.
** HCPE-University Hospital "Pedro Ernesto".

Table 3. *Hepatic vein catheterization in hepatosplenic form of Schistosomiasis mansoni*

Case identification	Splenic pressure mm Hg	WHVP mm Hg	FHVP mm Hg	WHVP-FHVP gradient mm Hg	Splenic-WHVP gradient mm Hg
1. PCC*/7116	27.2	13.0	7.0	6.0	14.2
2. PCC/7102	27.9	25.0	13.0	12.0	2.0
3. PCC/6161	35.7	22.4	12.9	9.5	13.3
4. PCC/6092	28.9	14.4	9.0	5.4	14.5
5. PCC/6145	32.3	10.8	6.8	4.0	21.5
6. PCC/2230	18.3	9.0	5.2	3.8	9.3
7. PCC/3822	19.1	20.1	7.0	13.1	zero
8. PCC/4679	22.0	12.9	8.8	3.1	9.1
9. PCC/5073	22.0	23.5	10.5	13.0	zero
10. PCC/5508	27.2	15.8	7.3	8.5	11.4
11. PCC/5710	16.9	14.1	7.6	6.5	2.8
12. PCC/6011	—	9.0	4.1	4.9	—
13. PCC/6012	—	12.9	9.4	3.5	—
14. PCC/6052	—	11.7	—	—	—
15. PCC/6192	33.8	10.1	2.9	7.2	23.7
16. PCC/6209	—	13.5	5.2	8.3	—
17. PCC/6348	22.7	7.6	1.0	6.6	15.1
18. PCC/6734	—	7.5	5.0	2.5	—
19. PCC/6485	27.2	7.0	5.5	1.5	20.2
20. PCC/7198	23.5	15.0	8.0	7.0	8.5
21. HCPE**/101.477	—	17.0	10.0	7.0	—
22. HCPE/104.118	—	18.0	7.6	11.4	—

* PCC-Tropical and Infections Diseases Clinic, University of Brazil.
** HCPE-University Hospital "Pedro Ernesto".

Two of these cases showed advanced lesions and in both WHVP was greater than 20 mm Hg.

Two out of the last 3 cases had only moderate lesions of the liver with WHVP of 13 and 14.4 mm Hg respectively.

The fifth case had very severe hepatic lesions and normal WHVP but this case had also portal vein thrombosis.

Correlation between splenomegaly and hepatic vein pressure is analysed in Table 9.

Table 4. *Results of hepatic vein catheterization in intestinal form of Schistosomiasis mansoni*

Categories	mm Hg
Pressure range	5—11
Mean WHVP	8.2
Mean FHVP.	4.6
Mean WHVP — FHVP gradient	36

Table 5. *Results of hepatic vein catheterization in 22 cases of hepatosplenic form of Schistosomiasis mansoni*

Patterns	mm Hg
I. 8 cases (36.4%) with WHVP within normal limits	
Pressure range	7—11
Mean WHVP	9.0
Mean FHVP	4.3
Mean WHVP — FHVP gradient	4.2
II. 14 cases 9 (63.6%) with elevated WHVP	
Pressure range	12.9—25
Mean WHVP	16.97
Mean FHVP	8.59
Mean WHVP — FHVP gradient	8.38
II. A) 10 cases (40.9%) with WHVP 14 mm Hg (mean)	
II. B) 4 cases (18.1%) with WHVP greater than 20 mm Hg	

Table 6. *Hemodynamic patterns of hepatosplenic Schistosomiasis mansoni*

Patterns	mm Hg
Group I	
Normal WHVP (8 cases)	
Mean FHVP	4.6
Mean WHVP — FHVP gradient	3.6
Mean splenic pressure	26.8
Mean intrasplenic — WHVP gradient	17.9
Group II	
WHVP between 12 and 20 mm Hg (10 cases)	
Mean WHVP	8.2
Mean WHVP — FHVP gradient	7.4
Mean splenic pressure	24.1
Mean intrasplenic — WHVP gradient	9.3
Group III	
WHVP greater than 20 mm Hg (4 cases)	
Mean FHVP	10.8
Mean WHVP — FHVP gradient	11.9
Mean intrasplenic WHVP gradient	3.7

Table 7. *Intrasplenic — WHVP gradient in hepatosplenic Schistosomiasis mansoni*

Patterns	mm Hg
I. 8 cases with normal WHVP	
5 cases analysed	
Mean intrasplenic pressure	26.8
Mean gradient	17.9
II. 14 cases with elevated WHVP	
10 cases analysed	
Mean intrasplenic pressure	25
Mean gradient	7.5
II. A) 10 cases with WHVP greater than 14 mm Hg	
8 cases analysed	
Mean intrasplenic pressure	26
Gradient	7.8
II. B) 4 cases with WHVP greater than 20 mm Hg	
4 cases analysed	
Mean intrasplenic pressure	26.1
Intrasplenic — WHVP gradient	

Table 8. *Pathological* and hemodynamic data in five cases of hepatosplenic Schistosomiasis mansoni*

Identification	WHVP mm Hg	FVHP mm Hg	WHVP FVHP Gradient mm Hg	Splenic pressure mm Hg	Splenic WHVP Gradient	Fibrosis	Granu-lomas	Angiomatoid	Lobular distortion	Observations
PCC**/711613		7.0	6	27.2	14.2	Coarse + +	+	+ +	Absent	Moderate degree o liver damage
PCC/7102	25	13.0	12	27.9	2.9	Coarse + + +	+	+ + + +	Absent	Focal liver cells necrosis, + + Extensive lympho-mono-cytic infiltration
PCC/6161	22.4	12.9	9.5	35.7	13.3	Coarse + + + +	+ + +	+ + +	In focal areas	Many binucleated cells
PCC/6092	14.4	9.0	5.4	28.9	14.5	Coarse + + +	Absent	+ +	Slight in focal areas	Extensive mono-nuclear infil-tration
PCC/6145	10.8	6.8	4.0	22.3	32.2	Coarse + + +	+	+ +	Focal areas	Septa + + +, Mononuclear in-filtration + + +; cellular alterations + +; portal vein thrombosis

* Surgical liver biopsies
** PCC-Tripical and Infectious diseases clinic, University of Brazil.

Table 9. *Spleen enlargement — WHVP relationship*

I. 7 cases with normal WHVP	
a — without splenomegaly	2 cases = 28.5%
b — Slight spleen enlargement	5 cases = 42.8%
c — Great spleen enlargement	1 case = 14.5%
II. 12 cases with WHVP greater than 12 mm Hg	
a — Moderate splenomegaly	4 cases = 16.5%
(up to 9 cm below costal margin)	
b — Great spleen enlargement	8 cases = 83.5%
(more than 9 cm below costal margin)	
III. 4 cases with WHVP greater than 20 mm Hg	
The greatest spleen enlargement of this series	
(12—15 cm below costal margins)	

Comments

The present series seems to warrant a classification of the hepatosplenic form of schistosomiasis mansoni in 3 distinct groups as shown in Table 10.

As one can conclude the degree of portal hypertension as measured by splenic pressure is about the same in all dree groups.

Clinico-pathological correlation seems to point to the fact that these groups are distinguished not by the degree of portal hypertension but rather by the degree of liver damage reflected in terms of the WHVP. As the liver damage progresses the hemodynamic pattern, quite distinctive in the mild forms, becomes very similar to that of cirrhosis of the liver. As a matter of fact these are not yet definite conclusions but previous assessments seem warranted in this series. Nothing could be found in the clinical examination to compare our 3rd group with that of complicated parenchyma-vascular form of schistosomiasis as described by Mousa [14].

Additional data from studies on liver blood flow measured by bromosulphalein [7] and last but not least by correlation measurements with splenoportography and hepatic venography [5] correlate quite well with the groups here described.

Table 10. *Clinical — pathological — hemodynamic patterns of hepatosplenic Schistosomiasis*

Group I: Mild forms
WHVP . . . .   normal
FHVP . . . .   normal
WHVP — FHVP gradient . . . .   normal
Splenic pressure   . . . .   elevated
Greatest intrasplenic — WHVP gradient (around 18 mm Hg)
Mild to moderate, occasionally absent, splenomegaly
Group II: Moderate forms
WHVP between 12—20 mm Hg
FHVP slightly elevated
WHVP — FHVP gradient slightly elevated
Moderate intrasplenic — WHVP gradient (around 7.5 mm Hg)
Great splenomegaly (9—12 cm below costal margin)
Moderate hepatic lesions (degree + ÷/+ + + +)
Group III: Severe forms
WHVP greatly elevated (more than 20 mm Hg)
                  "cirrhotic levels"
FHVP moderately to greatly elevated
Greatest WHVP — FHVP
Mean intrasplenic — WHVP gradient mild (around 3 mm Hg), or absent
Greatest spleen enlargements (12—15 cm below costal margin).
Advanced hepatic lesions, occasionsally with focal lobular distortion.
This hemodynamic pattern is quite similar to that found in portal cirrhosis

Summary

The clinical, pathological and hemodynamic studies in 8 cases of intestinal and 22 cases of hepatosplenic schistosomiasis mansoni have been reported. Wedge hepatic vein pressure (WHVP) and free hepatic vein pressure (FHVP) were normal in patients with intestinal form of bilharziasis.

36.3% of the patients with the hepatosplenic form showed normal WHVP and FHVP while 63.7% showed abnormally high values.

On the basis of WHVP, FHVP, splenic pressure, clinical and pathological studies, the authors were able to distinguish three degrees of liver damage in hepatosplenic form of schistosomiasis mansoni, namely, mild, moderate and severe forms. Mild forms show normal WHVP, FHVP and WHVP-FHVP gradient, enlarged splenic pressure gradient between splenic and WHVP pressure around 18 mm Hg and mild or occasionally absent splenomegaly. Moderate forms show WHVP between 12—20 mm Hg, FHVP slightly elevated, a slight WHVP-FHVP gradient, an intrasplenic — WHVP gradient around 7.5 mm Hg, a moderate splenomegaly and a severe degree (++/++++) of liver damage.

Severe forms show WHVP greater than 20 mm Hg, FHVP moderately to greatly elevated, the greatest WHVP-FHVP gradient, mild or more frequently absent intrasplenic — WHVP gradient, the greatest spleen enlargements and the severest liver damage. This hemodynamic pattern corresponds to that found in portal cirrhosis.

References

[1] AUFSES, A. H. JR., F. SCHAFFNER, W. S. ROSENTHAL, and B. E. HERMAN: Portal venous pressure in „pipestem" fibrosis of the liver due to schistosomiasis. Amer. J. Med. 27 807-810, (1959).

[2] BECKER, S., J. J. PUIGBO, P. BLANCO, V. CASOLTA, R. SALOMON, C. G. YEPEZ, e J. J. VALENCIA-PARPARCEN: Estudio hemodinamico del sindrome de hiper tension portal con especial referencia a la manometria simultanea intraesplenica y suprahepatica. G.E.N. 16, 251 (1961).

[3] BRADLEY, S. E.: Clinical aspects of hepatic vascular physiology in liver injury. In Transactions of the 9th Conference on Liver Injury. 2: 71—90. New York: Jesiah Macy JR. Foundation 1951.

[4] — F. J. INGELFINGER, A. E. GROFF, and G. P. BRADLEY: Estimated hepatic blood flow and hepatic venous oxygen content in cirrhosis of the liver. Proc. Soc. Exp. Biol. 67, 206—207 (1948).

[5] COUTINHO, A.: Patologia da esquistossomose, Mesa Redonda na Segunda Jornada Braziliera da Esquistossomose. Belo Horizonte: Imprensa Official 1955.

[6] — A hipertensão porta na síndrome hepatê-esplênica esquistossomótica. Estudío clínico e hemodinâmico. Tese. Fac. Med. Recife 1960.

[7] Alterações hemodynâmicas na esquistossomose mansônica hepato-esplénica. J. Bras. Med. 8, 299—308 (1964).

[8] — I. CAVALCANTI, and G. THOMPSON: Cateterização de uma veia hepática na sondrome hepatosplênica esquistossomótica. Pressão da vein hepática ocluida. An. Fac. Med. Recife 19, 157—159 (1959).

[9] DA SILVA, J. R.: Discussion on A. D. Coutinho's paper "Hemodynamic patterns of schistosomiasis mansoni hepato-splenic form". In: Proceedings Seventh Internat. Congr. Trop. Med. Mal. 2, 104. Lisbon 1958.

[10] HELLEMS, H. K., F. W. HAYNES, J. F. GOWDY, and L. DEXTER: The pulmonary capillary pressure in man. J. Clin. Invest. 27, 540 (1948).

[11] LAGERLÖF, H., and L. WERKÖ: Studies on the circulation of blood in man; pulmonary capillary venous pressure in man. Scand. J. Clin. Lab. Invest. 7, 147—161 (1949).

[12] LEEVY, C. M., G. R. CHERRICK, and C. S. DAVIDSON: Portal hypertension. New Engl. J. Med. 262, 397—403 (1960).

[13] — — — Portal hypertension (concluded). New Engl. J. Med. 262, 451—455 (1960).

[14] MOUSA, A. H.: Clinico-pathological haemodynamics studies and management of hepato-splenic bilharziasis in Egypt. In: Proceedings Sixth Internat. Congr. Trop. Med. Mal. 2, 104, Lisbon 1958.

[15] MYERS, J. D., and W. J. TAYLOR: An estimation of portal venous pressure by occlusive catherization of an hepatic venule. J. Clin. Invest. 30, 662—663 (1951).

[16] PATON, A., T. B. REYNOLDS, and S. SHERLOCK: Assessment of portal hypertension by catheterization of hepatic vein. Lancet 1, 918—921, 1953.

[17] RAMOS, O. L.: Contribuição para o estudo la hemodinamica do figado na fibrose hepática da esquistossomos mansônica esua repercussão sôbre as condicões funcionasi do Lepatocito. Tese. Escola Paulista de Medicina. Sao Paulo, 1961.

[18] SAAD, F. and W. P. LESER: Portal hemodynamics and liver cell function in hepatic schistosomiasis. Gastroenterology 47, 241—247 (1964).

[19] SHERLOCK, S., A. G. BEARN, B. H. BILLING, and J. C. S. PATERSON: Splanchnic blood flow in man by the bromosulfalein method: the relation of peripheral plasma bromosulfalein level to the calculated flow. J. Lab. Clin. Med. 35, 923—932 (1950).

[20] WARREN, J. V., and E. S. BRANNON: A method of obtaining blood samples directly from the hepatic vein in man. Proc. Soc. Exp. Biol. (N. Y.) 55, 144—146 (1944).

[21] WELCH, G. E., R. EMMETT, C. C. GRAIGHEAD, G. HOEFFLER, D. C. BROWN and I. ROSEN: Simultaneous pressure measurements in the hepatic venule and portal venous system in man. Amer. J. Med. Sci. 228, 643—645 (1954).

Schistosomiasis mansoni: Lesions Produced by Dead Worms in the Liver and Lungs

HUMBERTO MENEZES*

With 6 figures

The lesions induced by dead worms in patients or animals infected with Schistosoma have been known since the first descriptions of the parasitosis. Very

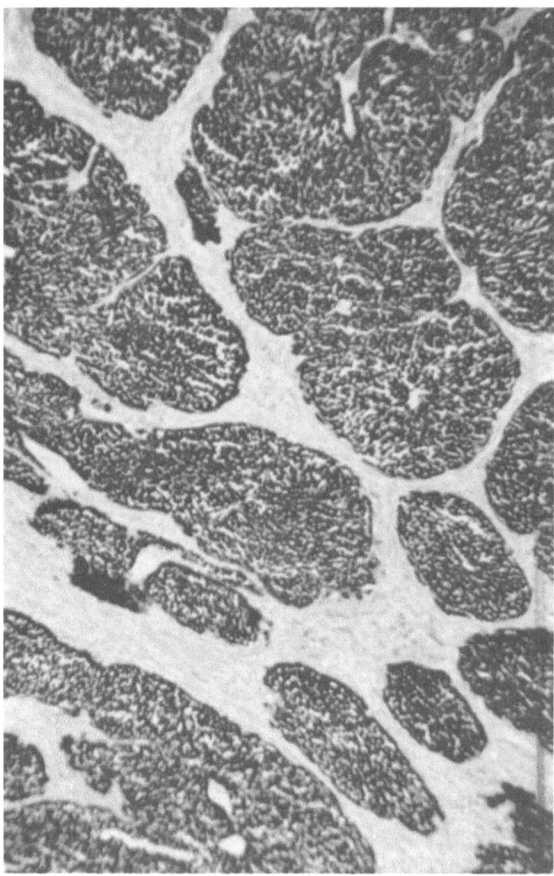

Fig. 1. Human case of hepatic bilharzial fibrosis

little attention was given to this fact and only few authors [11, 21] tried to establish some correlation between such lesions and the pathological manifestations of the disease.

* Department of Pathology, Faculty of medicine. University of Sao Paulo, Ribeirão Preto, Brazil.

In mansonial schistosomiasis two organs are particularly prone to manifest the sequelae of the presence of dead worms: the liver, because of its special situation in the course of the portal circulation and of its being the natural habitat of the parasites; and the lungs, because they constitute a transient habitat for the worm during its life cycle and also because in later stages, through a little knows mechanism, ova and/or adult worms may be found in the pulmonary arterial bed.

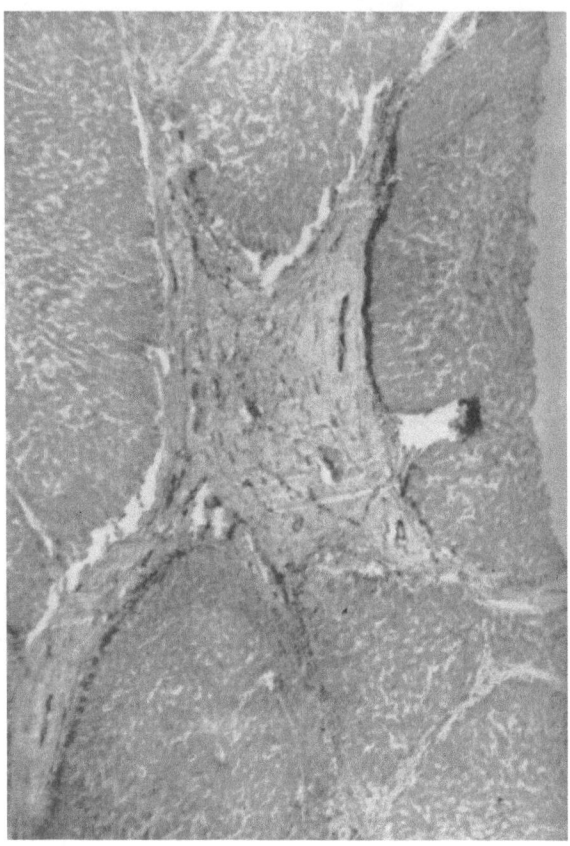

Fig. 2. Hepatic fibrosis induced in rabbit by portal embolization with adults *Schistosoma mansoni*

The majority of authors who have studied the pathogenesis of the hepatic fibrosis in cases of bilharziasis mansoni, have accepted the granulomatous lesions produced by the deposition of ova as the cause of the characteristic Symmers' fibrosis [3, 12] . Some others, however, have been unable to correlate the granulomatous lesions, due to the ova, with the hepatic fibrosis and have invoked the action of the metabolites of the parasite, hypothetical "toxins" and the phenomenon of sensitization to explain this important lesion [14, 16].

In 1944, COUTINHO, TAVARES and MENEZES [8], reporting the findings in a boy who died during antimonial treatment, emphasized the role of the dead worms in the genesis of the major hepatic lesions. SOROUR [26] first called attention to the proliferative endothelial phlebitis produced by the dead worms as the cause of the hepatic fibrosis. GIRGES [11] and MOLINA [21] emphasized the mechanical action of the dead worms in obstructing the lumen of the vessels and later inducing the appearance of the hepatic fibrosis.

TAVARES and MENEZES [27] published the first experimental work correlating the lesions produced by the dead worms with the hepatic fibrosis. They infected

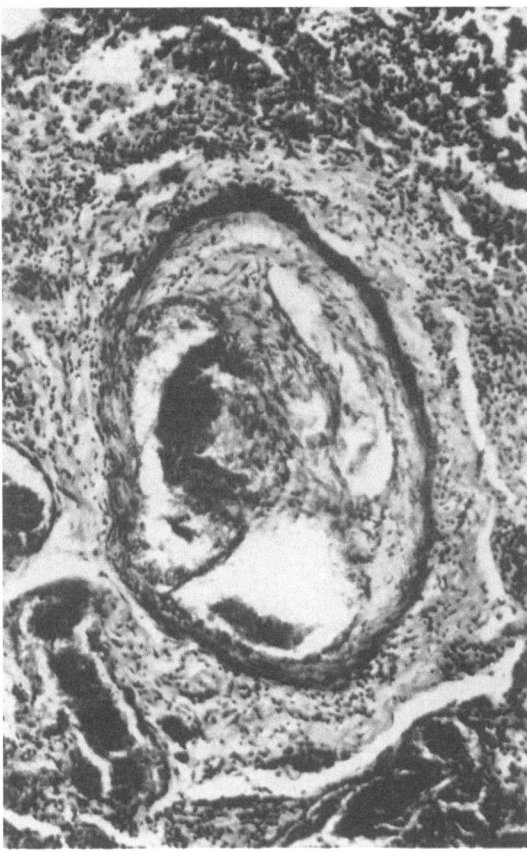

Fig. 3. Human case of "schistosomotic pulmonary arteritis"

guinea pigs with cercariae of *S. mansoni* and after 45 days treated the animals with antimonials. They found that dead worms promoted necrosis of the liver parenchyma. The necrotic lesions were initially invaded by eosinophiles and later encapsulated and replaced by fibrous tissue. These findings were confirmed in 1949 by COELHO, MENEZES and MAGALHÃES FO [6].

In 1960 MAGALHÃES FO., MENEZES and COELHO, [18] injecting the portal veins of human cases of schistosomiasis, described the vascular alterations in the advanced stages of the disease and compared them with severe cases of septal cirrhosis and normal human livers (Fig. 5 and 6). In addition to the dilatation of the hepatic branches of the portal vein in Symmers' fibrosis described by some authors

[2, 23], MAGALHÃES FO., MENEZES and COELHO [18] called attention to the obstruction of the vein with subsequent recanalization.

Correlating both the gross and the microscopic findings in their cases these authors concluded that the hepatic lesions are the result of repeated episodes that follow the occlusion of the intra-hepatic portal branches by dead worms.

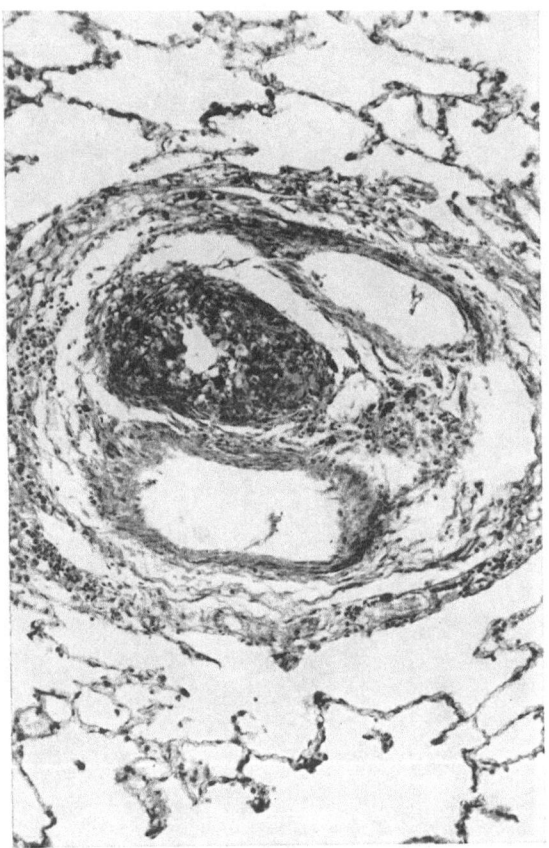

Fig. 4. Experimental schistosomotic lesions produced by the embolization of adults S. mansoni in the pulmonary artery of dog

It should be emphasized that the worms not only obstruct the vascular lumens, but cause destruction of the vessel walls, inducing an inflammatory reaction with proliferation of the sub-intimal connective tissue which extends to the fibrous tissue of the portal triad. This is the reason for the portal location of the fibrosis and the difficulty of finding the thrombosis.

The portal fibrosis is mainly due to the inflammatory reaction induced by the dead adult parasites and to the proliferation of the connective tissue. The deposition of ova in the newly opened capillaries only contributes to the increase of fibrosis.

The author has demonstrated experimentally that the body of the parasite disintegrates and disappears during the first two weeks after the embolisation. At the end of this period what was a large vessel is transformed to a great number of small capillaries. This fact can be easily recognized in autopsy cases if the arterial and the corresponding venous branches are carefully examined. Generally the latter cannot be seen because, as already stated, they are replaced by a number of small vessels, but when they are present they are dilated since they are distal to the obstruction.

The retraction of the portal connective tissue and the increase in the blood pressure in the portal system, of the occluded areas, are responsible for the

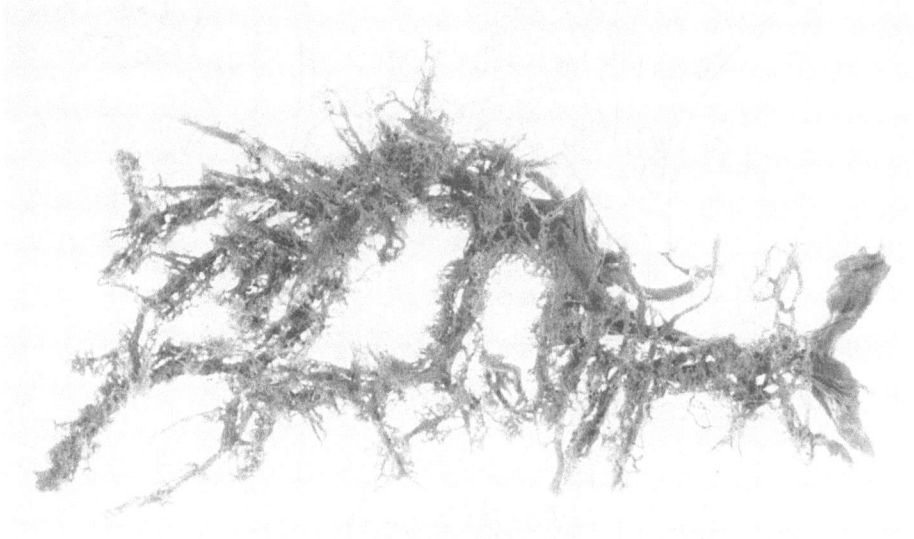

Fig. 5. Symmers' fibrosis. Human liver injected (portal vein and hepatic artery) with vinilyte. We can see the great reduction in the size of the portal branches of medium size that are dilated, tortuous and surounded by a network of new capillaries

hydrostatic hypertension, for the opening of the small adventitial portal capillaries and for the dilatation of the distal vessel segment.

The development of the adventitial portal capillaries is a typical feature of Symmers' fibrosis but can be seen in cases of intra-hepatic portal occlusion of any etiology (venous occlusive disease of the liver, old portal thrombosis).

A comparison of the plastic models of the portal bed in the schistosomial and normal livers shows a pronounced reduction of the smaller branches of the vascular tree with dilatation of the distal segments involved by an anastomotic capillary net.

The mechanism of reticular network collapse in the areas of atrophy and/or hepato-cellular destruction with resultant approximation of portal tracts, is similar to that described by POPPER and ELIAS [22] in the genesis of the post-collapse cirrhosis.

Schistosomial hepatic fibrosis can be included among lesions produced by massive collapse of areas of hepatic parenchyma except that the areas of collapse are always in relationship to a portal triad, since it in this zone that the veno-occlusive phenomenon, necrosis of the vascular walls and of the peri-portal parenchyma, takes place. After these events, Kiernan's space, with the portal venous segment recanalized, acts as a center of attraction of the adjacent collapsed areas of parenchyma. This results in planes of traction that are arranged radially, going beyond the areas of affected hepatocytes and inducing other vascular disturbances.

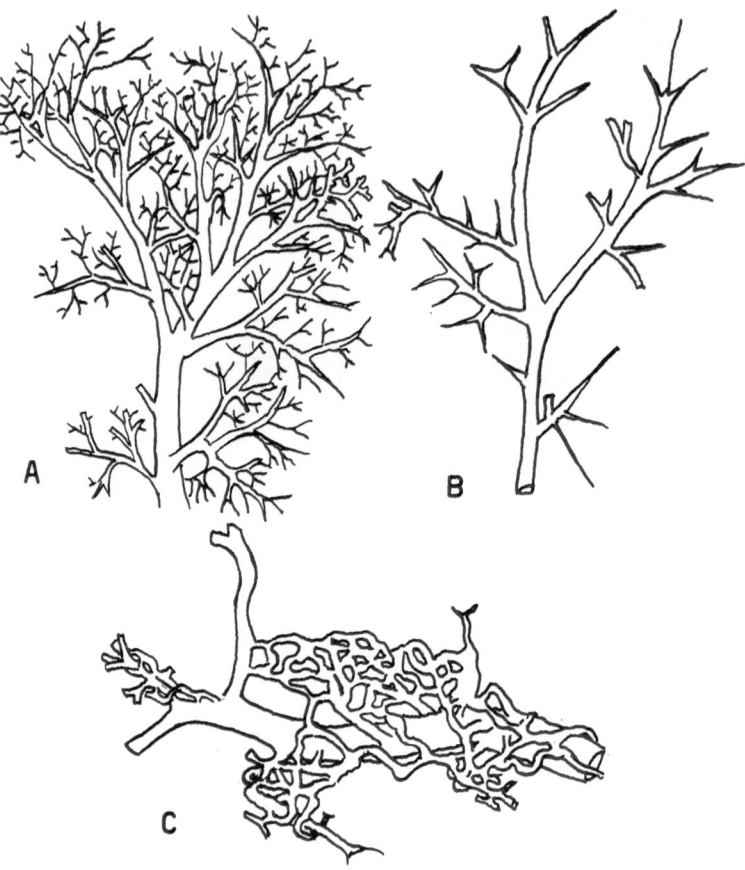

Fig. 6. Drawing from cases of human livers injected with vinilyte (portal vein). A — Normal liver, B — Septal cirrhosis, C — Bilharzial fibrosis

Experimentally these observations could be reproduced, first in rats and later in rabbits [19, 20] (Fig. 2).

The injection of dead worms into the portal system of these animals, especially the rabbit, which has a portal circulation more like that of man [9], promotes many alterations ending in a gross and microscopical pattern similar to that seen in man.

In the rabbit, we have often observed an early proliferative endophlebitis. The venous obliteration follows invasion of the portal connective tissue by leucocytes and later by hyperplasia of the fibrous tissue. Even in the absence of hepatic necrosis in the rabbit the connective tissue proliferates and invades the hepatic parenchyma, producing pseudo-lobulation. The only explanation offered by the author to this proliferative stimulation is the diffusion of substances from the parasites body through the histiocytes-vessel walls barrier.

Pulmonary lesions

SHAW and GHAREEB [25] in their well known paper on pulmonary schistosomiasis call attention to the role of this parasitosis in the genesis of a particular type of cor pulmonale.

These authors and almost all pathologist who have studied this subject, consider the ova as the principal etiologic agent of the socalled "chronic schistosomial cor pulmonale" [4, 5, 7, 15]. JAFFÉ [13], BARROS et al. [1] believe the vascular lesions to be the result of allergic mechanism, while FARIA [10] interprets alterations such as diffuse endarteritis, hyaline and fibrinoid degeneration of the vessel walls as being due to toxic or allergic reactions. These lesions would increase the permeability of the blood vessel walls, resulting in a serous and fibrinous inflammation of the intima. MAGALHÃES Fo. [17] emphasizes the primary lesions produced by the schistosomula in their migration through the lungs, before reaching the portal circulation.

It should be emphasized that the incidence of the misnamed bilharzial pulmonary arteritis or bilharzial cor pulmonale is relatively low in relation to the number of infected people. It must be also remembered that pulmonary involvement by schistosomiasis does not necessarily indicate arterial lesions.

Pseudo-tubercles without signs of arterial or arteriolar involvement are the most common lesions.

In 282 patients with schistosomiasis, SHAW and GHAREEB [25] found that 33% had pulmonary lesions and only 2.1%, diffuse vascular damage.

In 297 cases observed by the author at the University of Recife, Brazil, 16.4% had pulmonary lesions but only 1.3% pulmonary arteritis.

The figures of the prevalence of the so-called idiopathic cor pulmonale (including the cases of bilharziasis) are almost the same in Recife, northeast Brazil, which is a high endemic area as in Ribeirao Preto, southwest Brazil, where the parasitosis does not exist. KENAWY [15] who considered the ova as the cause of cor pulmonale, stated that "the syndrome is not an uncommon cause of rught-sided heart failure in Egypt but it is definitely less common than rheumatic heart disease which is prevalent among the Egyptians."

It is the author's opinion that the majority of the cases described as primary bilharzial pulmonary arteritis are cases of pulmonary hypertension induced by some other causes, complicated by schistosomial infection. Experimentally the embolization of the pulmonary arteries of dogs, by dead worms, promotes a proliferative endarteritis with recanalization that reproduces some of the pictures seen in "bilharzial cor pulmonale" (Fig. 4). The fundamental lesions are obtained in this way, lacking only the later complication by the ova.

These observations support the author's concept of the pathogenesis of the syndrome, that the arteriolar branches of the pulmonary artery are occluded by some type of emboli (including dead worms) and later are recanalized.

With the increase of the hydrostatic pressure in the blood vessels, "venous like" structures develop permitting the ova to lodge in them to produce the granulomatous lesions erroneously described as micro-aneurysm of the artery. The proliferating connective tissue of these structures invades the arteriolar lumens and further reduces the vascular diameter increasing the hydrostatic pressure.

Recanalization takes place at the level of the emboli and the newly formed capillaries will retain the ova, giving the false impression that the pseudo-tubercles are the cause of the vascular obstruction instead of the result.

It must be recalled that only in exceptional cases, an endarterial proliferation induced by an ovum, has been demonstrated in the intima of an arteriole. What is generally seen is the granulomatous lesions at the level of capillaries where the vascular lumen is smaller than the diameter of the ovum.

To find the ova in a large vessel it is necessary to have an early occlusion and recanalization, as previously mentioned.

In conclusion, it is important to emphasize that none of the vascular lesions described in the bilharzial arteritis are typical of this parasitosis. They also occur in cases of pulmonary hypertension of any etiology [24].

References

[1] BARROS, O. M., F. G. GIANNONI, E. MARIGO, and F. J. FRIZZO: „Cor pulmonale" e mio-cardite esquistossomoticas. Arch. Hosp. S. Casa S. Paulo 2, 33—72 (1956).

[2] BOGLIOLO, L.: Sobre o quadro anatomico do figado na forma hepato-esplenica da esquistossomose mansonica. Hosp. (Rio de J.) 45 283—306 (1954).

[3] — Segunda contribuicao ao conhecimento do quadro anatomico do figado na esquistossomose mansonica hepato-esplenica. Hosp. (Rio de J.) 47, 507—542 (1955).

[4] — Pathological changes in mansoni bilharziasis. Rev. Anat. Pat. Oncol. 23, 269—297 (1963).

[5] CHAVES, E.: Cor pulmonale cronico esquistossomotico. II Alguns aspectos das lesoes vasculares pulmonares causadas pelos ovos de S. mansoni. Rev. Inst. Med. Trop. S. Paulo 2, 163—170 (1960).

[6] COELHO, B., H. MENEZES, and Fo. A. MAGALHÃES: Esquistosomiase mansoni experimental Lesoes hepaticas de cobaios infestados e submetidos a tratamento pelo tartarato de sodio e antimonila. Rev. Bras. Med. 6, 378—383 (1949).

[7] COELHO, R. B., and J. A. M. CARVALHO: Lesoes arteriais pulmonares na esquistossomose mansonica. Anais III Reuniao Bienal Soc. Brasil. Patologistas. 71—101. Parana: Imprensa Universitaria 1962.

[8] COUTINHO, B., L. TAVARES, and H. MENEZES: Lesoes hepaticas no tratamento da esquistosomiase atribuidas aos vermes mortos. Rev. Bras. Med. 1, 660—662 (1944).

[9] ELIAS, H., and H. POPPER: Venous distribution in livers. Arch. Path. 59, 332—340 (1955).

[10] FARIA, J. L.: Histopatologia da endarterite pulmonar esquistossomotica (S. mansoni). S. Paulo. Brasil Emprêsa Grafica da Revista dos Tribunais 1952.

[11] GIRGES, R.: Schistosomiasis mansoni. Lancet 1, 816—819 (1929).

[12] HASHEM, M.: The aetiology and pathogenesis of the endemic form of hepato-splenomegaly "Egyptian splenomegaly". J. Roy. Egyp. Med. Ass. 30, 48—79 (1947).

[13] JAFFE, R.: Communicaciones sobre bilharziosis pulmonar. Gac. Méd. Caracas 46, 390—393 (1939).

[14] — Anatomia patologica y patogenia de la bilharziosis mansoni en Venezuela. Arq. Venezuelanos Patol. Trop. y Parasitol. Med. 1, 32—62 (1948).

[15] KENAWY, M. R.: The syndrome of cardio-pulmonary schistosomiasis (cor pulmonale). Amer. Heart J. 39, 678—696 (1950).

[16] KOPPISCH, E.: Studies in S. mansoni in Puerto Rico. J. Pub. Hlth. Trop. Med. 18, 1—54 (1937).

[17] MAGALHÃES, Fo, A.: Pulmonary lesions in mice experimentally infested with S. mansoni. Amer. J. Trop. Med. Hyg. 8, 527—535 (1959).

[18] — H. MENEZES, and B. COELHO: Patogenese da fibrose hepatica na esquistossomose mansoni (estudo das alteraces vasculares portais mediante modelo plastico). Rev. Ass. Med. Bras. **6**, 284—294 (1960).

[19] MENEZES, H.: Experimental intrahepatic portal embolism induced by adult Schistosoma mansoni. Amer. J. Trop. Med. Hyg. **12**, 741—744 (1963).

[20] — Embolizacao experimental dos ramos intra-hepaticos da veia porta de coelhos porexemplares adultos de Schistosoma mansoni. Rev. Inst. Med. Trop. S. Paulo **5**, 70—74 (1963).

[21] MOLINA, R. R.; Schistosomiasis mansoni, cirrhosis of the liver with splenomegaly and macrocytic anemia. Bol. Assoc. Med. Puerto Rico 28, 119—120 (1936).

[22] POPPER, H., and H. ELIAS: Histogenesis of hepatic cirrhosis studied by the three dimentional approach. Amer. J. Path. **21**, 405 (1955).

[23] RASO, P.: Lesoes vasculares intra-hepaticas na forma hepato-esplenica da esquistossomose mansonica. Hosp. (Rio de J.) **52**, 517—550 (1957).

[24] ROSSAL, R. E., and H. THOMPSON: Formation of new vascular channels in the lungs of a patient with secondary pulmonar hypertension. J. Path. Bact. **76**, 593—598 (1958).

[25] SHAW, A. F. B., and A. A. GHAREEB: The pathogenesis of pulmonary schistosomiasis in Egypt with special reference to Ayerza's disease. J. Path. Bact. **46**, 401—429 (1938).

[26] SOROUR, M. F.: Bilharziasis of the blood vessels. Proc. Roy. Soc. Med. **23**, 1369—1370 (1930).

[27] TAVARES, L., and H. MENEZES: Estudo experimental das lesoes hepaticas no tratemento da esquistosomiase mansoni, atribuidas aos vermes mortos. Rev. Bras. Med. **2**, 455—458 (1945).

The Pathogenesis of Schistosomiasis Mansoni

L. Bogliolo*

With 10 figures

Pathogenesis is taken to indicate formal genesis of lesions provoked by an etiologic agent and, in the present case, the mechanisms by which *Schistosoma mansoni* causes lesions. It is evident that the anatomical and clinical forms in which the disease presents itself will depend upon these mechanisms. It is also clear that the mechanisms will be multiple and will vary qualitatively, quantitatively, and chronologically through the influence of various factors. Nonetheless, nearly all classifications of schistosomiasis limit themselves to grouping the clinical or anatomo-clinical forms in which the disease can be seen on the basis of symptomatology, parasitologic criteria (phase of invasion, maturation and post-maturation) or static anatomic lesions already fully developed and characterized. Such classifications do not consider the mechanisms by which the etiologic agent provokes the lesion.

Except for the classification of Girges [11], who speaks of "phases" of the disease in an attempt to establish the diverse manifestations of schistosomiasis in a causal context, no interpretations seem to exist to explain the disease as a single entity or to outline its natural history. In particular, these interpretations do not attempt to clarify the interrelationships between the state of reactivity of the organism and the states of general and local reactivity of the host. This interrelation determines the clinical-anatomical forms in which diseases present themselves, evolve and heal, anatomically or clinically.

In other words, there is no interpretation which attempts to define the initial reactions provoked by *Schistosoma mansoni*, their evolution, the modifications, the constituents, the successor, their interrelationships with the manifestations in the tissue and, therefore, with the development of the anatomical and clinical forms of the disease. It is clear that many other factors may modify the general reaction of the host and the inflammatory response. These variables might include the strain of the parasite, the intensity of infections, reinfections and the interval between reinfections, the nutritional state of the host and of the parasite, and others. It is permissible to predict, however, that the same mechanisms and principles which influence the interrelationships between the general and local reactivity of the host in other prolonged infections are also active in schistosomiasis. Theories that invoke the action of parasitic toxins, the effects of unisexual infections, dead worms or local reaction to eggs etc. do not satisfactorily explain these interactions. Nor do they explain the appearance of the diverse types of local reactions or the manifestations in different clinical-anatomical forms.

In fact, many anatomical and clinical phenomena can only be explained if one admits that the response of the host to the parasite: a) is already qualitatively and

* Department of Anatomical Pathology, Faculty of Medicine, University of Minas Gerais. Belo Horizonte, Brazil.

quantitatively established in the first or invasive phase of the infection; b)manifests itself through the interactions of general and local sensitivity, also qualitatively and quantitatively variable; and c) is subject to modification during the course of the disease: at first by the maturation of the worms and later by the presence of eggs, their penetration and destruction, or persistence in the tissue. It is also possible that the state of viability or maturation of the eggs interferes, in part, with the nature and intensity of the local and general responses. Subsequent modification of the response may be affected by new infections or by the death of eggs and worms through treatment, etc.

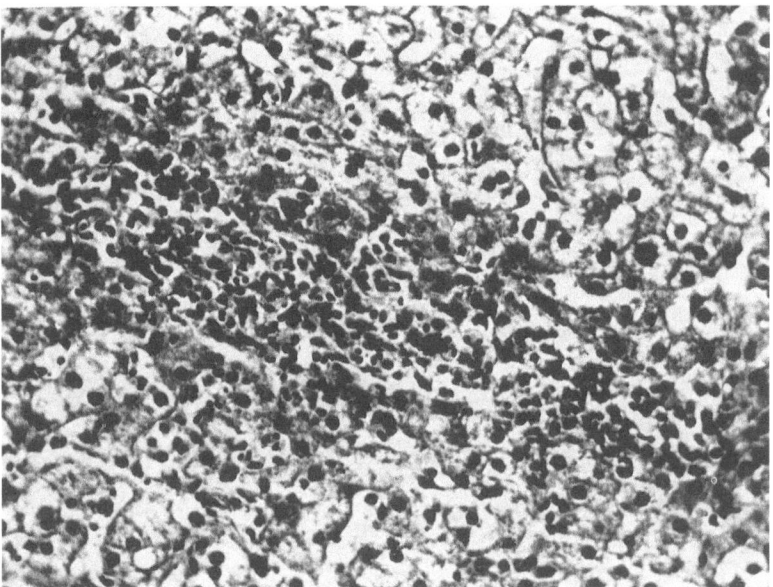

Fig. 1. *Acute toxemic mansonic schistosomiasis in man.* Intense acute focal hepatitis, not related topographically with schistosomulae. Needle biopsy 23 days after the infection

There exists certain observations of the evolution of *S. mansoni* infections which cannot be intelligently interpreted in the context of present theories, and which should be re-analized in the light of the above concepts. The following well known facts may be cited:

1. Beginning of the toxemic form – at times explosively 15–25 days after exposure and therefore prior to maturation of the worms or deposition of eggs. We have had occasion to observe needle biopsies of the liver in human cases 22, 23 and 25 days after exposure and again between 45 and 60 days [9, 10]. A more or less intense hepatitis already exists in the pre-postural phase, in foci which do not contain schistosomulae.

2. The nature of the hepatitis changes and it becomes more severe, clinically and anatomically, after the inception of oviposition. Besides the presence of granulomas, which have certain distinct characteristics to be described later, the intralobular and extralobular infiltrates become more extensive.

3. Splenomegaly is noted on the 15th to 25th day of the infection, before oviposition, and becomes more marked after egg laying. In our experience with

8 autopsies, the spleen showed the characteristics of acute infectious splenitis. Except for the almost constant presence of intense focal eosinophilic infiltrates, this splenitis was essentially identical to that encountered in the majority of acute, toxic infectious diseases.

4. Intestinal symptoms begin before the phase of oviposition, and are characterized by abdominal colic and diarrhea which is more or less intense but rarely bloody. In all cases, these symptoms become worse after the initiation of egg laying, and the feces become bloody. Most importantly, as demonstrated in autopsied cases [9, 10], the type of the intestinal lesions is entirely different from

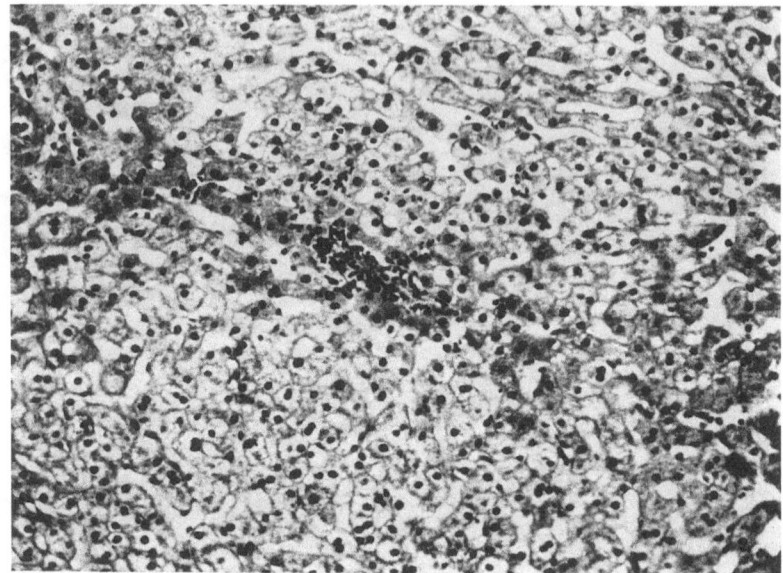

Fig. 2. *Acute toxemic mansonic schistosomiasis in man.* Acute focal hepatitis not related topographically with schistosomulae. Needle biopsy 25 days after exposure

those of the "intestinal form" of schistosomiasis. The lesions of the acute stage are characterized by numerous small superficial necrotic and hemorrhagic ulcerations of the intestinal mucosa, including that of the jejunum and ileum. The number of ulcers is far out of proportion to the number of eggs seen in the mucosa and, in fact, the majority of the eggs and granulomas are localized on the serosal surface. From the purely morphological point of view, the lesions are analagous to those seen in the intestine in the Shwartzman phenomenon [9].

5. Immunologically competent cells are seen in inflammatory infiltrates in the liver before oviposition. After it, these cells become more abundant, aggravating the hepatitis.

6. The serum gamma globulins remain at nearly normal levels during the pre-oviposition phase, when hepatitis and acute infectious splenitis already exist. The gamma globulin becomes abnormally high, frequently with inversion of the albumin/globulin ratio, after egg laying, as the hepatitis and splenomegaly become more marked [10].

7. The toxemic form of the disease, unequivocal in its clinical and anatomical (confirmed by autopsy) manifestations, has been noted in an individual infected many years previously and with hepato-splenic schistosomiasis and Symmers' fibrosis [12, 14]. This fact indicates that, at a certain moment, a change or modification occured of the already existing sensitivity or reactivity.

8. The necrotic and exudative types of reaction to the eggs, minimal at times and extremely intense at others, are not always related to the state of eggs maturation. Thus Andrade speaks of hypoergic, normergic and hyperergic reactions, referring to the granulomas [2]..

9. The systematized periportal fibromas and vascular neoformation, which characterize the lesions of Symmers' fibrosis [17], are noted in only a small fraction of infected people, and it has long been recognized that the fibrosis is out of proportion to the number of eggs and granulomas encountered and to the always relatively slight, though persistent, inflammatory reaction. Symmers' lesion could perhaps be best described as hyperplastic, and slowly progressive, even after the disappearance of granulomas.

10. In a certain percentage of cases with the chronic intestinal form of the disease, the formation of polyps also represents excessive, hyperplastic neoformation, disproportionate to the small number of eggs or worms encountered and to the usually slight inflammatory reaction.

11. When eggs are found in ectopic or unusual locations, such as the mesentery, the intestinal serosa, the retroperitoneal tissues etc., the same hyperplastic connective tissue reaction is seen, also out of proportion to the quantity of eggs, immature worms or inflammatory reaction [1, 3, 7]. The tumor-like neoformations produced may be of considerable size, and we have seen one weighing more than four kilograms.

12. In the chronic intestinal form, bouts of hemorrhagic necrosis of the intestinal mucosa, similar to those of the toxemic form, have been noted [8]. This reactivation of the anatomical lesion is accompanied by acute crisis of the clinical symptomatology.

13. In rare cases in which eggs are localized in the brain, there may occur lesions of the vascular wall which are disproportionate to the few eggs and the modest inflammatory reaction present. We have seen such a case in a man of 22 in whom there were various hemorrhagic episodes, terminating in massive cerebral hemorrhage [16] demonstrated at autopsy. The necrotic vascular lesions could not be related to any other cause than schistosome infection, despite the great reluctance to admit the existence of such relationship.

Having examined some of the phenomena which occur in the course of schistosome infections, we must now attempt to see if the information available is sufficient to explain the means by which the etiologic agent *(S. mansoni)* determines the various types of lesions (anatomo-clinical forms) in the course of human infection. The lesions may assume different types, corresponding to different anatomico-clinical forms. In an infected person, at a given moment, the form of reaction may vary; for example, the acute toxemic state may develop in a chronically infected patient with hepatosplenic schistosomiasis.

The information derived from experimental schistosome infections can be applied to human pathology only in the initial phases of the infection. At least, in the acute phase, the findings in small laboratory animals and man before and soon after ova deposition appear comparable. Although the opposite opinion is held by some authors, the chronic forms have not been demonstrated in laboratory animals, where no examples have been seen of hepatosplenic schistosomiasis with Symmers' fibrosis, of the intestinal polypoid type and of the cardiopulmonary form. This could perhaps be explained in part by the short life span of these

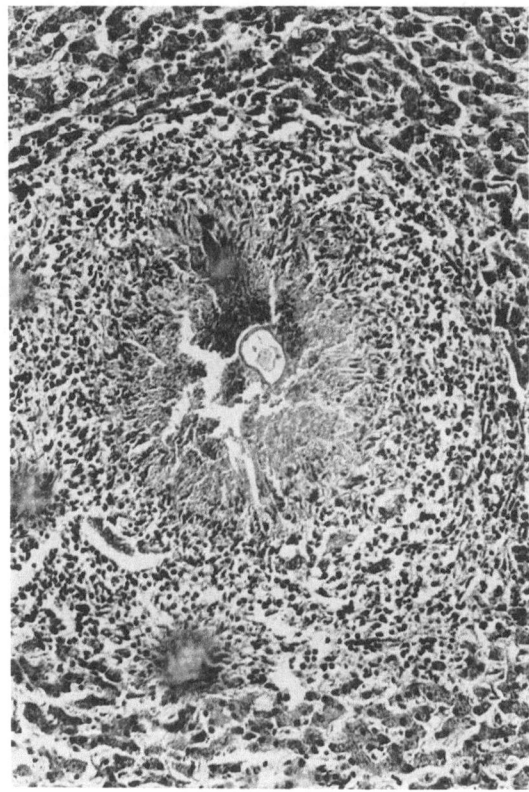

Fig. 3. *Acute toxemic mansonic schistosomiasis in man.* Large necrotic zone and intense eosinophilic infiltrate around an egg. Approximately 3 months after exposure

animals and in part by differences in the reaction of the human and animal host to the infection. On the other hand, information is available concerning the reactions of reinfected small animals but similar data from man are scarce.

We would provisionally summarize the available data as follows:

1. Reactions and lesions which appear before maturation of the worms, excluding the period immediately after penetration of the carcariae (i. e. after the 7th to 10th days).

Developing between the 15th and 25th days these consist principally of acute infectious splenomegaly and intralobular and extralobular hepatitis. The inflammatory foci in the liver are not topographically related to schistosomulae. In the mouse and rat this reaction is constant, and a certain number of animals may succumb. The presence of the reaction in man has been confirmed by needle biopsy of the liver but it is not known whether this is constant. In laboratory animals there is hyperplasia of reticuloendothelial cells in the liver and spleen, together with an initial increase in plasma cells. In the human liver, the hyperplasia of reticuloendothelial cells is slight. The nature of histologic changes in other organs is not known, since autopsies have not been done in this phase. In man, gamma globulin levels are normal.

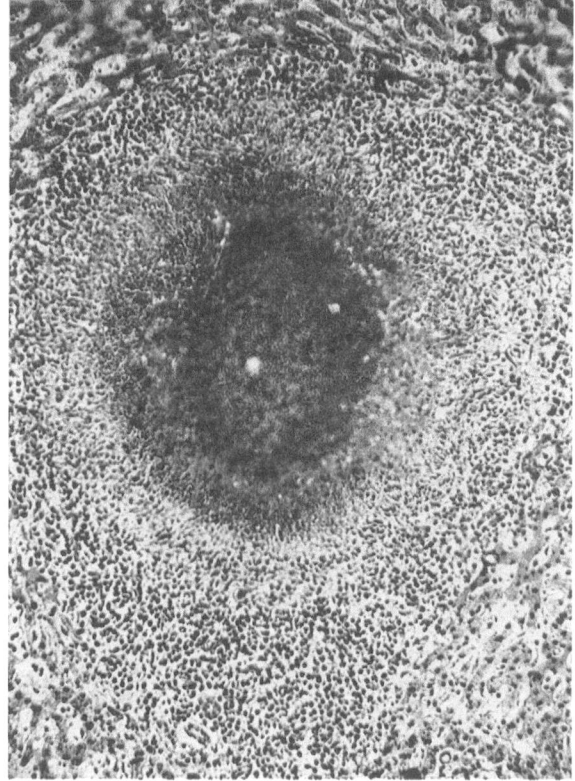

Fig. 4. *Acute toxemic mansonial schistosomiasis in man.* Explanations as in Fig. 7

A general host reactivity, with concomitant anatomical lesions in various organs (spleen, liver, and perhaps lungs) is indicated by hepatosplenomegaly and the frequently sudden onset of general symptoms such as fever, joint pains, headache, dry cough etc. At times these symptoms are preceeded by generalized urticaria, which is independent of the cutaneous reaction produced by cercarial penetration. It is not known if this reaction is constant in man, indeed the spectrum of variations in the intensity of the reactions is unknown since the only cases studied were those with evident clinical symptomatology. It is therefore legitimate to conjecture that the type of host reaction to the parasite is conditioned by the initial reaction, which may in part determine subsequent reactions and consequently the anatomico-clinical forms in which the disease manifests itself.

2. In a certain number of cases, the hepatitis and splenomegaly become more marked after egg deposition and are accompanied by slight generalized lymphadeno-

190   L. BOGLIOLO:

pathy. The clinical syndrome may also be aggravated, at times after a period of
remission, and may present clearly toxic features. In certain cases, there is diffuse
necrotizing ulcerative enteritis with characteristics analogous to the Shwartzman
phenomenon. This development coincides with a marked destruction of eggs, while
the granulomas which develop, may show intense necrosis and eosinophilic
infiltrate. Eosinophilia is almost constant and the eosinophilic infiltration of

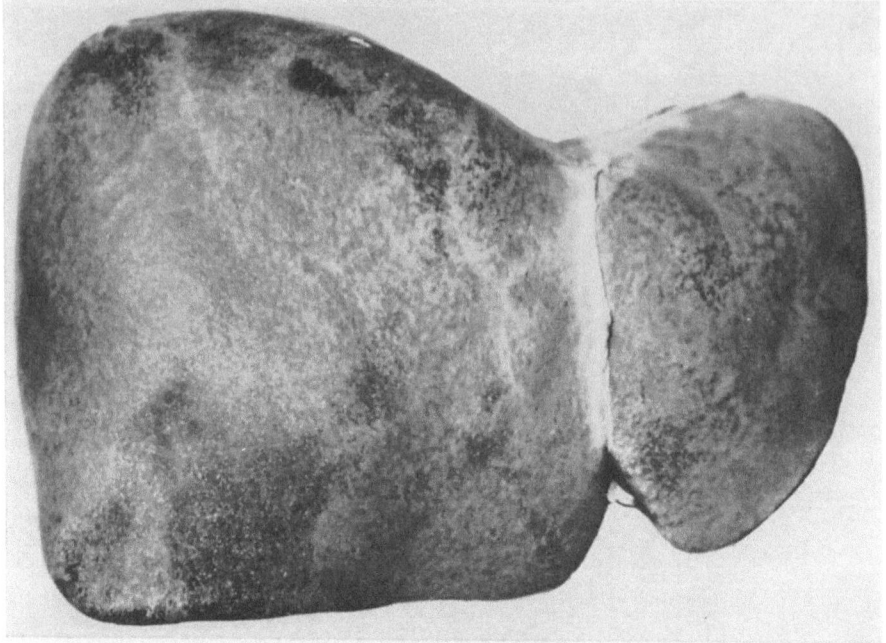

Fig. 5. *Acute toxemic mansonic schistosomiasis in man.* Massive dissemination of schistosomatic granulomas in the liver
3 months after exposure

the spleen is frequent. The reticuloendothelial reaction is intense, and abundant
plasmocytes appear. In man, plasmocytosis is noted especially in the lymphnodes.
In this phase there is an increase of serum alpha and gamma globulins and inversion
of the albumin globulins ratio.

In man, these phenomena were observed only in symptomatic cases and in a
few autopsied cases. It is reasonable to suppose that they exist, to a variable
degree, in a larger number of infected patients. In mice and rats the reaction is
almost constant, and also of variable intensity. In these animals the presence of
an antibody reaction has been noted around the eggs, and this is accentuated upon
disintegration of the eggs[2]. In the spleen there is an increase in the acid phosphatase and in the secretion of gamma globulins [2].

Taken together, these phenomena indicate that in a certain number of infected
persons there is a sudden change in host reactivity after oviposition, perhaps partly
conditioned by disintegration of eggs. This change is towards a state of general and
local hyperreactivity, or a state of hypersensitivity.

3. Development of the acute toxemic form of schistosomiasis in the course of
chronic infection.

The human cases in which this change has been satisfactorily documented are rare and to our knowledge no specific information exists on this phenomenon in experimental animals. In the only case observed by us, the chronic infection was documented by the existence of the typical lesions of hepato-splenic schistosomiasis, with Symmers' fibrosis and granulomas already in the fibrotic stage. The

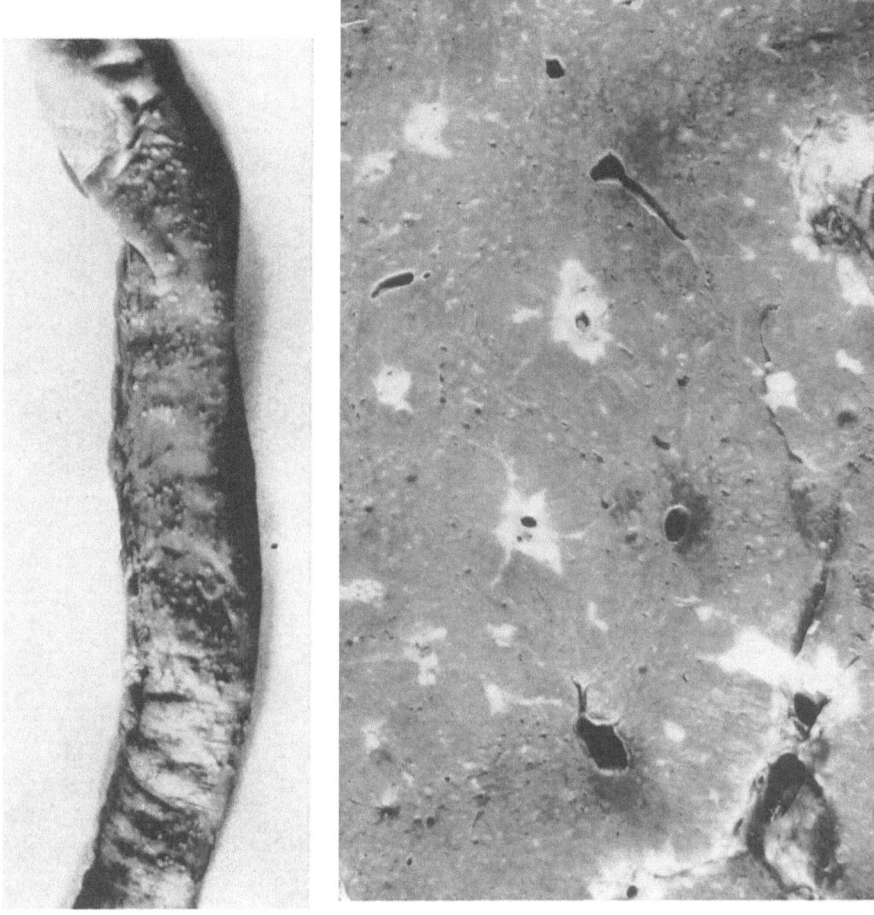

Fig. 6   Fig. 7

Fig. 6. *Acute toxemic mansonic schistosomiasis in man*. Massive dissemination of schistosomatic granulomas in the serosa of the small intestine 3 months after exposure

Fig. 7. *Acute toxemic mansonic schistosomiasis in the course of chronic infection (hepato-splenic form)*. Symmers' fibrosis of the liver

clinical history in this case indicated that reinfection was responsible for the toxemic form, and at autopsy, in addition to the lesions of chronic infection, the anatomic signs of recent infection were present. These included massive miliary dissemination of granulomas of nearly the same age, all in the necrotic-exudative phase, and with the characteristics previously noted. In the other organs also, the combination of acute and chronic lesions was noted. Specifically, the acute lesions of the toxemic phase in the spleen were associated with fibrocongestive changes.

The following conclusions seem warranted: a) protection against reinfection, documented in laboratory animals and probably existing in man, fails to occur in a number of individuals. b) Manifestations of the acute toxemic form which represent a form of hyperreactivity may occur in reinfected persons. In fact, the case cited had Symmers' fibrosis which, as we have already indicated and will elaborate later, seems to be conditioned by a peculiar state of chronic

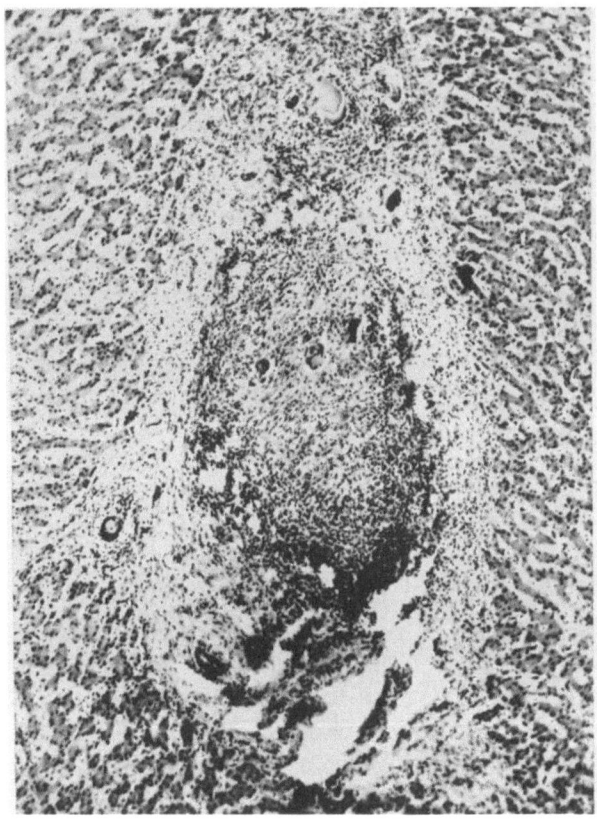

Fig. 8. *Same case as Fig. 9.* Death 130 days after the second exposure. Observe the recent acute granulomas

hyperreactivity. c) Thus a hypersensitivity reaction may occur in at least two different situations — 1) in the initial infection and, 2) occasionally in individuals already hypersensitive because of previous infection. One cannot therefore exclude the possibility that an analogous condition of hypersensitivity could arise in a chronically infected individual because of the changes in the nature of the immune reaction, independent of reinfection. d) One can also not exclude the possibility that in certain cases of reinfection this hypersensitivity reaction is not due to infection with a different strain of schistosome to which the first strain did not offer sufficient resistence.

4. The generalized formation of hyperplastic fibro-vascular tissue about the portal branches which characterizes Symmers' fibrosis, the typical and most

frequent form of hepatic fibrosis produced by *S.mansoni*, seems to be the result of an excessive local tissue reaction, in other words, of a local hyperactivity. In fact, worms, eggs and granulomas are encountered in the liver in almost all schistosome-infected patients, the eggs usually being found in the smaller portal branches, which they obliterate through production of intravascular granulomas. However, the obstruction of a certain number of these vessels is not accompanied by the generalized formation of fibrovascular tissue characteristic of Symmers' fibrosis, nor by disurbances of the portal circulation or clinical presentation of the hepatosplenic form of the disease. Hepatosplenic schistosomiasis mansoni is found almost exclusively in cases with Symmers' fibrosis. On the other hand, Symmers' fibrosis is seen in only a minority of infected patients. In Symmers' fibrosis, two types of lesions are encountered: a) intravascular or perivascular granulomas with or without obliteration of the vascular lumen, as we have emphasized and as is clearly shown in the studies of RASO [15]; b) the generalized formation of new fibrovascular tissue in the portal spaces. Only the latter is exclusively and characteristically pathognomonic of Symmers' fibrosis, and therefore of the absolute

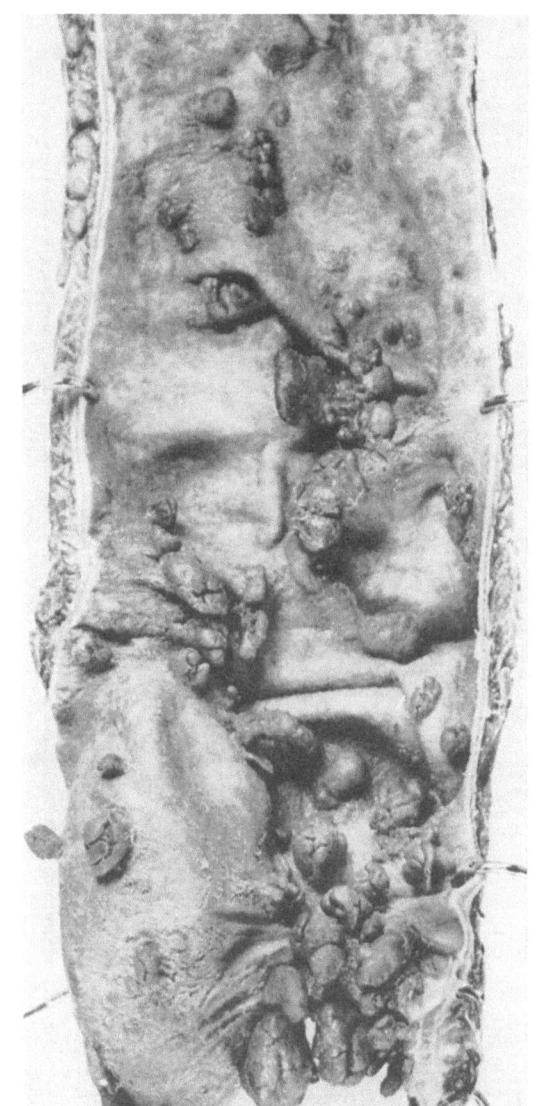

Fig. 9. *Chronic intestinal mansonial schistosomiasis.* Polypous form

majority of patients with hepato-splenic schistosomiasis mansoni. The first lesion is common to all infected persons; it does not seem to be accompanied by grave disturbances in the portal circulation, at least in the great majority of cases. The generalized formation of new connective tissue about the portal branches is not satisfactorily explained by lesions of the hepatic parenchyma, which in Symmers' fibrosis are always few and focal and never generalized. We should also consider that in massive infections as in the acute toxemic form, when the number of eggs and of granulomas in the liver is enormous, one does not find excessive new formation of the periportal connective tissue. One cannot therefore always attribute the excessive formation of connective tissue in Symmers' fibrosis to massive infections, nor to the mere phenomenon of fibrous replacement of destroyed hepatic parenchyma. We must find another explanation for its development and maintenance, more precisely, a factor which stimulates and conditions a hyperreactivity of the periportal connective tissue sheath. It is reasonable to think that this factor is a modification of the normal mode of reactivity to eggs and worms encountered in the majority of infected persons. Thus, Symmers' fibrosis also becomes an allergic rather than a normergic form of reactivity to schistosomiasis. It must be admitted that the mechanisms which lead to this modification of local tissue reactivity are not clearly understood.

5. The same consideration may be applied to the hyperplastic reactions (polyps etc.) of the chronic intestinal form and to the excessive formation of connective tissue sometimes seen when eggs and worms are localized in ectopic or unusual sites, such as the intestinal serosa, mesentery, retroperitoneum etc., where the tissue reaction may be disproportional to the intensity of infection. These lesions are also seen in only a minority of infected patients. For the same reasons previously cited, these manifestations should be considered as allergic rather than normergic.

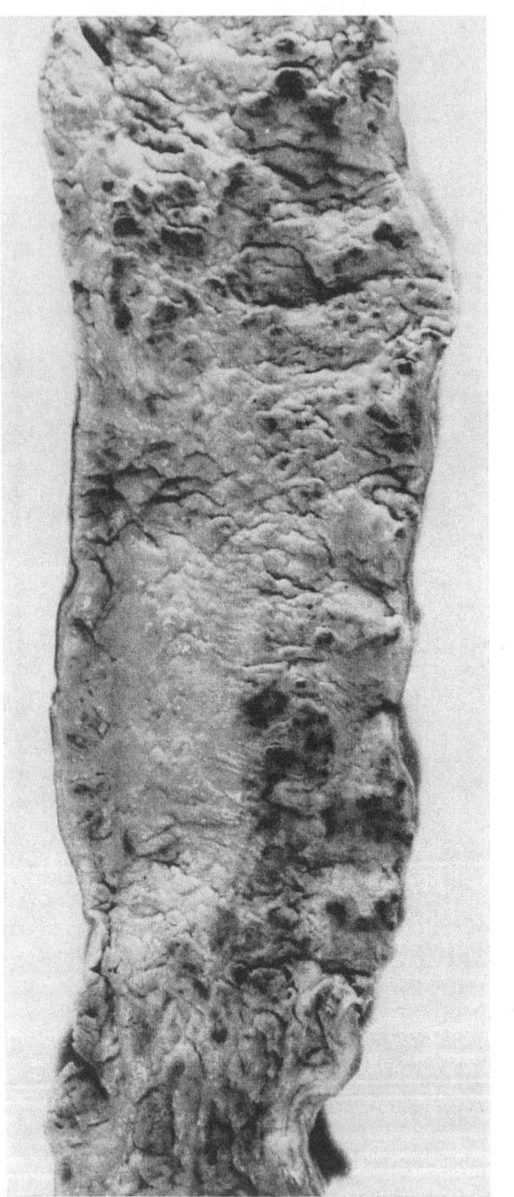

Fig. 10. *Acute eruptions in chronic intestinal mansonic schistosomiasis in man.* Superficial hemorrhagic acute ulcerations

6. Necrotic lesions, especially of blood vessels, as encountered in the rare case of cerebral schistosomiasis with massive hemorrhage, must also be considered to be other than normergic reactions. In the majority of infected persons with lesions of the brain or spinal cord seen by us or reported in the literature, the reaction to the eggs in surrounding tissues was not qualitatively or quantitatively different from that in other organs. We are forced to admit that in our case another factor may have changed the reaction to a different or local allergic type.

7. Finally, even the granulomas around schistosome eggs may be of different types not solely explained by the stage of the egg which provoked the lesions, lending support for Andrade's [1] concept of hypoergic, normergic and hyperergic granulomas. We have already indicated that in the acute toxemic forms the granulomas are frequently exaggerated, as compared to the usual reaction, and necrotic and exudative features corresponding to the hyperergic reaction of Andrade are present.

These observations indicate that the pathogenetic mechanisms in schistosomiasis are complex and cannot be explained only by the local action of schistosomules, dead worms or eggs. In our present state of understanding, we are forced to admit that the reactivity of the host, general and local, varies in different cases. Thus the anatomical and clinical forms in which the disease presents itself must be characterized not only by the stage of development of the parasite [2] in the organ most severely affected by the schistosomulae, mature worms or eggs; but also by the type and form of general and local reactivity. *Any proposed classification must consider the simultaneous interactions of these three factors if the natural history of the disease is to be understood.*

Summary

At the moment the known facts of the human and experimental pathology of schistosomiasis allow the following observations:

a) one type of reactivity of the host is established in the invasive phase, before maturation of the parasite, probably between the 15th and 25th days after the infection. In this phase, in the first infections, only schistosomulae are present. Thus it must be these, or more correctly, the products of their destruction, which condition the first type of reactivity of the host and in turn, determine the successive general and local reactions, i.e. those occurring after oviposition. In some individuals this reactivity will be abnormal, i.e. different from the general and local reactivity exhibited by the majority of infected patients. At the moment, the best known of these "abnormal" reactions is the acute toxemic form of the initial infection.

b) abnormal reactions may also occur in reinfections, the acute toxemic form having been noted in a patient with chronic hepato-splenic schistosomiasis.

c) therefore, in man reinfections are not always manifestated clinically because of acquired relative immunity.

d) abnormal local reactivity may also be seen in chronic forms of the disease, chiefly in the following forms: 1) the more common, predominantly hyperplastic form to which would belong Symmers' hepatic fibrosis, intestinal polyps and the pseudo tumors found in certain unusual sites; and 2) the predominantly necrotizing or necrotizing and exudative lesions as observed in the brain of one case.

To understand these last forms, one should perhaps consider each egg penetrating the tissues as a new infection, certainly as a new contact of the antigen with the sensitized tissue to result in a certain form of reaction.

References

[1] ANDRADE, Z. A., and G. RODRIGUES: Manifestacões pseudo-neoplásicas da esquistossomose intestinal. Arch. Bras. Med. **44**, 437—444 (1954).

[2] —, and T. BARKA: Histochemical observations on experimental schistosomiasis in mouse. Amer. J. Trop. Med. Hyg. **11**, 12—16 (1962).

[3] BICALHO, S. A.: Sôbre as neoformações conjuntivo-hiperplasticas pseudotumorais na esquistossomose mansoni. Organo Official de la Sociedad Venezolano de Gastroenterologia, Endocrinologia y Nutricion (G.E.N.) **19**, 256—271 (1965).

[4] BOGLIOLO, L.: Sôbre o quadro anatômico do fígado na forma hépato-esplênica da esquistossomose mansônica. Hospital (Rio de J.) **45**, 283—306 (1954).

[5] — Segunda contribuição ao conhecimento do quadro anatômico do fígado na esquistossomose mansônica hépato-esplênica. Hospital (Rio de J.) **47**, 507—542 (1955).

[6] — The anatomical picture of the liver in hepato-splenic schistosomiasis mansoni. Ann. trop. Med. Parasit. **51**, 1—14 (1957).

[7] — Patologia da esquistossomose mansônica. Rev. Bras. Malar. **11**, 359—424 (1959).

[8] — Pathological changes in mansonic bilharziasis. Riv. Anat. Pat. **23**, 269—297 (1963).

[9] — Subsídios para o estudo da anatomia patológica da forma aguda toxêmica da esquistossomose mansônica. G.E.N. **9**, 157—236 (1964).

[10] —, and J. NEVES: Ocorrência de hapatite na forma aguda ou toxêmica da esquistossomose mansônica, antes da maturacão dos vermes e da postura dos ovos, com algumas considerações sôbre a forma aguda ou toxêmica da esquistossomose. An. Fac. Med. (Lima) (in press).

[11] GIRGES, R.: Schistosomiasis (Bilharziasis) p. 529. London: J. Bale, Sons & Danielson Ltd. 1934.

[12] KATZ, N., and D. BITTENCOURT: Sôbre um caso de provável forma toxêmica no decurso da forma hepato-esplênica da esquistossomose mansônica. Hospital (Rio de J.) **67**, 847—858 (1965).

[13] KOPPISCH, E.: Studies on schistosomiasis mansoni in Puerto Rico — Morbid anatomy of the disease as found in Puerto Ricans. Puerto Rico J. Publ. Hlth. **16**, 395—455 (1941).

[14] NEVES, J., and P. RASO: Estudo anatomo-clínico de um caso de forma toxêmica da equistossomose mansônica que evoluiu para a forma hepatoesplênica em 130 dias (fibrose hepática tipo Symmers). Rev. Inst. Med. Trop. S. Paulo **74**, 256—266 (1965).

[15] RASO, P.: Lesões vasculares intra-hepáticas na forma hépato-esplênica de esquistossomose mansônica. Hospital (Rio de J.) **52**, 517—550 (1957).

[16] — W. L. TAFURI, N. DE ALMEIDA JR., J. A. RODRIGUES, J. M. SANTIAGO, and L. F. ROCHA: Hemorragia cerebral maciça devida ao schistosoma mansoni. Hospital (Rio de J.) **65**, 537—551 (1964).

[18] SYMMERS, W. ST. C.: Note on a new form of liver cirrhosis due to the presence of the ova of Bilharzia hematobia. J. Path. Bact. **9**, 237—239 (1904).

Radiological Pathology and Methods of Investigation in Schistosomiasis

J. H. MIDDLEMISS*

With 10 figures

It is unusual for any radiological examination to produce conclusive evidence of schistosomiasis, though calcification in the bladder wall due to a cause other than S. haematobium infection is so rare as to make this appearance of significant of diagnostic value in endemic areas. Of far greater value is the ability to demonstrate graphically structural changes in the organs and viscera of individuals known to have a schistosomal infection, and thus provide criteria for the clinical assessment of such cases. At the present time the life history of individuals with schistosomiasis is so little known or understood that graphic illustrations of pathological states and of structural organic changes are of the utmost value in the prognosis of those individuals and in the assessment of the effect of infection. Further, in areas of the world where schistosomiasis is endemic, in the investigations of individuals with specific symptoms and signs, the demonstration of certain structural changes may lead to a positive diagnosis which in other circumstances would have been delayed. Indeed, in some circumstances during life, a positive and firm diagnosis of schistosomiasis may be so difficult to establish that such indirect data as can be provided by radiological means may, when added to that obtained from other laboratory methods, be of considerable significance in establishing the diagnosis and its effects.

In the following section S. haematobium, S. mansoni and S. japonicum are considered separately, except for the radiological discussion of cardiopulmonary disease, the manifestations of which appear to be identical irrespective of the form of schistosomiasis.

S. haematobium infections

Radiological investigation in the first instance consists of plain radiography of the urinary tract and excretion urography. The abnormalities that may be noted are:

1) Calcification in the bladder wall. This is a relatively late feature in the natural history of the infection. Eggs deposited in the mucosa and submucosa of the bladder wall cause a cellular reaction, ulceration, and haemorrhage followed by fibrosis. Though eggs continue to be passed many remain lodged in the fibrous tissue in the bladder wall and these entombed eggs eventually become necrotic and calcify. At first this is seen as a thin intermittent line of calcification in the bladder wall but subsequently it shows as a pencil-line of calcification round the entire bladder, sometimes becoming very dense (Fig. 1). This often extends to outline the lower ureters where eggs have been similarly entombed. Occasionally

---

* Department of Radiology, United Bristol Hospitals. Department of Radiodiagnosis, University of Bristol, England.

the whole ureter, or the seminal vesicles or even the posterior urethra may be thus demonstrated (Fig. 2). Sometimes, clusters of ova have been encased in mounds of granulation tissue and when they calcify they show as undulations in the bladder wall, possibly simulating calculi, but distinguishable from calculi in that they do not change position with change of posture (Fig. 3). This calcification does not affect the muscle coat and so can be observed to distend and contract with filling and emptying of the bladder. Occasionally a space-occupying lesion interrupting the smooth calcific edge of the bladder and projecting into its cavity can be

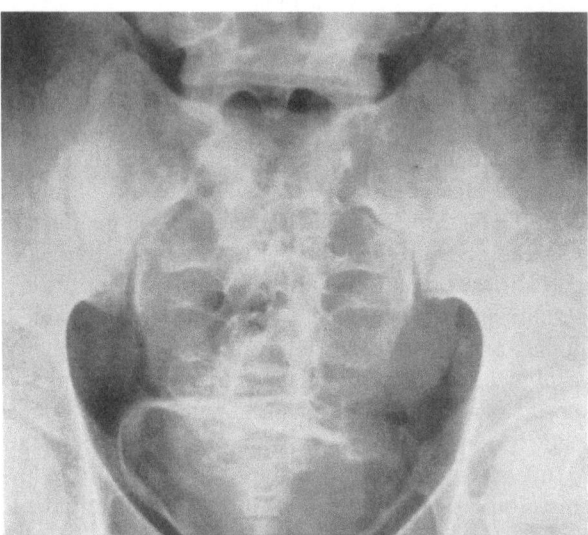

Fig. 1. Calcification in the wall of a bladder still retaining its normal contours

tentatively diagnosed as carcinoma. Examples of this latter feature have been seen by the writer in Egypt and Rhodesia. Similarly urinary calculi will occasionally be demonstrated. They appear to occur with greater frequency in Egypt than elsewhere. They may be in the bladder or sometimes in the lower end of the ureter, held up there by stenosis at the lower end of the ureter.

2) At excretion urography, ureteric narrowing, hydro-ureter, hydronephrosis, non-functioning kidney or filling defects in the lower ureter and bladder, may be demonstrated. The actual mechanism or underlying pathological cause of some of these features is at present incompletely understood.

If ureteric narrowing is demonstrated it is usually in the lower third. It may show merely as the ureter tapering to a point and not being visualised beyond this point, or as a narrow segment. It is not known if this early radiological feature is due to fibrotic stenosis or merely due to reactive oedema and swelling of the ureteric mucosa, though in advanced cases of ureteric schistosomiasis fibrosis is a well recognised condition; in this latter condition however there is usually impairment of kidney function and radiological demonstration is poor or is not achieved by excretion urography.

Quite often hydro-ureter is seen. The early stage of hydroureter may be difficult to assess, for in the normal adult during passage of urine or contrast medium down the ureter, this structure may distend to a radiographic diameter of as much as one centimetre (Fig. 4), though usually it is not so wide, and usually only one spindle is thus demonstrated, commonly the middle third of the ureter. The demonstration of a ureter as wide as this on a single film may, therefore, be a normal feature or due to pathology, and must be assessed with care. If it is due to

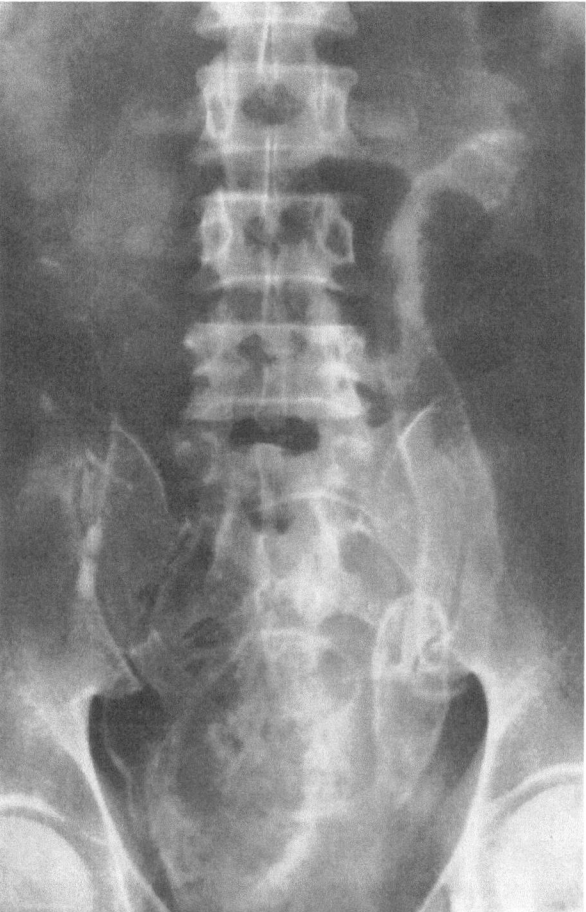

Fig. 2. Calcification in the bladder wall and along the lengths of both ureters

pathology it is likely to persist in more than one film and to affect more than the middle third of the ureter; in gross cases the ureter may be enormously dilated.

Similarly hydronephrosis may be demonstrated. In the normal kidney the minor calyces appear as well cupped structures. In the early stage of hydrone-phrosis this cupped shape appears "blunted". This proceeds to loss of the cupping and thence to dilatation of the calyces, (Fig. 5), and such dilatation can reach immense proportions relative to the normal size. At the same time as the develop-ment of advanced calyceal dilatation there is usually also dilatation of the renal pelvis. Concurrent with this structural change in the upper urinary tract there is usually also impairment of concentration, and excretion of contrast medium by the affected kidney is therefore less good. Finally the function of a kidney may be so disturbed that little information about its structural state is obtained from this examination. The kidney merely shows as a "nephrogram"; this is to say the renal outline shows more densely than on the preliminary film due to intra-vascular

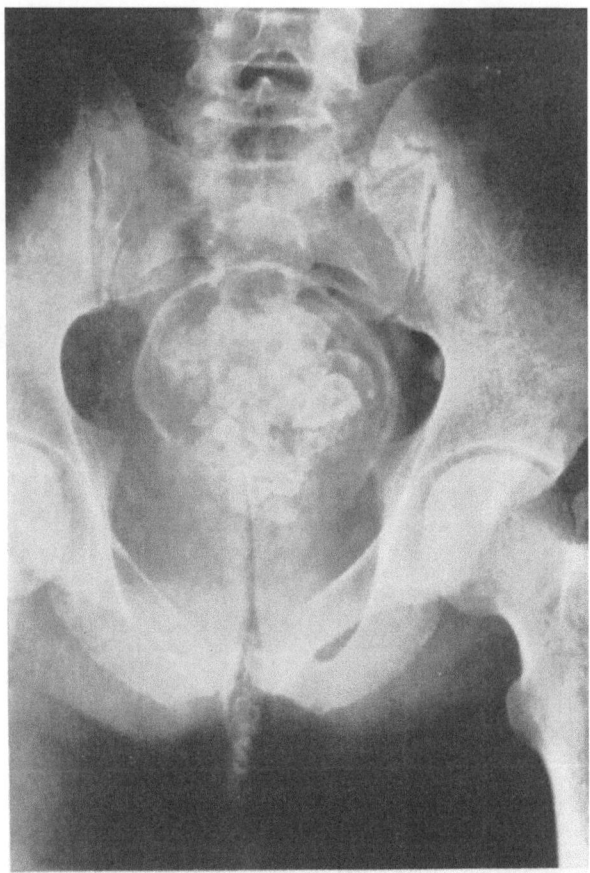

Fig. 3. Calcification in the bladder wall and in mounds of granulation tissue, as well as in the posterior urethra

contrast medium and thus appears to "blush". Renal damage however may be so great that not even this feature is shown, and radiologically the organ is a "non-functioning" kidney.

The effects on the upper urinary tract may occur in young persons, these changes having been observed from the age of six upwards. They are more common in boys than in girls, and may be unilateral or bilateral [11]. At present it is not clear to what extent these changes in the upper urinary tract are due to obstruction and to what extent they are due to ureteric reflux during micturition, though it must be stated that very little conclusive evidence, if any, has been put forward from any source to suggest that ureteric reflux has a large part to play in the earlier stages of the natural history of the disease. The conditions here described have been observed in East Africa, in Rhodesia and in Egypt. Curiously, to date, they have not been observed to any great extent in West Africa where S. haematobium infection also is common. In the present state of our knowledge the natural history of these upper urinary tract lesions is not known, and it can not be stated authoritatively whether they are progressive or may regress to any extent.

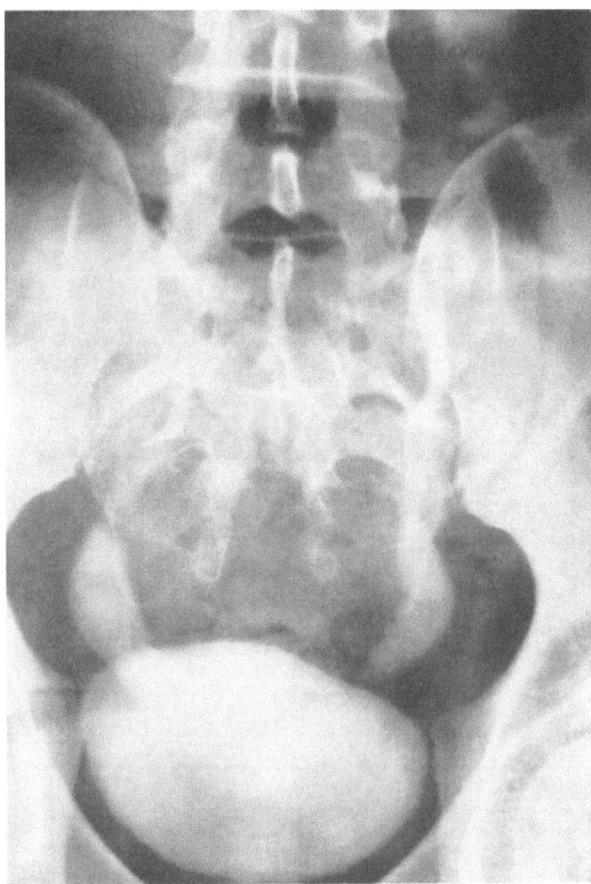

Fig. 4. Dilatation in the lower ends of both ureters

In the assessment of individual cases the technique of infusion of pyelography as described by SCHENKER [19] probably gives the greatest anatomical detail of the upper urinary tract. Further, in the assessment of the natural history of these lesions in individual cases, it is probable that the affected individual, commonly a young person, will be subject to more than one, possibly serial, urographic examinations and so a modified form of urography should be employed in order to limit the dose of radiation.

In Nigeria bladder lesions have been shown at excretion urography in this condition. These take the form of filling defects, "mounds" 1—3 cms in diameter protruding into the bladder cavity. Similar mounds smaller in size may be seen in the lower third of the ureter, particularly its terminal part. These lesions have not at the time of writing been observed cystoscopically, so their true nature is not known. They have been observed in symptomless children and young persons in community surveys assessing the incidence and significance of schistosomal infection.

The term "granuloma" has been applied to them but as they have been observed radiologically subsequently to resolve it seems possible that they are more in the nature of reactive oedema than true granulomatous masses [6].

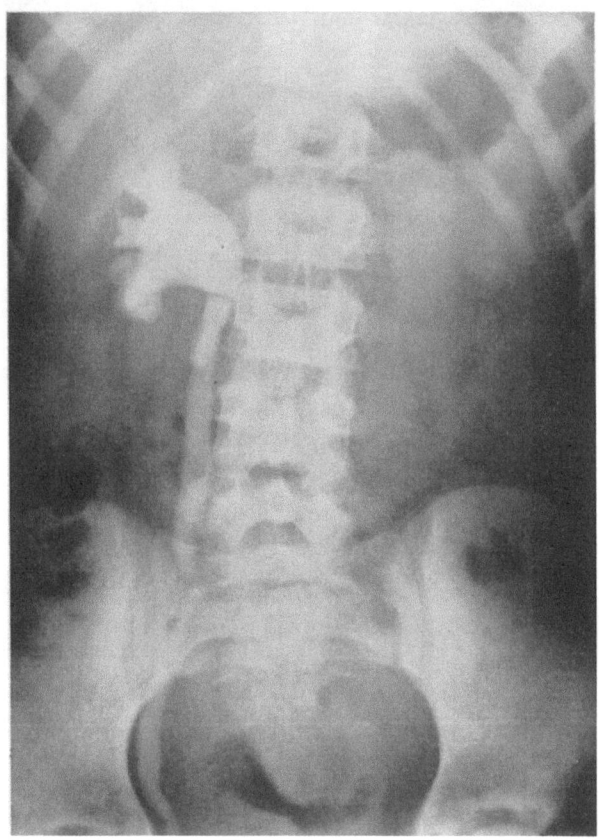

Fig. 5. Hydro-ureter of the whole right ureter with loss of "cupping" of the calyces of the right kidney. There is no evidence of function by the left kidney. The patient was an 8 year old girl whose only complaint was haematuria

In the later stages of the disease in the urinary tract bladder pathology is common, and this is often complicated by chronic secondary infection. Cystoscopy will often cause an acute flair-up of the infection. Plain radiography will often, as already described, assist in establishing the diagnosis, but two further radiological techniques, one of which can be employed without bladder instrumentation may provide further useful information regarding the interior of the bladder:

1) *Micturating cystography*. The bladder can be filled by the per-urethral method using a Knuttson clamp [24]. The bladder is then observed during micturition fluoroscopically and spot films taken. Ureteric reflux can thus be demonstrated. This procedure has been employed in Egypt in advanced cases

and reflux commonly demonstrated [15, 22], but to date no large series of relatively early cases of infection in young persons has been published.

Retrograde cystography by this method may also demonstrate filling defects in the contrast-filled bladder due to carcinoma. It is not the purpose of this paper to discuss the causal relationship between schistosomiasis and bladder carcinoma, but where the two are coincident this method of investigation may provide a positive diagnosis by a less traumatic means than cystoscopy, it having been shown [3] that growths with a diameter greater than 2 cm are like lyto be demonstrated.

2) Double contrast cystography by the technique of DOYLE [9]. This has been employed in advanced cases in Egypt by SINNA [22]. By this method he has been able to demonstrate, in addition to small growths, schistosomal ulcers on the bladder wall.

S. mansoni infections

Radiological investigation in the first instance consists of plain radiography of the abdomen and chest. This may confirm a clinical diagnosis of hepatomegaly and splenomegaly. Enlargement of the liver may be apparent by elevation of the right dome of the diaphragm or the soft tissue shadow of the lower edge may be seen low in the abdomen, displacing downwards colonic gas and faecal shadows. Spleen enlargement may be seen as a large soft tissue mass under the left dome of the diaphragm projecting downwards and medially in the abdomen. It frequently displaces the stomach gas bubble medially, and occasionally if the renal outlines are detectable, the left kidney may be seen to be displaced downwards.

Of the simpler X-ray examinsations this is the most frequently performed. However examination of the alimentary tract may provide valuable data especially in the colon, though at the present stage of our knowledge there would seem to be an excellent case for small bowel examinations to be carried out by a barium follow through technique. It is known that in S. mansoni infections eggs may be passed in large numbers from the small bowel. It would be surprising if the passage of such large numbers of eggs did not have some effect on bowel motility or absorption. The radiological diagnosis of malabsorption states is now a well-established procedure and the investigation of infected persons by this method may be fruitful. Such demonstrations would not necessarily contribute to a diagnosis of schisto-somiasis, but they may well enhance our knowledge of the effect on the individual of the infection.

Similarly examination of the colon by barium enema using the modern technique of incorporating a colonic adjuvant and followed by air insufflation is surprisingly not commonly undertaken. Yet by this method changes in bowel mucosa if they are relatively severe can be demonstrated. In S. mansoni infections when eggs ulcerate the mucous membrane healing takes place by fibrosis and subsequent crops of eggs may become entombed, producing an irritative reaction round which a granulomatous reaction may occur. This process can produce an alteration in the lumen of the bowel and in its mucosal surface — at sigmoidoscopy the wall may appear as a glistening granulation tissue or there may be actual blebs and polyps visible. Polyps can be demonstrated, both their size and the extent of bowel affected, by barium enema examination as was first demonstrated by RAGHEB [18] and subsequently by DIMMETTE and SPROAT [8]. They appear as mul-tiple small filling defects, most profuse in the sigmoid colon and are best seen

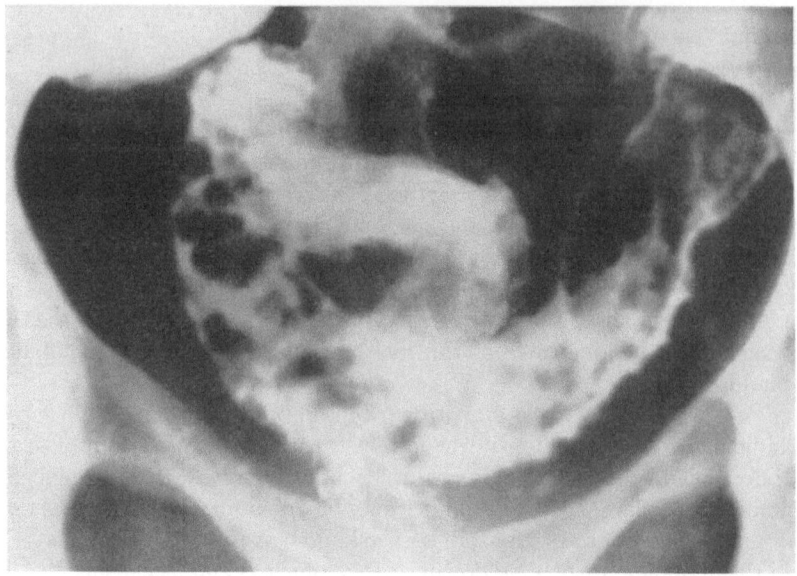

Fig. 6a. Polyps in the sigmoid colon of an adult with S. mansoni infection

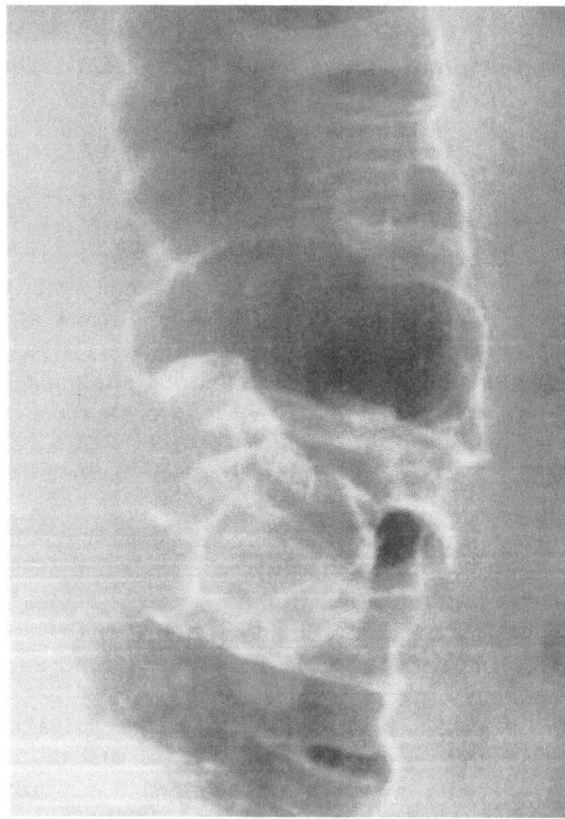

Fig. 6b. Granulomatous mass in the descending colon due to S. mansoni infection simulating carcinoma and causing
obstructive symptoms

in films taken after evacuation and preferably with air insufflation (Fig. 6a). Occasionally these parasitic granulomas assume large proportions, projecting into the bowel, narrowing the lumen and producing obstructive symptoms. These lesions have been reported from Brazil [23] and more recently from Porto Rico [20]. Radiologically they are indistinguishable from carcinoma (Fig. 6b); even

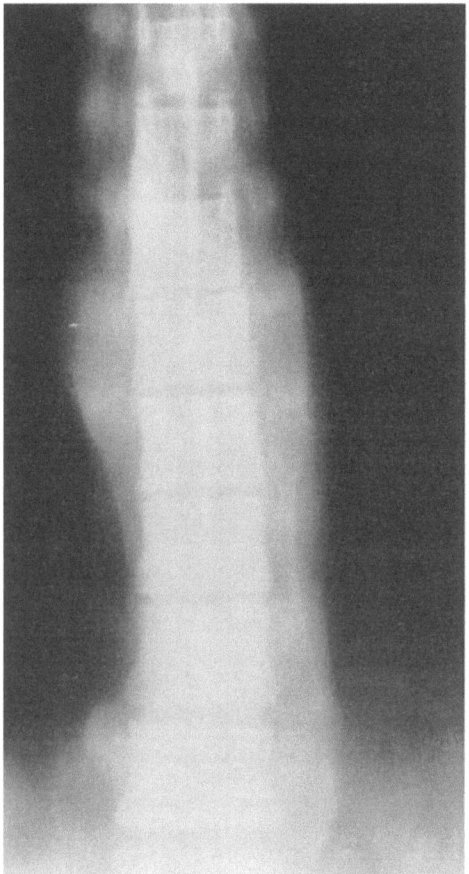

Fig. 7. Widening of both right and left paravertebral shadows due to varicosities in the azygos and hemi-azygos systems

after surgical resection, macroscopically they may appear to have the features of neoplasm, only histological examination showing their true nature.

When portal hypertension develops consequent upon the fibrotic changes in the liver radiological investigations can be undertaken to demonstrate the collateral circulation and to confirm that the increased resistance to the outflow of portal venous blood is due to an intra-hepatic obstruction. Collateral circulation develops where the portal blood can be diverted into systemic channels and this occurs most frequently round the oesophagus and the gastric fundus, retro-peritoneally and in the falciform ligament. The examinations that may help are:

1) Chest. A well penetrated chest film may show enlarged azygos and hemi-asygos veins if they are involved in the collateral circulation. The azygos vein is

normally seen as a small elliptical shadow adjacent to the right main bronchus. If it is distended it may reach a diameter on the radiograph of up to 2 cm [10]. The hemi-azygos vein is not seen on normal radiography but if it becomes varicose it can cause considerable widening of the left paravertebral shadow above the diaphragm (Fig. 7).

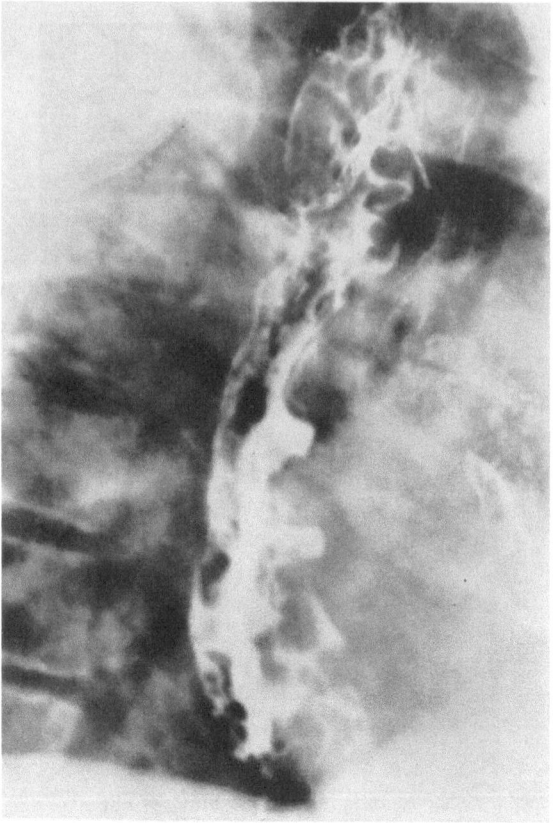

Fig. 8. Large oesophageal varices in a case of schistosomiasis with portal hypertension

2) Barium examination of the upper alimentary tract. Gastric varices are best demonstrated by coating the fundus with barium and then bringing the patient into the erect or prone position so that a double barium/air contrast of the fundus is obtained. The varices appear as lobulated or rounded filling defects in the fundus and upper part of the lesser curve. They may produce a large mass difficult to distinguish from carcinoma.

Oesophageal varices can only be demonstrated on good mucosal pattern films of the oesophagus, and may be difficult to demonstrate. The least useful position is the erect, the prone position being commonly the best, with the respiratory phase midway between inspiration and expiration. Small varices produce some thickening of, and small rounded projections on, the borders of the mucosal folds of the lower end of the oesophagus, and also filling defects on the oesophageal outline. Large varices produce linear, globular or worm-like filling defects of varying sizes and produce complete distortion of the mucosal pattern (Fig. 8). They may involve only the lower end or extend right up into the neck. Claims varying from 14%–87% of the accuracy of demonstrations of known varices have been made, but selection of cases probably accounts for this difference. Probably in the hands of an experienced radiologist an accuracy rate of 70–75% is a fair expectation.

3) Portal venography. The object of this examination is to demonstrate the state of the portal vein, the site of the obstruction, the collateral circulation and the

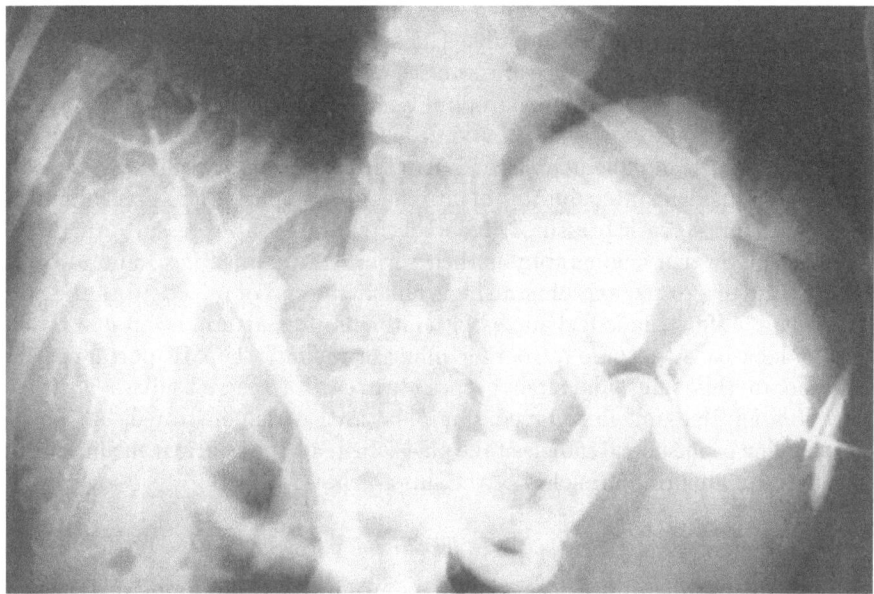

Fig. 9. Portal venogram in a case of schistosomiasis with portal hypertension showing a collateral pathway along the left gastric vein and large gastric varices

presence or absence of thrombi in the portal vein if any form of surgical portocaval anastomosis is contemplated. The usual method is by percutaneous trans-splenic injection. If splenectomy has been performed this cannot be carried out, and portal venography can then only be undertaken at operation by injection into a tributary of the superior mesenteric vein such as a jejunal vein. By the percutaneous method, using a wide-bore needle for splenic puncture (after which the splenic pulp pressure can be read with a manometer), 30 ml of contrast medium is injected rapidly into the spleen and serial films taken in rapid succession [16]. The normal portal venogram shows the splenic vein and portal vein.

The commencement of the portal vein is identifiable due to the streaming effect of blood from the superior mesenteric vein mingling with the contrast column. Within the liver it divides into left and right branches, which again divide into smaller branches, by simple forking, diminishing in size progressively as they pass to the periphery. Finally the contrast medium reaches the sinusoids and produces a "blush" i.e. a hepatogram. Where the obstruction is intra-hepatic as in S. mansoni infections the splenic and portal veins are patent, though the splenic vein may exhibit various degrees of tortuosity. Various collateral pathways are shown by retrograde flow of contrast medium along them, e.g. the left gastric vein often leads to varices in the fundus of the stomach, and these latter may also be filled from the short gastric veins (Fig. 9). These varicosities usually lead on to peri-oesophageal and oesophageal varices above the diaphragm. Inferior and superior mesenteric veins may be filled by retrograde flow and occasionally a large para-umbilical vein fills from the left branch of the portal vein. In the normal individual the spleen-to-liver time is usually 2—3 seconds. In intra-hepatic portal obstruction this time may be increased up to 6—7 sec. Within the liver distortion of the portal radicles may be shown. The main branches are often dilated and run a tortuous course, tapering rapidly. The smaller branches may be sparser than usual [1, 2]. It is in such cases rare to see a hepatogram.

4) Wedge hepatic vein angiography. Using the technique described by Sher-lock [21], Rodrigues da Silva and his colleagues [7] have recently been employing this technique in cases of S. mansoni infection. A catheter is introduced by the right median antecubital vein into the supra-hepatic vein. Free inferior vena cava and supra-hepatic pressures, and wedged supra-hepatic pressures are recorded. Wedge hepatic vein angiography is then performed by injecting 15 ml of contrast medium in 10—20 sec exposing a single film at the end of injection. In the normal individual a fan shaped shadow without definite pattern is produced in the sinusoidal area. Also some retrograde filling of the intra-hepatic portal radicles in relation to this sinusoidal area occurs. In cases of schistosomiasis with portal hypertension the same fan-shaped sinusoidal area is demonstrated, but no retrograde filling of the portal radicles take place. Instead the contrast medium returns through neighbouring branches of the supra-hepatic veins.

S. japonicum

The clinical manifestations of S. japonicum infection simulate those of S. mansoni. Radiological aid, therefore, in the investigation of cases is identical. Hepatomegaly and splenomegaly may be recorded by plain radiography of the abdomen. Oesophageal varices and gastric varices may be demonstrated by barium examination. Portal venography will demonstrate any structural changes in the portal circulation. These investigations and appearances have been well described by Chikiamco [5].

It is interesting to note also that the massive colonic granulomata that may occur in S. mansoni infections have also been demonstrated as occasionally occurring in S. japonicum infections [4].

Chest disease

Cardio-pulmonary disease may arise in all forms of schistosomiasis. In S. haematobium infections this is easy to comprehend for the worms are already in the systemic circulation. In S. mansoni and S. japonicum infections where the worms are in the portal circulation it is clear that ova are unlikely to reach the pulmonary circulation until some degree of portal hypertension has arisen and a collateral pathway has been provided to allow the passage of ova to the lungs.

Schistosomal ova thus reaching the pulmonary circulation may cause obstruction of pulmonary arterioles, where they set up an arteritis followed by fibrosis, which may produce marked restriction of the vascular bed. This gives rise to raised pulmonary artery pressure with consequent hypertrophy and eventual failure of the right ventricle i.e. cor pulmonale. In certain instances it appears that the arteritis produces destruction of part of the arteriolar wall through which deficiencies blood can escape into endothelial lined vascular spaces which communicate with the pulmonary venous circulation, and these shunts together with

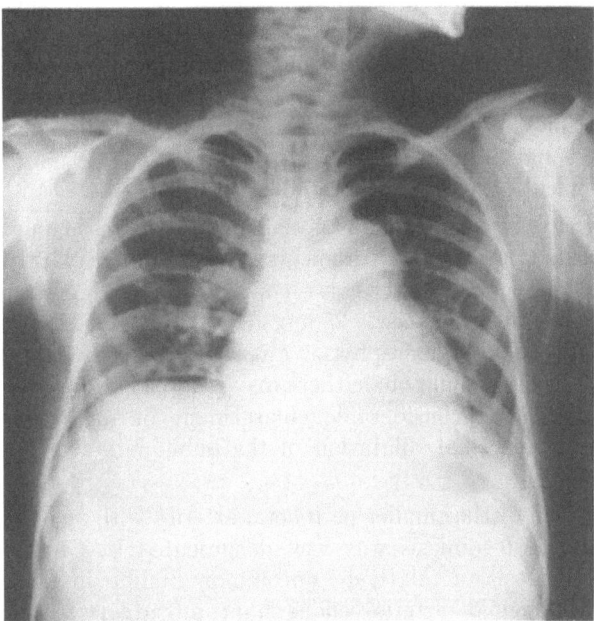

Fig. 10. Pulmonary hypertension in a case of schistosomiasis. The pulmonary artery is dilated, the main branches of the pulmonary artery are engorged and the peripheral vessels are small

the fibrotic restriction of the vascular bed and a degree of thrombotic occlusion of the vessels are the genesis of the pulmonary hypertension [14]. Once the stage of cor pulmonale is reached the disease is progressive and fatal.

Cor pulmonale is defined as hypertrophy of the right ventricle resulting from diseases affecting the function or structure of the lung. The diagnosis is established on clinical, radiological and E.C.G. findings, sometimes supplemented by cardiac catherisation, and can only be made by considering all the data together. Clinically there may be a systolic thrust, a loud pulmonary second sound, a gallop rhythm and jugular venous pulsation. There are E.C.G. deviations from the normal usually regarded as indicative of right ventricular hypertrophy.

Radiologically there may be no observable cardiac abnormality in the straight chest film though enlargement of the right ventricle, indicating dilatation and not necessarily hypertrophy, may be seen in the lateral film of the same patient. Similarly increase in the transverse diameter of the heart in the P.A. film indicates chamber dilatation and not necessarily hypertrophy. Filling in or actual convexity of the left heart border in the pulmonary artery segment on the P.A. film, or convexity in the right anterior oblique film may be regarded as dilation of the outflow tract of the right ventricle. Dilatation of the pulmonary artery and of its main branches with narrowing of the smaller peripheral branches is related to altered haemodynamics and indicates pulmonary hypertension (Fig. 10). Fluoroscopy will often show pulmonary artery pulsation at the hila, and will confirm the presence of right ventricular enlargement. Pulmonary angiography, performed by cardiac catheterisation and introduction of the catheter into the pulmonary artery, produces an impressive graphic demonstration of the marked dilatation of the central pulmonary arteries and the constriction of the smaller peripheral branches. The change from the dilated branches to the constricted branches is abrupt — a sort of "cut-off". Relating such angiography films to the conventional preliminary ones it is also possible to demonstrate this "cut-off" on the routine films. It is possible therefore on routine radiological examination of conventional films to suspect and pick up instances of pulmonary hypertension before gross cardiac enlargement has taken place.

Cardiac catheterisation is needed for diagnostic purposes in only a few patients. Cardiac output and pressure measurements should be made with the patient in a steady state. Pulmonary hypertension is considered to be present when the mean pulmonary artery pressure exceeds 25 mms Hg at rest. This examination can be followed by pulmonary angiography, as already described, if deemed necessary. In the later stages of cor pulmonale there may be great increase in the transverse diameter of the heart, considerable enlargement of the right ventricle and enormous, even aneurysmal, dilatation of the pulmonary artery and its central branches.

The constriction of the smaller peripheral arteries with associated pulmonary hypertension in schistosomiasis was well documented by Girgis [13], and the association of cyanosis, a relatively uncommon finding in schistosomal heart disease, with the "angioid" arterio-venous shunts already described, was shown by Lopes de Faria et al. [14]. This group of workers demonstrated by pulmonary angiography an unusual change in the peripheral lung fields in this type of case. There was a persistence of the contrast medium for a far longer period than usual. A fine "lacework pattern" causing a granular appearance in the lung fields was noted, presumably due to pooling of contrast medium in the "angioid" spaces that were subsequently noted at autopsy.

It is not at present clear how frequently the cardio-pulmonary disease here described occurs. It has been described in association with S. haematobium, S. mansoni and S. japonicum. It appears to have been noted most commonly in Egypt and in South America. Gelfand [12] however has found it but infrequently in Central Africa. There is undoubtedly scope for further work here, and it would seem that careful scrutiny of community chest X-ray surveys in endemic areas may provide further data in this field.

In addition to the cardio-pulmonary disease thus far described, much has been written [12, 17] about interstitial pulmonary fibrosis occurring as a result of ova deposition in the lungs. If, however, this does occur as an entity demonstrable radiologically, there are no specific features that render it recognisable as such, and it must indeed be rare. Palmer [17] detected no case fulfilling previous radiological descriptions in a series of over 15,000 chest X-ray examinations in an endemic area in Central Africa.

References

[1] BERGSTRAND, I., and C. A. EKMAN: Percutaneous lieno-portal venography. Acta Radiol. 43, 377—392 (1955).

[2] BIBAWI, E., A. A. EL-DEEB, and M. M. MAHFOUZ: Portal circulation in hepatic fibrosis associated with bilharziasis. Amer. J. Trop. Med. Hyg. 4, 913—922 (1955).

[3] BRABAND, H.: The incidence of urographic findings in tumours of the urinary bladder. Brit. J. Radiol. 34, 625—629 (1961).

[4] CH'EN, M. C., and S. C. WANG CH'EN: Acute colonic obstruction in schistosomiasis japonica; a clinical study of 40 cases; 14 associated with carcinoma. Chin. Med. J. 75, 517—532 (1957).

[5] CHIKIAMCO, P.: Schistosomiasis Japonica. In: Tropical Radiology, pp. 107—114. MIDDLEMISS, J. H. (Ed.) London: Heinemann 1961.

[6] COCKSHOTT, P.: Personal communication. Ibadan, Nigeria.

[7] COUTINHO, S. G., E. A. SAAD, and J. DA SILVA RODRIGUES: Segmental Hepatic Angiography. W. H. O. Document BILH/WP/2765 (restricted).

[8] DIMMETTE, R. M., and H. F. SPROAT: Rectosigmoid polyps in schistosomiasis; general clinical and pathological considerations. Amer. J. Trop. Med. Hyg. 4, 1057—1067 (1955).

[9] DOYLE, F. H.: Cystography in bladder tumours. A technique using "steripaque" and carbon dioxide. Brit. J. Radiol. 34, 205—215 (1961).

[10] — A. E. READ, and K. T. EVANS: The mediastinum in portal hypertension. Clinical Radiol. 12, 114—128 (1961).

[11] FORSYTH, D. M., and G. MACDONALD: Urological complications of endemic schistosomiasis in school children. I. USAGARA School. Trans. Roy. Soc. Trop. Med. Hyg. 59, 171—178 (1965).

[12] GELFAND, M.: Cor-pulmonale and cardiopulmonary schistosomiasis. Trans. Roy. Soc. Trop. Med. Hyg. 5, 1 533—540 (1957).

[13] GIRGIS, G.: Pulmonary heart disease due to bilharzia: bilharzial cor pulmonale; clinical study of 20 cases. Amer. Heart J. 43, 606—614 (1952).

[14] LOPES DE FARIA, J., J. CZAPSKI, M. O. RIBEIRO LEITE, D. DE O. PENNA, T. FUJIOKA, and A. B. DE U.CONTRA: Cyanosis in Manson's schistosomiasis. Role of pulmonary schistosomatic arteriovenous fistulas. Amer. Heart J. 54, 196—204 (1957).

[15] MAKAR, N.: Urological aspects of bilhariziasis in Egypt. Cairo: Societe Orientale de Publicite Press 1955.

[16] MIDDLEMISS, J. H., and F. G. ROSS: Portal hypertension and its radiological investigation. Postgrad. Med. J. 39, 299—307 (1963).

[17] PALMER, P. E. S.: Pulmonary manifestation of schistosomiasis. In: Tropical Radiology, pp. 103—107. MIDDLEMISS. J. H. (Ed.) London: Heinemann 1961.

[18] RAGHEB, M.: Radiological manifestations in bilharziasis. Brit. J. Radiol. 12, 21—27 (1939).

[19] SCHENCKER, B.: Drip infusion pyelography. Indications and applications in urologic roentgen diagnosis. Radiology 83, 12—21 (1964).

[20] SEAMAN, W.: Radiology (In press).

[21] SHERLOCK, S.: Diseases of the liver and biliary system. 3d ed. Philadelphia: F. A. Davis 1963.

[22] SINNA, A. M. A. A.: M. D. thesis. 1963. Cairo University.

[23] SOBRINHO, J., and F. O. KELSCH: Aspectos tumorais da esquistossomose do colon. Rev. Bras. Radiol. 2, 1—5 (1959).

[24] WALDRON, E. A.: Urethrocystography. J. Fac. Radiol. 4, 54—63 (1952).

Geographic Pathology of Schistosomiasis Mansoni*

Studies on Liver Injury

DOMINGOS DE PAOLA** and DONALD J. WINSLOW***

With 10 figures

The interpretation of the structural damage to the liver in schistosomiasis and the relationship of this damage to pathogenesis are still subject to considerable disagreement [1, 5, 10, 12, 22, 24, 31]. Although a relatively large amount of research, especially in the fields of immunology and immuno-pathology has been carried out [2, 11, 27, 28, 29, 30, 32, 40], the results, unfortunately, are not entirely comparable with human pathology. Man is a more complex host and subject to many factors, some of which have not yet been completely evaluated. There can be no question, however, that in the pathogenesis of the fibrotic schistosomal liver, the basic lesion consists of confluent granulomas surrounding the ova [5, 13]. Their peculiar intraluminal position causes venous obstruction. The experimental evidence for these facts is irrefutable [11, 15, 27, 28, 40].

Symmers' fibrosis depends upon repeated oviposition [6, 14, 25]; a single infection produces rare granulomas which, in their natural evolution are healed by fibrosis [12, 15]. In most cases one can find Symmers' fibrosis with rare eggs and granulomas [5, 13, 17, 25]; however, in a few cases, one can detect severe inflammatory infiltration in the portal tracts with destruction of liver cells in the periphery of the lobules ("piece-meal necrosis") without correlation with the parasitic elements [3, 13]. This advanced picture, in the opinion of some researchers [3, 13] is responsible for distortion of lobular architecture and a more severe clinical evolution. In the interpretation of these findings, ANDRADE et al. [3] suggest a possible autoimmune mechanism with perpetuation of the process of liver cell destruction, terminating in a picture of focal cirrhosis. Nevertheless, in this situation, the possibility of association of schistosomiasis and other factors should not be overlooked. Schistosomiasis, viral hepatitis and malnutrition have similar geographic distribution [9, 39].

These problems led us to study the general mechanism of liver injury produced by Schistosoma mansoni, particularly their different "strains" [17, 18, 26, 33], according to the geographic distribution.

Material and Methods

One hundred cases of hepatic schistosomiasis registered at the Armed Forces Institute of Pathology (U.S.A.) and the Department of Tropical Diseases (Uni-

* This paper was partially supported by the U.S. Public Health Service Research grant AI 00518801. National Institutes of Health, Bethesda, Md. U.S.A.

** Department of Tropical Diseases, National Faculty of Medicine, University of Brazil. Rio de Janeiro, Brazil.

*** Armed Forces Institute of Pathology, Washington, D.C. 20305.

versity of Brazil) were examined. This material came from various regions of the world, distributed as follows:

Region	Number of Cases	Region	Number of Cases
Puerto Rico	8	Mauritius	1
Surinam	3	Congo	36
Brazil	30	French Congo	12
Egypt	10		

The tissue was obtained mostly by autopsy and in a few, from surgical biopsy, and each case was represented by one to a few stained sections by haematoxylin-eosin; in one third of cases it was possible to examine several sections stained by different methods. The abstract of the clinical history included age, race, laboratory tests and therapeutic data. The lack of uniformity in the clinical information limited our analysis to histopathology.

Results

The summary of the histological findings correlated with the geographical site of origin in the 100 studied cases is given in Table 1.

Forty one cases were from the American continent and fifty nine from Africa. The full spectrum of the changes was seen ranging from minor alterations with rare granulomas with or without eggs to typical Symmers' fibrosis, including advanced forms with angiomatoid, piece-meal necrosis and active hepatitis Fig. 1—10. As might be expected the cases obtained by surgical biopsy, mostly from Brazil, were patients with Symmers' fibrosis in which surgical correction of portal hypertension had been attempted. It is not intended to analyze statistically the different degrees of incidence of liver injury, but rather to consider the significance of some of the findings. Thus in the eight cases from Puerto Rico, an advanced form of Symmers' fibrosis was found showing severe mononuclear infiltration in portal tracts and in the intralobular portion. In seven cases schistosomal granulomas were found; in one an adult worm. Pigmentation was seen in only three cases.

In one of the three cases from Surinam a large necrotic area resembling tuberculoid structure was found surrounding ova. Such a necrotic granuloma is an unusual finding. It was associated with old granulomas and even with portal fibrosis.

The thirty cases from Brazil all had portal hypertension and Symmers' fibrosis; although in a few we could identify only a thin perilobular fibrosis. This is probably due to the limitations of surgical biopsy as a sample of the whole organ. In at least 14 cases it was possible to detect angiomatoids in portal tracts enlarged by fibrosis. In 23 cases schistosomal granulomas were found; in 12, pigment and in only 3, adult worms. Symmers' fibrosis coexisted in 5 cases with severe inflammatory infiltration in the perilobular and intralobular portions, together with focal necrosis in lobular periphery. Fatty degeneration was described only in a single case.

Among the 10 cases from Egypt, there were 6 of Symmers' fibrosis; 4 of these showed angiomatoids and 2 focal necrosis and active hepatitis. Schistosomal granuloma was identified in 6, adult worm in only 1 and pigment in 4 cases.

DOMINGOS DE PAOLA and DONALD J. WINSLOW:

Table 1. *Correlation of Histological Findings in Schistosomiasis with the Geographic Location*

Explanation of Abbreviations

(AFIP)	— Armed Forces Institute of Pathology	Gran	— granulomas
(DTD)	— Department of Tropical Diseases	Pig.	— pigment
		PMN	— "piece-meal necrosis"
Geogr.	— geographic region	AH	— active hepatitis
LD	— lobular distortion	Deg.	— liver cell degeneration
P	— lobular periphery	Reg.	— liver cell regeneration
		F.D.	— fatty degeneration

KC	— Kupffer cell proliferation
PT	— portal tract
F	— fibrosis
II	— inflammatory infiltration
Pyc.	— pyknosis
Sy.	— Symmers' fibrosis
A.	— "angiomatoid"

Registry	Geogr.	LD	Gran/Egg	Worm	Pig.	PMN	AH	Deg.	Reg.	KC	PT
152.784 (AFIP)	P. Rico	—	+/—	—	+	—	—	—	—	—	—
114.557 (AFIP)	P. Rico	+ P	+/—	—	—	—	+	—	—	+	Sy/II/A
212.058 (AFIP)	P. Rico	—	+/+	—	—	—	—	—	—	—	—
302.978 (AFIP)	P. Rico	—	+/+	+	—	—	—	—	—	—	II
333.799 (AFIP)	P. Rico	—	+/—	—	—	—	—	—	—	—	F
171.042 (AFIP)	P. Rico	—	+/+	—	—	—	—	—	—	—	—
507.509 (AFIP)	P. Rico	—	+/+	—	++	—	—	—	—	—	—
540.592 (AFIP)	P. Rico	—	+/+	—	+++	—	—	—	—	—	—
1065.459 (AFIP)	Surinam	—	+/+	—	+++	—	—	—	—	+	F/II
1065.460 (AFIP)	Surinam	—	+/+ ++	+	—	—	—	—	—	+	F/II
1065.531 (AFIP)	Surinam	—	+/+	—	—	—	—	—	—	+	II
92 (DTD)	Brasil	—	+/+ ++	—	+++	—	—	—	—	+	F/II
219 (DTD)	Brasil	—	+/+ ++	—	—	—	—	—	—	+	F/II/A
577 (DTD)	Brasil	—	+/+ +	+	+	—	—	—	—	+	F/II
10.277 (DTD)	Brasil	+ P	+/+	—	—	—	+	—	—	+	F/II/A
35.443 (DTD)	Brasil	—	+/+	—	—	—	—	—	—	—	Sy/II/A
126.300 (DTD)	Brasil	—	—	—	+++	—	—	—	—	+	Sy/II
127.402 (DTD)	Brasil	+ P	+/+	+	+	—	—	—	—	+	Sy/II/A
132.058 (DTD)	Brasil	—	+/+	—	+++	+	+	—	—	+	Sy/II
135.042 (DTD)	Brasil	+ P	+/+	—	—	+	+	—	—	+	Sy/II
151.981 (DTD)	Brasil	—	+/+ ++	—	+	—	—	Pyc.	—	+	Sy/II/A
155.142 (DTD)	Brasil	—	+/+	+	—	—	+	—	—	+	Sy/II
156.320 (DTD)	Brasil	+ P	+/+	—	+	—	—	—	—	+	Sy/II
181.694 (DTD)	Brasil	—	+/—	—	—	—	—	FD	—	—	Sy
207.846 (DTD)	Brasil	+ P	+/—	—	+	++	+++	—	—	+	Sy
216.728 (DTD)	Brasil	—	+/+	—	+	++	+++	Pyc.	—	+++	Sy/II/A

Case No.	Source	Location	Class	1	2	3	4	5	6	7	8	9	10
226.987	(DTD)	Brasil	Sy/II	+	−	Pyc.	+	−	−	−	+/+		−
247.293	(DTD)	Brasil	Sy/II	+	−	−	−	+	−	+	+/+	P	+
251.859	(DTD)	Brasil	Sy/II/A	++	−	Pyc.	+	+	+	−	+/+		−
256.476	(DTD)	Brasil	F/II	+	−	−	−	−	−	−	−		−
260.487	(DTD)	Brasil	Sy/A	+	−	−	−	−	+	−	−		−
265.492	(DTD)	Brasil	Sy/II/A	+	−	−	−	−	+	−	++		−
272.071	(DTD)	Brasil	Sy/II	+	−	−	++	−	−	−	++		−
274.371	(DTD)	Brasil	Sy/II	+	−	−	++	−	−	−	++/+	P	+
274.379	(DTD)	Brasil	Sy/II/A	+	−	−	−	−	+	−	+/+	P	+
278.534	(DTD)	Brasil	Sy/II/A	+	−	−	−	−	−	−	+/+		−
291.417	(DTD)	Brasil	Sy/II/A	++	−	−	+	−	+	−	+/+	P	+
297.158	(DTD)	Brasil	Sy/II/A	+	−	Pyc.	−	−	−	−	+		−
304.276	(DTD)	Brasil	Sy/II/A	−	−	Pyc.	−	−	−	−	+		−
310.148	(DTD)	Brasil	Sy/II	−	−	−	−	−	−	−	+		−
312.268	(DTD)	Brasil	Sy/II/A	+	−	−	−	−	−	−	+/+	P	+
818.883	(AFIP)	Mauritius	II	−	−	−	−	−	++	+	+/+		−
616.168	(AFIP)	Egypt	Sy/II/A	+	−	Pyc.	+	+	++	−	++/+		+
616.169	(AFIP)	Egypt	—	−	−	FD	−	−	+	+	+/+		−
616.273	(AFIP)	Egypt	F/II	−	−	−	+	−	++	−	++/+	P	−
644.797	(AFIP)	Egypt	F	+	−	−	+	−	+	−	+/+	P	+
644.800	(AFIP)	Egypt	Sy/A	+	−	−	++	−	+	−	++/+	P	+
679.304	(AFIP)	Egypt	Sy/II/A	+	−	−	−	−	−	−	++/+	P	+
684.901	(AFIP)	Egypt	Sy/II	+	−	FD	+	−	+	−	+/+		−
686.735	(AFIP)	Egypt	Sy/II	+	−	Pyc.	++	−	−	+	+/+		−
772.067	(AFIP)	Egypt	Sy/II/A	−	−	−	−	−	−	−	+/+		−
772.071	(AFIP)	Egypt	II	−	−	−	−	−	−	−	−		−
562.206	(AFIP)	Congo	F/II	+	−	−	+++	−	+	−	++/+		+
565.866	(AFIP)	Congo	F/II	+	−	−	+++	+	+	−	++/+		−
565.868	(AFIP)	Congo	II	+	−	−	+++	+	+	−	++/+		−
565.869	(AFIP)	Congo	II	+	−	−	+++	+	+	−	+/+		−
565.874	(AFIP)	Congo	F/II	+++	−	−	+	+	+	−	++/+	P	+
569.883	(AFIP)	Congo	Sy/II/A	+	−	Pyc.	+	+	+	−	++/+		−
574.732	(AFIP)	Congo	F/II	+	−	−	−	−	−	−	−		−
576.187	(AFIP)	Congo	II	+	−	−	−	−	+	−	−		−
576.188	(AFIP)	Congo	II	−	−	−	+	+	−	−	+/+	P	+
580.882	(AFIP)	Congo	F/II	+	−	−	+	+	−	−	+/+		−
594.595	(AFIP)	Congo	Sy/II/A	++	−	−	+	−	+	−	++/+		+
614.985	(AFIP)	Congo	II	+	−	Pyc.	−	−	+	−	+/+		−
606.772	(AFIP)	Congo	Sy/II	++	−	Pyc.	+	−	−	+	++/+	P	+
615.319	(AFIP)	Congo	II	+	−	−	+	−	−	−	++/+		−

Table 1. (Continued)

Registry	Geogr.	LD	Gran/Egg	Worm	Pig.	PMN	AH	Deg.	Reg.	KC	PT
662.626 (AFIP)	Congo	+ P	—	—	++	—	—	—	—	++	II
690.260 (AFIP)	Congo	—	+/+	—	++	—	—	—	—	++	II
615.325 (AFIP)	Congo	—	+/+/+	—	—	—	—	—	—	+	F/II
700.023 (AFIP)	Congo	—	+/+/+	—	—	—	—	—	—	—	II
700.028 (AFIP)	Congo	—	+/+/+	—	—	—	—	—	—	—	II
706.518 (AFIP)	Congo	+ P	+/+/+	—	—	+	+	—	—	+++	Sy/II/A
742.028 (AFIP)	Congo	—	+/+	—	++	—	—	—	—	—	II
755.083 (AFIP)	Congo	—	+/+	—	++	—	—	—	—	—	II
760.560 (AFIP)	Congo	—	—	—	++	—	++	—	—	+	II
766.215 (AFIP)	Congo	—	+/+	—	—	—	++	Pyc.	—	++	F/II
770.583 (AFIP)	Congo	—	+/+/+	—	—	—	+++	Pyc.	—	++	F/II
770.584 (AFIP)	Congo	+ P	+/+/+	—	+	—	+	FD	—	+	Sy/II
787.742 (AFIP)	Congo	—	+/+/+	—	—	—	—	—	—	—	II
722.311 (AFIP)	Congo	—	+/+/+	—	—	—	—	—	—	—	II
747.521 (AFIP)	Congo	—	+/+/+	—	—	—	—	—	—	+	II
787.741 (AFIP)	Congo	+ P	+/+/+	—	—	+	++	Pyc.	—	+++	Sy/II/A
795.539 (AFIP)	Congo	—	+/+/+	—	—	—	—	—	—	—	F/II
819.399 (AFIP)	Congo	—	+/+	—	—	—	—	—	—	—	II
825.723 (AFIP)	Congo	—	+/+	—	—	—	—	—	—	—	II
850.707 (AFIP)	Congo	—	+/+	—	—	—	—	—	—	—	F/II
853.422 (AFIP)	Congo	—	+/+	—	—	—	—	—	—	+	II
865.711 (AFIP)	Congo	—	—	—	—	—	—	FD	—	—	Sy/A
813.477 (AFIP)	Fr. Congo	+ P	+/+/+	—	—	++	++	—	—	++	Sy/II/A
860.952 (AFIP)	Fr. Congo	+ P	—	—	—	—	—	Pyc.	—	—	Sy/A
860.954 (AFIP)	Fr. Congo	+ P	+/+/+	—	—	—	—	—	—	+	F/II
860.960 (AFIP)	Fr. Congo	—	+/+/+	+	++	—	—	—	—	++	II
922.252 (AFIP)	Fr. Congo	—	+/+/+	—	—	—	—	—	—	—	II
813.484 (AFIP)	Fr. Congo	—	+/—/+	—	—	—	—	FD	—	—	F
829.484 (AFIP)	Fr. Congo	—	+/+/+	—	—	—	—	—	—	—	II
860.955 (AFIP)	Fr. Congo	—	+/+/+	—	—	—	—	—	—	—	Sy/II/A
838.967 (AFIP)	Fr. Congo	+ P	+/+/+	—	—	—	—	—	—	—	II
889.054 (AFIP)	Fr. Congo	—	+/+/+	—	—	—	—	—	—	—	II

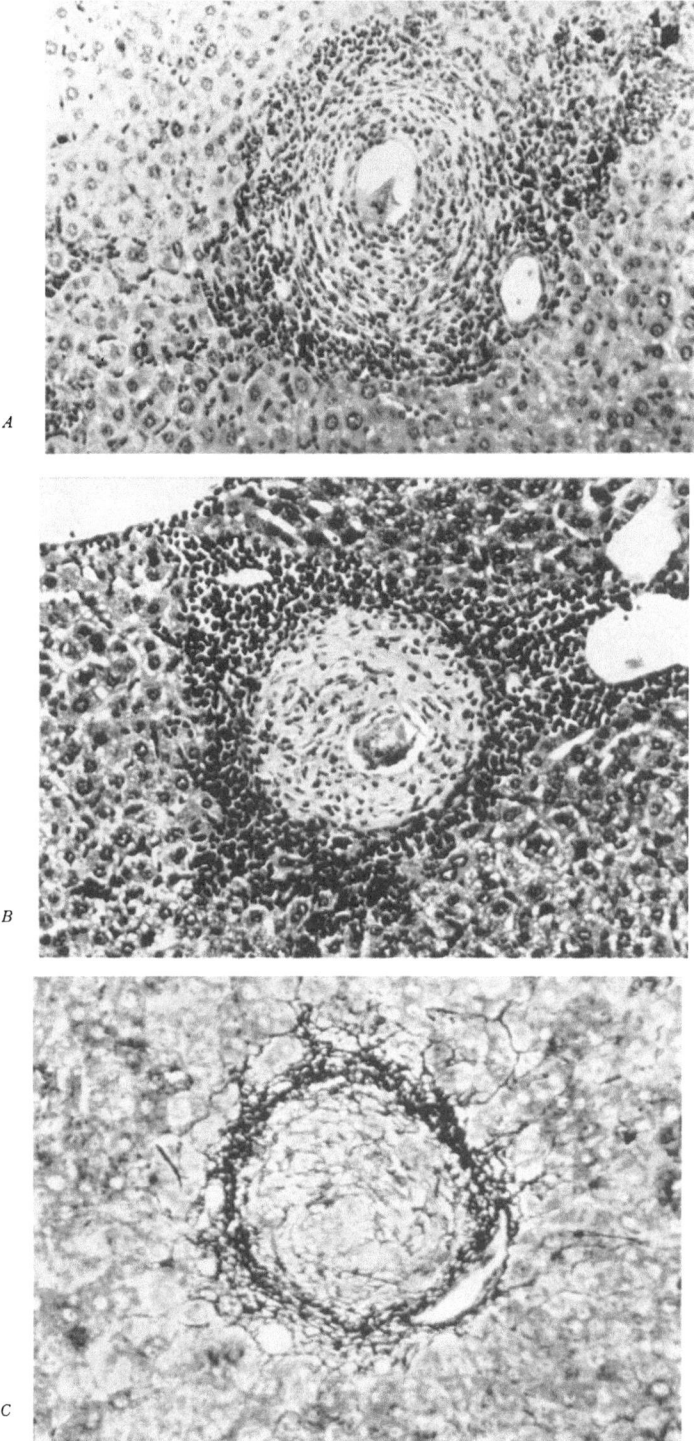

Fig. 1. Evolution of schistosomal granuloma to scar. H. & E., *A*; Gomori trichromic, *B*; and reticulin stains, *C*. 150 X

Of the 36 cases from the Congo, 6 showed Symmers' fibrosis, 4 with angiomatoids. Schistosomal granuloma was detected in 30, adult worm in 1 and pigment
in 14 cases. A single case showed a large area of necrosis around eggs (AFIP 614.985).

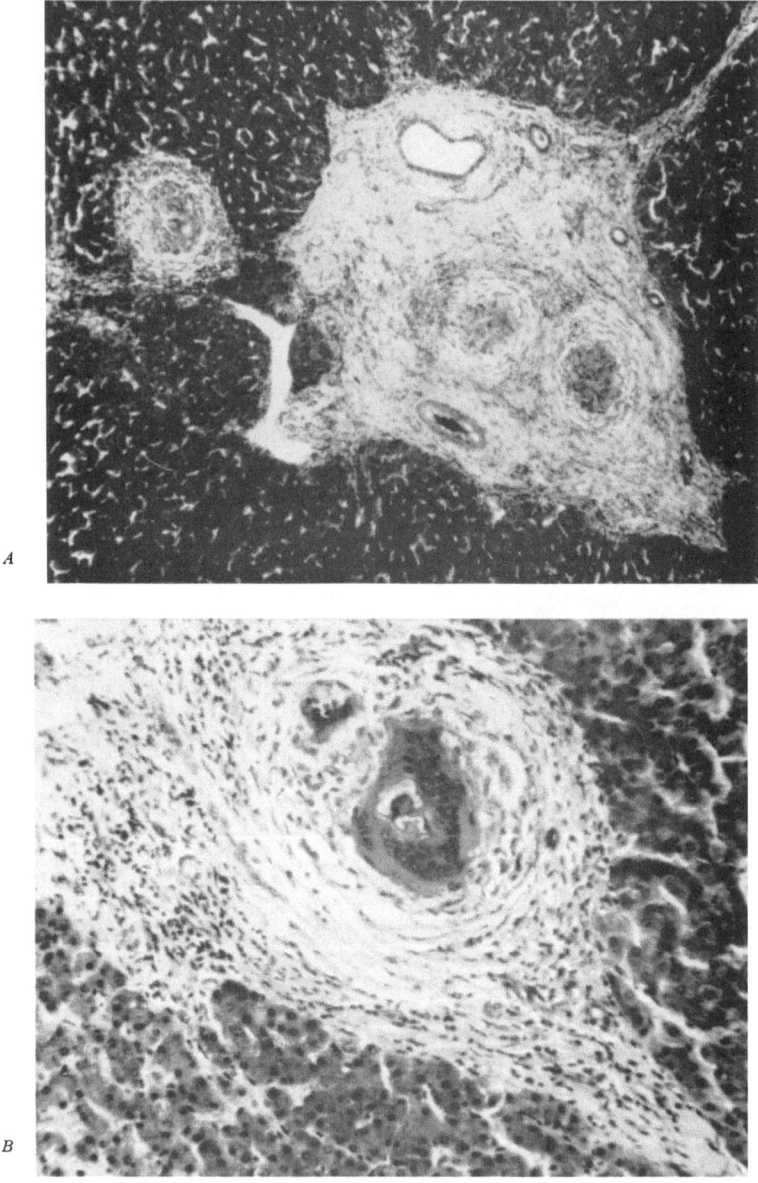

Fig. 2. *A*: fibrous enlargment of portal tract due to confluent granulomas (Symmers' fibrosis). *B*: schistosomal granulom
in the perilobular portion. Gomori trichromic stain. 60 X and 150 X

In 7 cases focal necrosis at the periphery of the lobule and active hepatitis were
observed. Among these 3 were associated with Symmers' fibrosis, 2 with fibrous
portal enlargement and 2 without fibrosis. In only 1 case fatty degeneration was

observed. In the 12 cases from French Congo, 4 had Symmers' fibrosis associated with angiomatoids. Granulomas were found in 11 cases, pigment in 2 and adult worm in only 1. Piece-meal necrosis and active hepatitis were found in only 1 case of Symmers' fibrosis. Fatty degeneration was detected in a single case.

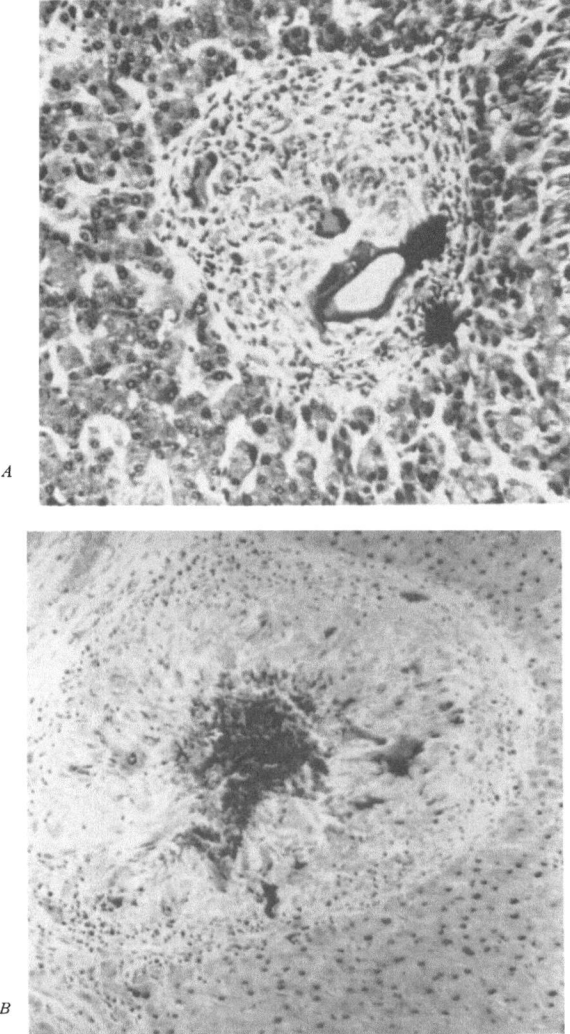

Fig. 3.*A*: intralobular granuloma;*B*: necrosis around adult dead worm. Gomori trichromic stain and H. & E.; 160 X and 100X

Comments

One hundred cases of schistosomiasis mansoni obtained from the main endemic areas of the world have been analyzed. Although the tissues were obtained from endemic areas of Africa and America with their diverse strains each with its own distinct physiological behavior, in general there was quite a similarity of the lesions.

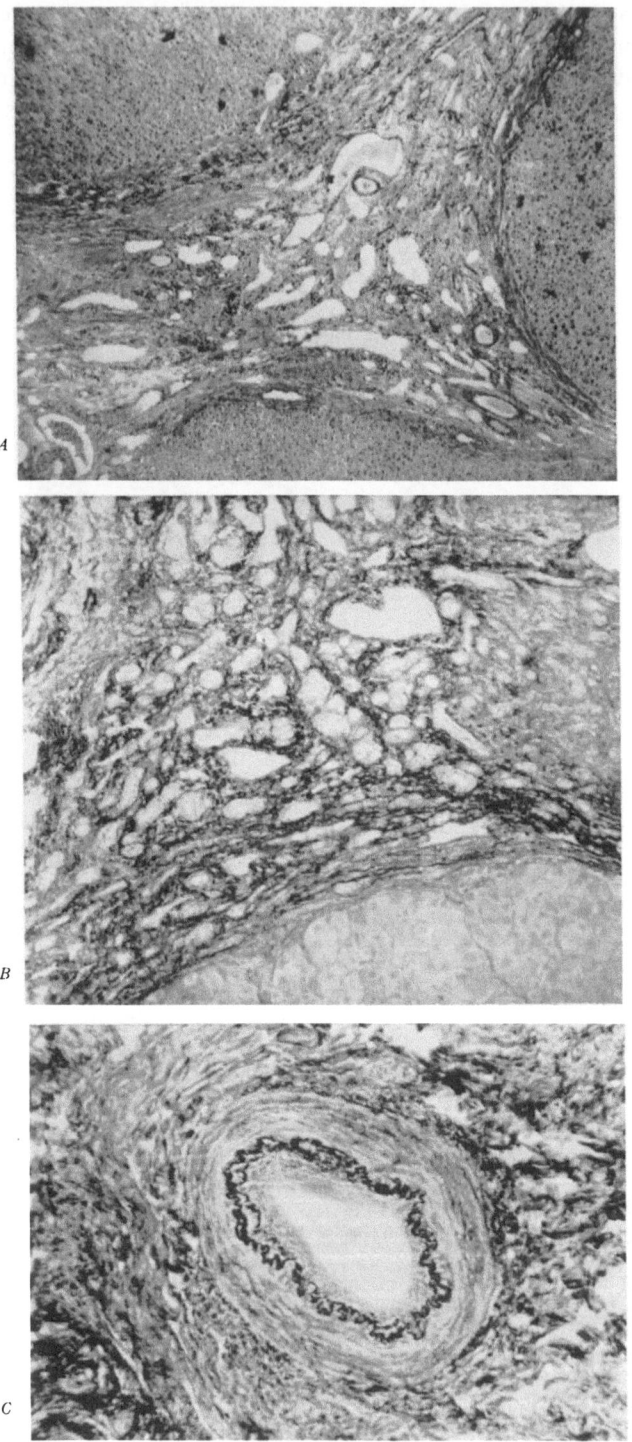

Fig. 4. *A* and *B*: Symmers' fibrosis with vascular proliferation ("angiomatoid"); *C*: mild fibrous thickening of arterial intima. H. & E. and Weigert stain. 100 X and 120 X

Since the hepatic lesions produced by the different stains were qualitatively similar, the general pathology was basically the same. In a single infection or limited exposure, the lesions are represented by a few granulomas diffusely distributed in the organ, with a natural tendency to scar transformation and

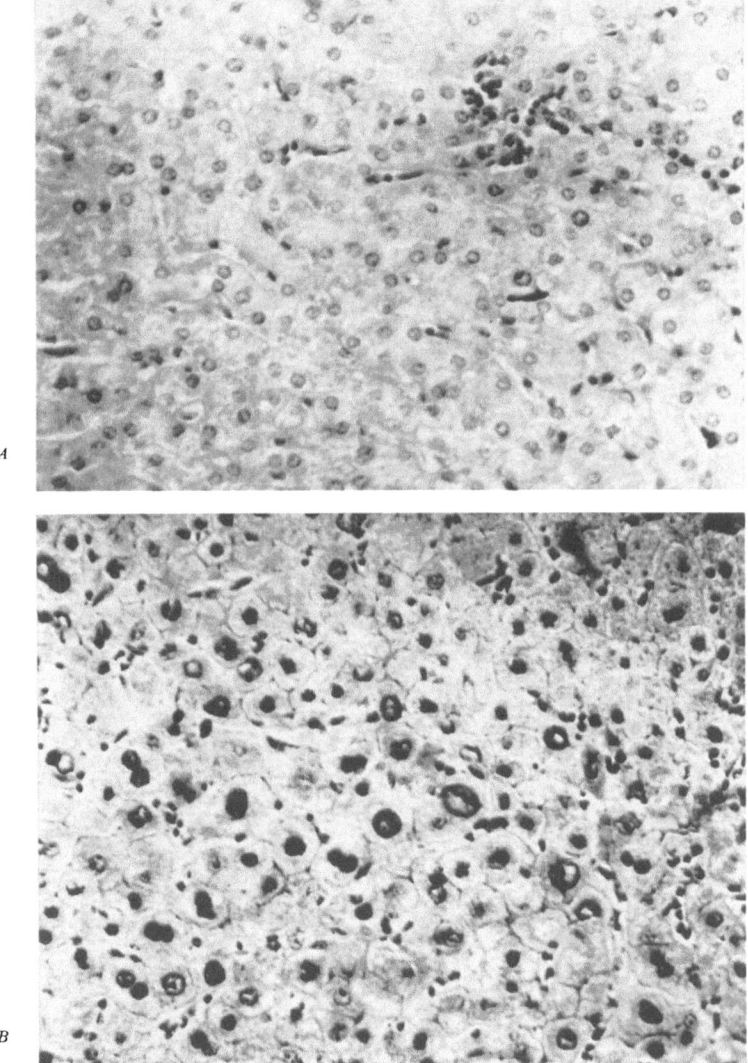

Fig. 5. *A* mild Kupffer cells proliferation; *B* intralobular mononuclear infiltration and liver cells pyknosis. H. & E. 160 X and 180 X

extinction of the disease. In repeated infections in patients from endemic areas, the granulomas are more numerous, but the natural evolution is still to fibrous scars [5, 38]. Experimentally, in sensitized animals the granulomas are of greater diameter [11, 28]. In a hypersensitive host the eggs are surrounded by large necrotic areas with eosinophilic infiltration.

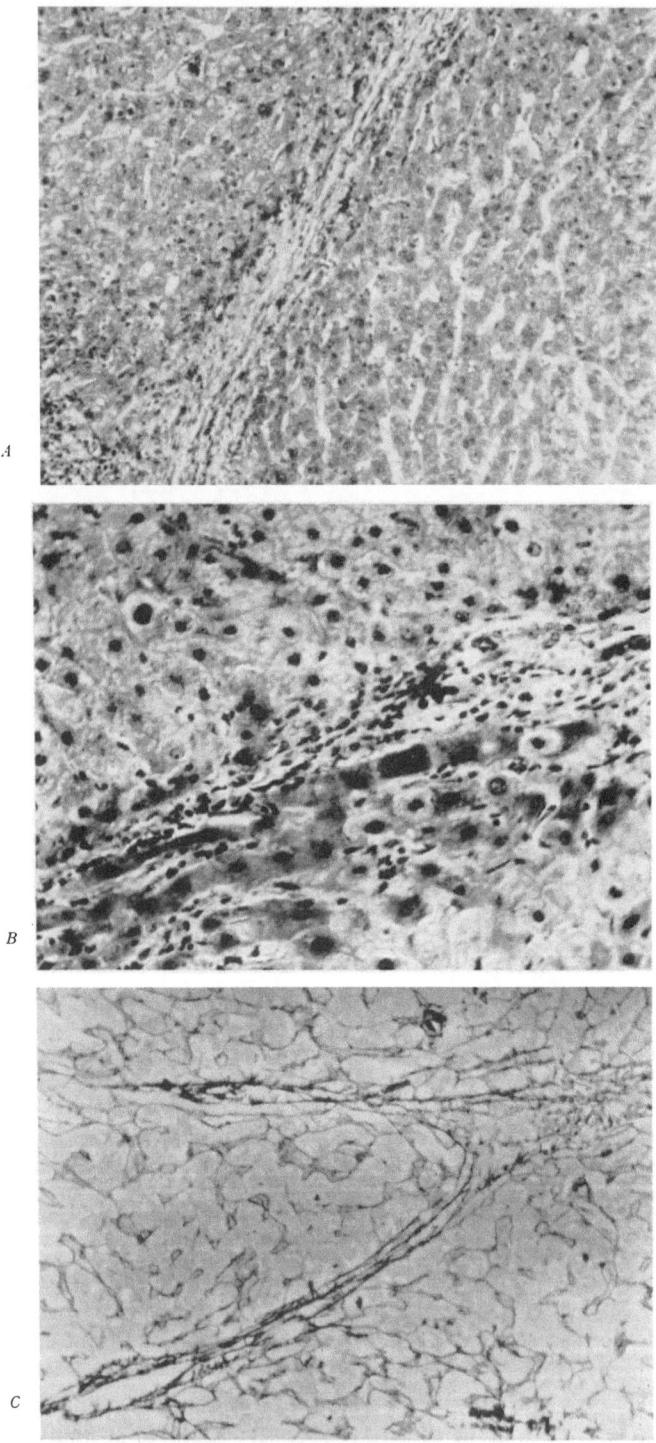

Fig. 6. Different aspects of intralobular connective tissue septa formation; observe liver cell degeneration in the periseptal limits. H. & E., *A*; Gomori trichromic, *B*; and reticulin stains, *C*. 100 X and 160 X

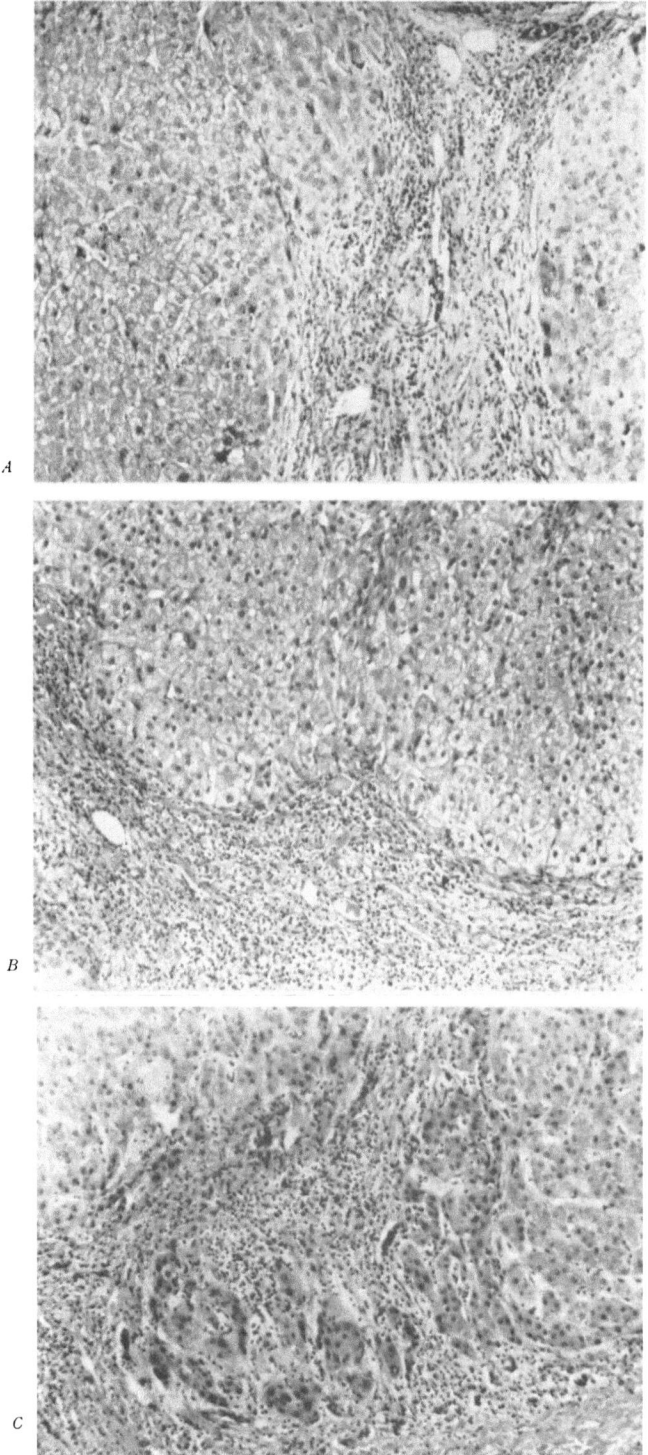

Fig. 7. Different aspects of lymphocytic and plasma cells infiltration (active hepatitis) and piece-meal necrosis. H. & E.
A, B and C 120 X and 160 X

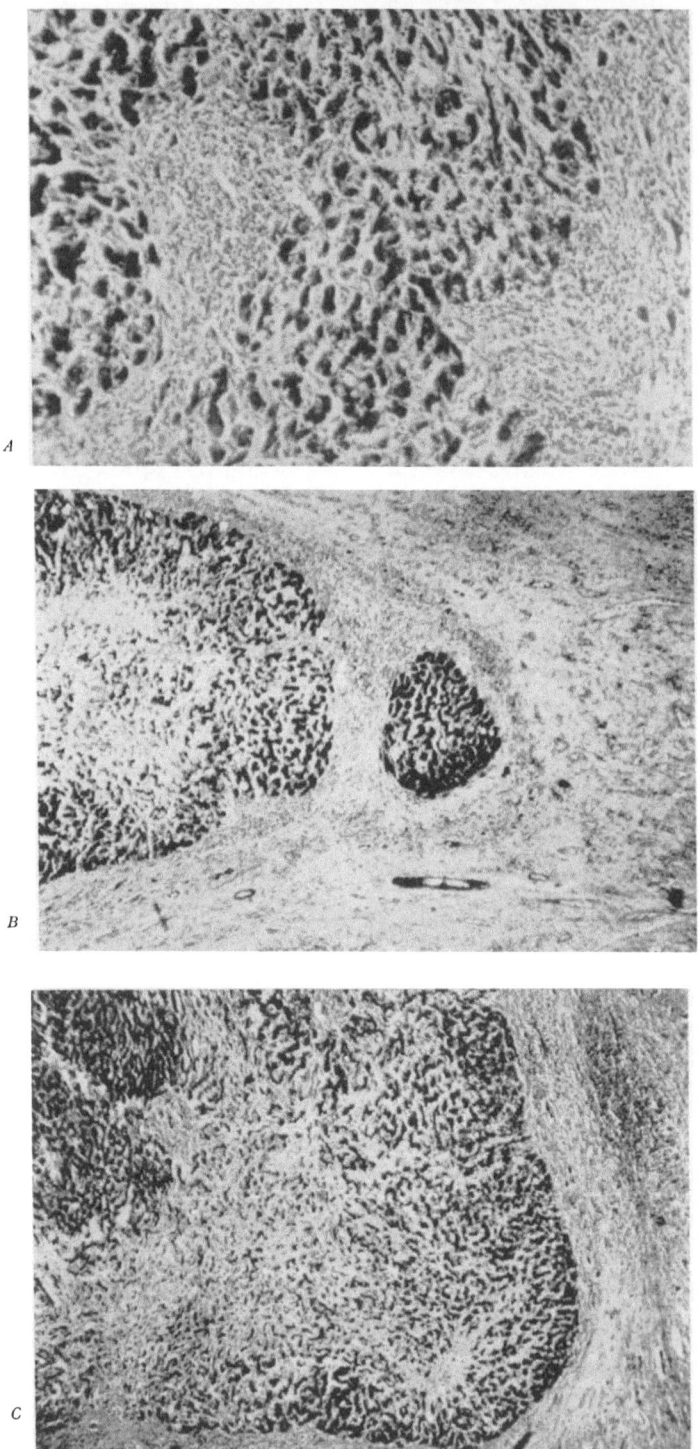

Fig. 8. *A* and *B*: advanced form of liver schistosomiasis with focal insulation of liver cells; *C*: centrolbular necrosis by anoxia due to hemorrhagic episode. Gomori trichromic stain. 80 X and 120 X

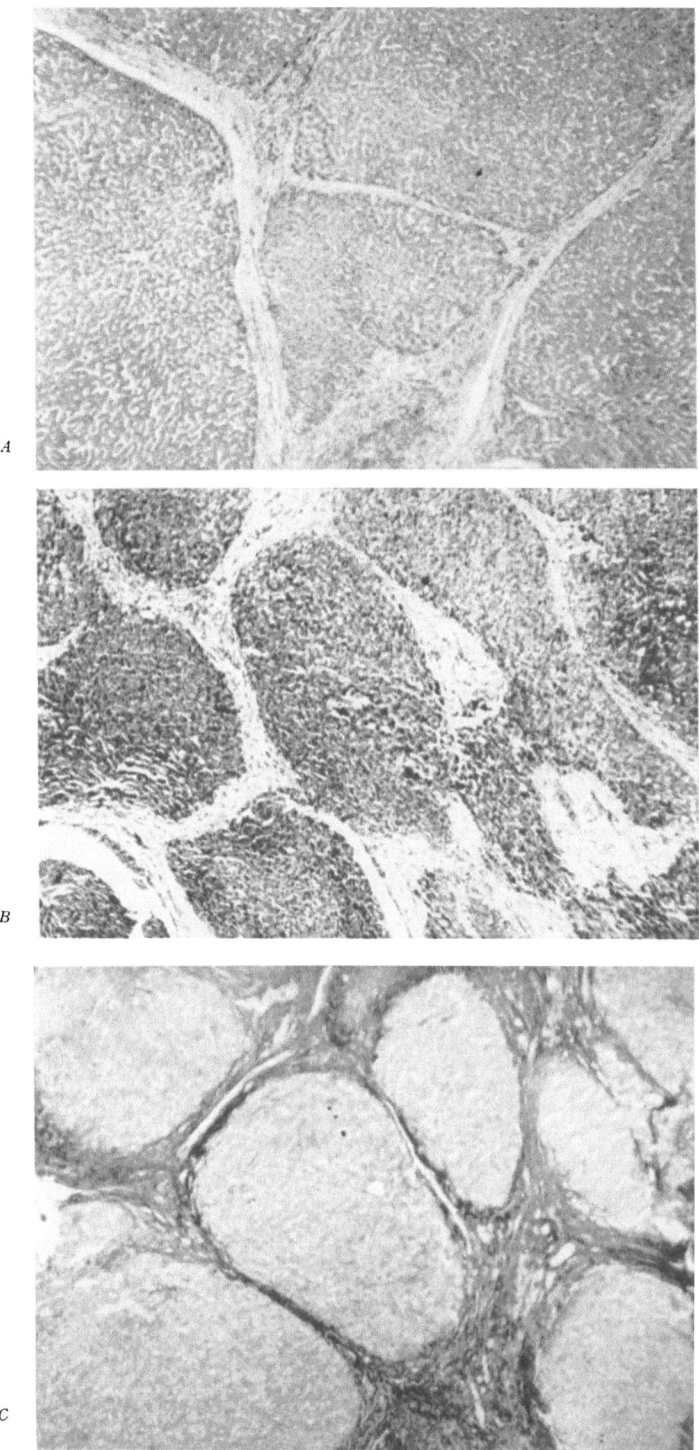

Fig. 9. Different degrees of focal lobular distortion in advanced form of Symmers' fibrosis. Gomori trichromic stain, 120 X
A, B and C

15   Bilharziasis

BRACKEN et al. [7] observed similar lesions in the S. japonicum infections of American soldiers in the Philippines and classified them as recent and acute. We have excluded this possibility on the basis of our analysis of the same material in the

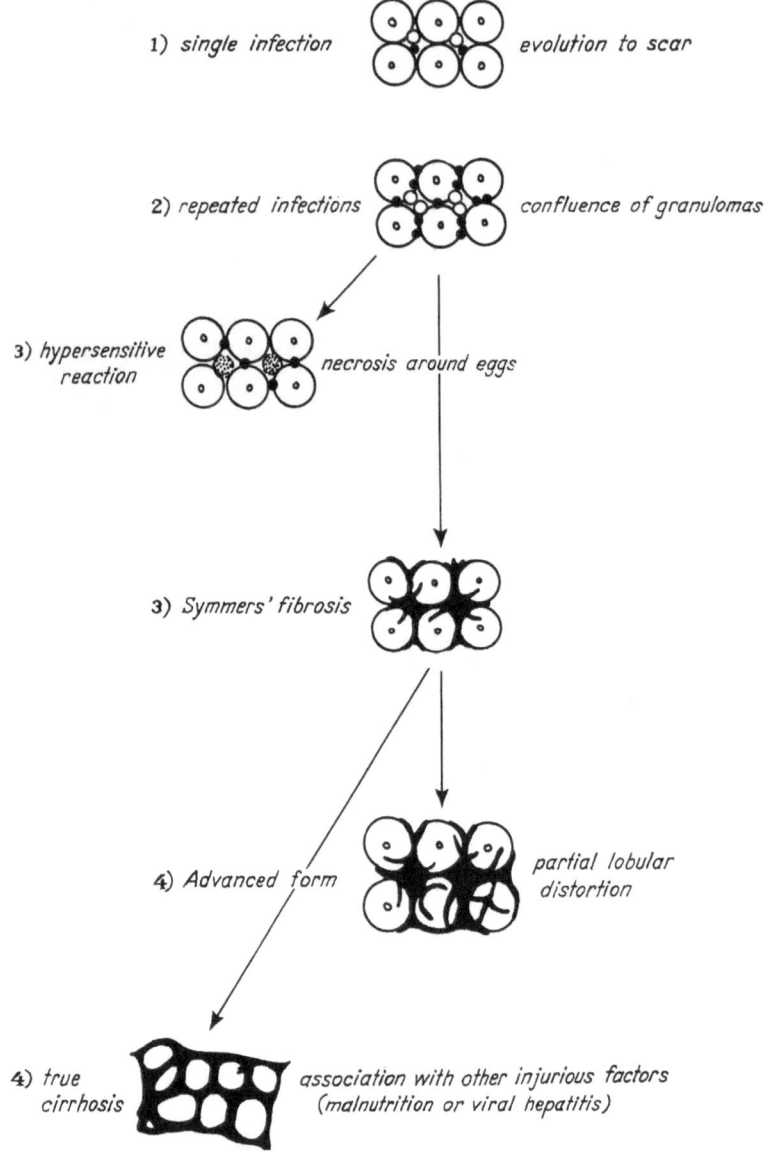

1) *single infection*   *evolution to scar*

2) *repeated infections*   *confluence of granulomas*

3) *hypersensitive reaction*   *necrosis around eggs*

3) *Symmers' fibrosis*

4) *Advanced form*   *partial lobular distortion*

4) *true cirrhosis*   *association with other injurious factors (malnutrition or viral hepatitis)*

Fig. 10

AFIP files and the finding of the coexisting old, scarred and necrotic granulomas. Experimentally [16, 24] and in human cases [6] in the so-called acute or toxemic form of the disease, the lesions are of the same morphology.

The repeated infections are, undoubtedly, responsible for the final picture of Symmers' fibrosis. Because of the angiomatoid appearance brought about by the newly formed vessels, this type of fibrosis must be considered specific of the hepato-splenic form of schistosomiasis, even though granulomatous structures are absent [5, 6]. In the periphery of the hepatic lobules of some types of hosts a lymphocytic and plasma cell infiltration can be found with pyknosis of liver cells or even necrosis ("piece-meal necrosis"). Experimentally, the immunofluorescence tech-nics show the existence of schistosomal antigen not only around the eggs and in the granuloma cells, but at times in small quantities in the periphery of the granuloma [2], although admittedly degenerating cells and necrotic tissue demon-strate non-specific fluorescence [32]. It is possible that all the stainable schistosoma antigen is not "sequestrated", but there is some diffuse antigen fraction, in "suffi-cient concentration", to be responsible for the liver cell injury [8, 21, 34] despite some recent observations to the contrary [35]. ANDRADE [4] believes that a "delay-ed type of hypersensitivity", represented by active hepatitis with no correlation between the intensity of the reaction and the number of parasitic elements, has a destructive character and progresses to fibrosis [19].

Thus, active hepatitis and "piece-meal necrosis" may produce formation of secondary connective tissue septae with partial distortion of the lobular architec-ture simply by separating the liver cells, but without nodular regeneration [21, 36]. On the other hand the analysis of our material has permitted the observation of active hepatitis and "piece-meal necrosis" in the early stages of the disease. Because of the strictly focal distribution of these lesions, the progression of the fibrous process cannot be justifiably attributed to viral hepatitis.

In our experience, it was not possible to prove the transformation of the advanced form of schistosomal fibrosis into a picture of true cirrhosis. Actually, in endemic areas, the association of schistosomiasis with malnutrution and viral hepatitis can produce a picture of cirrhosis [20, 37]. However, in some areas, one frequently finds a nutritional or post hepatitis cirrhosis with incidental schistosomal granulomas [23, 37]. These observations make critical judgment very difficult.

Although the venous obstruction is irreversible, the granuloma, in most cases, has a natural tendency to scar. Because of the segmental distribution of the lesions and the fact that destruction is limited to the peripheral liver cells, it is difficult to believe that Symmers' fibrosis can be transformed into true cirrhosis.

Summary

The authors reviewed 100 cases of liver schistosomiasis proceeding from different regions of the world. The structural damages that have been found were of similar pattern. The correlation between experimental data and human patho-logy has permitted to suggest a sequence of events. In advanced forms of Symmers' fibrosis, partial lobular distortion may occur, but true cirrhosis occurs only in association with other liver injury factors.

References

[1] AMBERSON, J. M., and E. SCHWARZ: On African Schistosomiasis. Trans. Roy. Soc. Trop. Med. Hyg. **47**, 451—502 (1953).

[2] ANDRADE, Z. A., F. PARONETTO, and H. POPPER: Immuno cytochemical studies in schistosomiasis. Amer. J. Path. **39**, 589—598 (1961).

228 DOMINGOS DE PAOLA and DONALD J. WINSLOW:

[3] ANDRADE, Z. A., F. SERGIO SANTANA, and E. RUBIN: Hepatic changes in advanced schistosomiasis. Gastroenterology 42, 393—400 (1962).
[4] — Immunopathology of Manson's Schistosomiasis. Rev. Inst. Med. Trop. S. Paulo 6, 181—187 (1964).
[5] BOGLIOLO, L.: The anatomic picture of the liver in hepato-splenic schistosomiasis mansoni. Ann. Trop. Med. Parasit. 51, 1—14 (1957).
[6] — Subsídio para o conhecimento da forma hepato-esplênica e da forma toxêmica da esquistossomose mansônica. Serv. Nac. Educ. Sanit. Minist. Saúde. Rio de Janeiro 1958.
[7] BRACKEN, M. M., W. R. BAILEY JR., and H. M. THOMAS: The lesions of schistosomiasis japonica. Amer. J. Path. 24, 611—623 (1948).
[8] BRUMPT, E., and P. CHEVALLIER: La rate et les spleno-hepatites des bilharzioses experimentals. Ann. Parasit. Hum. Comp. 9, 15—67 (1931).
[9] CHANDLER, A. C.: Interrelations between nutrition and infectious diseases in the tropics. Amer. J. Trop. Med. 6, 195—208 (1957).
[10] CARTER, R. A., and S. SHALDON: The liver in schistosomiasis. Lancet 1959 II, 1003—1008.
[11] CHEEVER, A.: Hepatic vascular lesions in mice infected with Schistosoma mansoni. Arch. Path. 72, 648—657 (1961).
[12] COELHO, B.: Morfogênese das lesões hepáticas na esquistossomose mansônica experimental. Publ. Avulsas. Inst. Aggeu Magalhães. Recife, Brazil 1, 61—98 (1952).
[13] DE PAOLA, D., and L. B. DIAS: Súmula da Anatomia Patológica da Esquistossomose. Bol. Cent. Estud. Hosp. Serv. Estado 16, 223—236 (1964).
[14] DESCHAMPS, S. H., J. L. REDMOND, and H. DELEEUW: Hepatic granulomas in Schistosomiasis. Gastroenterology 28, 990—1015 (1955).
[15] DIAS, L. B., D. DE PAOLA, and J. RODRIGUES DA SILVA: Esquistossomose experimental no camundongo. Histogênese do granuloma esquistossomótico. Rev. Inst. Med. Trop. S. Paulo 4, 140—148 (1962).
[16] FAIRLEY, N. H.: A comparative study of experimental bilharziasis in monkeys contrasted with the hitherto described lesions in man. J. Path. Bact. 23, 289—314 (1920).
[17] FILES, V. S.: A study of the vector-parasite relationships in Schistosoma mansoni. Parasitology 41, 264—269 (1951).
[18] —, and E. B. CRAM: A study on comparative susceptibility of snail vectors to strains of Schistosoma mansoni. J. Parasit. 35, 555—560 (1949).
[19] GELL, P. G. H.: Cytologic events in hypersensitivity reactions. In: Cellular and humoral aspects of the hypersensitive states. LAWRENCE, H. S. (Ed.). pp. 43—88. New York: Hoeber Inc. 1959.
[20] GILLET, J., and J. WOLFS: Les bilharzioses humaines au Congo Belge et au Ruanda Urundi. Bull. Wld Hlth Org. 10, 315—419 (1954).
[21] GÖNNERT, V. R.: Schistosomiasis-Studien. IV. Zur Pathologie der Schistosomiasis der Maus. Z. Tropenmed. Parasit. 6, 279—336 (1955).
[22] HASHEM, M.: The aetiology and Pathogenesis of the endemic form of Hepato-splenomegaly "Egyptian splenomegaly". J. Egypt Med. Ass. 30, 48—79 (1947).
[23] JAFFE, R.: Was lehrt uns die Bilharzia-Zirrhose in bezug auf die Probleme der Leber-Zirrhose? Schweiz. Med. Wschr. 72, 1149—1154 (1942).
[24] KOPPISCH, E.: Studies on schistosomiasis mansoni in Puerto Rico. IV. The pathological anatomy of experimental schistosomiasis mansoni in the rabbit and albino rat. Puerto Rico. J. Publ. Hlth Trop. Med. 13, 1—114 (1937/38).
[25] — Studies on schistosomiasis mansoni in Puerto Rico. VI. Morbid anatomy of diseases as found in Puerto Ricans. J. Publ. Hlth Trop. Med. 16, 395—455 (1941).
[26] KUNTZ, R. E., G. M. MALAKATIS, and W. H. WELLS: Susceptibility of laboratory animals to infection by Egyptian "strains" of Schistosoma mansoni, with emphasis on the albino mouse. In: Proceedings V Cong. Internat. Med. Trop. Palud. Istanbul 2, 374—391 (1954).
[27] LICHTENBERG, F. V.: Host response to eggs of S. mansoni. I. Granuloma formation in the unsensitized laboratory mouse. Amer. J. Path. 41, 711—731 (1962).
[28] — Studies on granuloma formation. III. Antigen sequestration and destruction in the schistosoma pseudotubercle. Amer. J. Path. 45, 73—94 (1964).

[29] Lichtenberg, F. v., E. H. Sadun, and J. I. Bruce: Tissue responses and mechanism of resistance in Schistosomiasis mansoni in abnormal hosts. Amer. J. Trop. Med. 11, 347−356 (1962).

[30] − − Parasite migration and host reaction in mice exposed to irradiated cercariae of Schistosoma mansoni. Exp. Parasit. 13, 256−265 (1963).

[31] Magalhães, Fo. A.: Aspectos da patologia da esquistossomose mansonica. VI. Comportamento patogênico do verme morto com especial referência às lesões hepáticas esquistossomóticas. An. Fac. Med. Recife 16, 153−160 (1956).

[32] − I. M. Krupp, and E. A. Malek: Localization of antigen and presence of antibody in tissues of mice infected with Schistosoma mansoni as indicated by fluorescent antibody technics. Amer. J. Trop. Med. 14, 84−99 (1965).

[33] Malek, E. A.: Susceptibility of the snail Biomphalaria boissyi to infection with certain strains of Schistosoma mansoni. Amer. J. Trop. Med. 30, 887−894 (1950).

[34] Meleney, H. E., D. V. Moore, H. Most and B. H. Carney: The histopathology of experimental schistosomiasis. I. The hepatic lesions in mice infected with S. mansoni, S. japonicum and S. haematobium. Amer. J. Trop. Med. 1, 263−286 (1952).

[35] Raslavicius, P. A.: Schistosomiasis in parabiotic mice. Histopathological comparisons in infected mice and their uninfected partners. Amer. J. Trop. Med. 14, 100−110 (1965).

[36] Perez, V., F. Schaffner, and W. H. Loery: Pathologic features of pipestem fibrosis of the liver due to schistosomiasis. J. Mt Sinai Hosp. 26, 544−552 (1959).

[37] Rodrigues da Silva, J.: Estudo clínico da esquistossomose mansônica. Thesis. Rio de Janeiro 1949.

[38] Schwetz, J.: Sur l'immunité clinique dans les bilharzioses humaines. Bull. Soc. Path. Exot. 49, 52−56 (1956).

[39] Symmers, D.: Pathogenesis of liver cirrhosis in schistosomiasis. J. Amer. Med. Ass. 147, 304−305 (1951).

[40] Warren, K. S.: The etiology of hepato-splenic schistosomiasis mansoni in mice. Amer. J. Trop. Med. 10, 870−876 (1961).

Histopathology of Schistosomiasis

Donald J. Winslow, M.D.*

With 9 figures

First phase of infection

The entrance of the bodies of cercariae through the skin of the definitive host marks the earliest stage of infection in Schistosomiasis. The success or failure of parasitism may be determined by the host-parasite relationship at this stage[9]. Those metacercariae (from species of schistosomes not pathogenic to man) which quickly die in human subcuticular tissue promote a prominent reaction by the host manifested clinically by severe pruritus whereas those metacercariae (pathogenic to man) which can survive in human tissue promote much less reaction and are able to enter lymphatics and blood vessels and progress in their development within the host. At this earliest stage of infection which also may take place through mucous membranes, the severity and time of onset of histologic changes is influenced not only by the adaptability of the parasite but also, in cases of acquired immunity, by the past experience of the host. Fundamentally, however, the metacercariae which are able to survive in the tissues of the host produce little if any cellular reaction. Various animal schistosomes, most of which have birds as their definitive host, are unable to develop in man [7]. As they die in the skin, an inflammatory response is produced. Polymorphonuclear neutrophiles, lymphocytes, larger mononuclear cells, plasma cells and eosinophils infiltrate the infected areas. Hyperemia, edema and clinical evidence of urticaria are associated with severe itching. In contrast to this "swimmer's itch", the invasion of the skin of man by pathogenic cercariae may produce little noticeable reaction [4]. For this reason, the patient may not realize when he was infected. This host-parasite relationship exists, however, for non-sensitized hosts. In endemic areas where man may be repeatedly exposed, a severe dermal reaction can take place even to pathogenic cercariae. In Japan the intense pruritus and erythema has been called "kabure", and in Puerto Rico, "piquina".

Second phase of Infection

The next phase of infection is the period of migration and development during which the metacercariae enter the blood stream and grow to adult male and female worms. During this phase there is little to be observed in the way of histopathologic changes unless some developing schistosomes die in vessels within an organ such as lung, liver or spleen. If this happens, the involved vessel becomes thrombosed and an intense inflammatory reaction takes place around the degenerating schistosome. It is possible, however, to obtain sections of mature or immature viable worms within blood vessels of liver, spleen, bladder, and other organs. Very little if any inflammatory reaction may be present around the viable worms. It appears that

---

* Armed Forces Institute of Pathology, Washington DC. 20305 USA.

the living healthy worm (insofar as we can observe in histologic sections) is somehow protected from host defense mechanisms and provokes little if any inflammatory reaction. The clinical manifestations, if any, during this phase of the infection (migration and development) are probably related to a significant parasite mortality or to toxic metabolic products of the developing schistosomes although there is little if any histologic evidence for the latter.

Third phase of infection

The third phase of the infection is the conjunction of male and female schistosomes in the abdominal or pelvic veins and the extrusion of fertilized ova from the females in order that they may pass through the bowel or vesical wall to the external environment for repetition of the evolutionary cycle outside the definitive host. It is during this stage that the imperfection of the host-parasite relationship becomes most apparent both clinically and pathologically. The ova may not successfully escape from the host, and wherever they are deposited in the tissues produce more or less inflammation with sequelae. In addition, due to chemotherapy or some unknown factor, the adults may wander back to the liver or into various other organs where they die and provoke a severe inflammatory reaction. This third stage may require weeks or months to become clinically manifest. Its severity is related to such poorly understood factors as host resistance, dosage of cercariae, single or repeated exposure, treatment and associated disease or conditions. In general it is a chronic disease (or host-parasite interaction) resulting in the loss of thousands of ova from the parasite and more or less deterioration of the host. The early third stage of the infection may, however, be associated with severe symptoms of acute schistosomiasis with allergic manifestations and high fever [3]. As the third stage enters the picture, a high-dose infection in a nonimmune patient may be associated with hyperemia, edema and hemorrhage from mucosal involvement by ova or metabolic products and may provoke a pulmonary and hepatic dysfunction. As immunity develops, eosinophilia decreases and fever subsides. In endemic regions, relatively immune persons may live for years with chronic schistosomiasis, but many will develop severe liver disease, gastrointestinal abnormalities or genitourinary alterations. Many will die of unassociated conditions, and some die of intercurrent infection probably precipitated by lowered resistance.

In some cases of schistosomiasis mansoni and hematobium the lungs are the site of numerous granulomas formed around schistosome ova [5,6]. The ova within the pulmonary arterioles are responsible for initiating a pulmonary endarteritis resulting in pulmonary circulatory obstruction and pulmonary heart disease. Involvement of the central nervous system may occur if ova reach the brain *(S. japonicum especially)* or spinal cord. In Egypt the schistosomiasis caused by *S. hematobium* produces extensive destruction to the genitourinary tract. Not infrequently, especially in men, the involved bladder is also the site of papillomas or invasive carcinomas. It is doubtful, however, that the schistosomiasis is directly causally related to these cancers although its role is still being investigated.

Host reaction as related to species of ova

The most important histologic alterations in human schistosomiasis are related to the hundreds or thousands of ova which become deposited in various tissues of the host. The lesions produced vary, depending on the time of deposition, the type of ovum (*S. mansoni, S. japonicum, S. hematobium,* rarely others), the number of ova (more numerous with *S. japonicum* and *S. hematobium*), and the degree of immunity or hypersensitivity of the host. Other factors such as nutritional status of the host, presence or absence of other diseases, and treatment are also of importance.

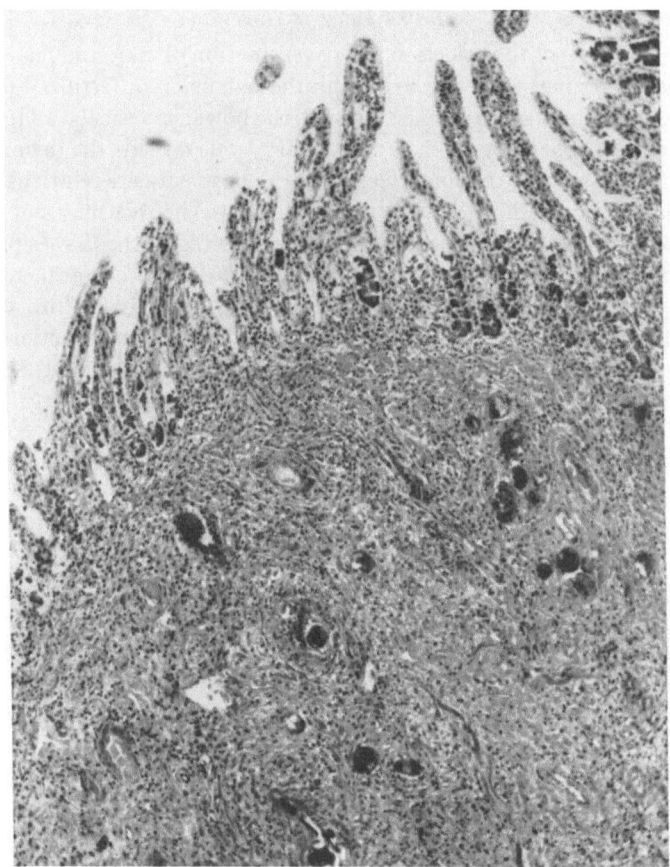

Fig. 1. Intestine, showing numerous ova of S. mansoni. H. & E. X 56. AFIP Neg. no. 65-4903

The time of deposition of the ova is related to the presence or absence of a host reaction and the type of reaction, if present. Ova of *S. mansoni* seem to be generally more active in stimulating an inflammatory reaction. Numerous ova of *S. mansoni* in the mucosa and submucosa of the intestine (Fig. 1). Practically all of the ova are in various stages of degeneration and there is a severe inflammatory reaction to them. The ovum of *S. mansoni* which is caught in an abnormal position undergoes degeneration, and a cellular reaction to the dying ovum or to its metabolic products takes place. The reacting cells consist of lymphocytes, larger mononuclear cells, plasma cells and some eosinophils. The larger mononudear cells form multinucleated giant cells which surround and also enter the degenerating ovum, consuming all of the ovum (Fig. 2). The shell of the ovum is the last to disappear and may be observed particularly well by the use of Periodic acid Schiff stain or silver stains. The lymphocytes and plasma cells represent the immunogenic component of the lesion and the eosinophils indicate a degree of hypersensitivity. The later lesions become fibrotic and a laminated fibrotic nodule is the end stage of a single lesion. Resolution of such lesions has

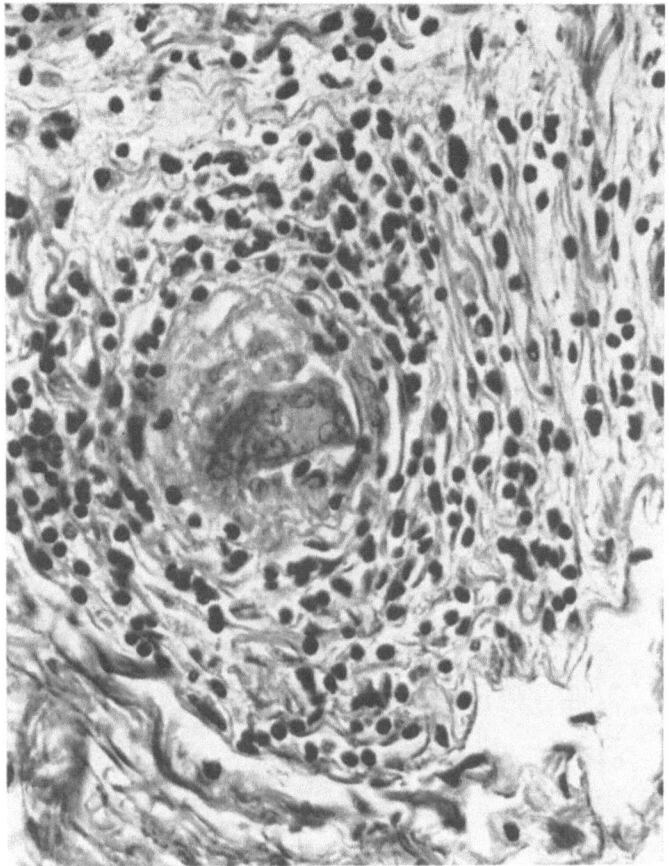

Fig. 2. Granuloma with central giant cell in wall of intestine. Same case as Fig. 1. H. & E. X 350. AFIP Neg. no. 65-4904

been demonstrated experimentally [1]. For some unknown reason the ova of *S. mansoni* do not have much tendency to calcify. This is in marked contrast to the ova of *S. japonicum* and *S. hematobium* which appear often to calcify without producing much or any antigenic stimulation. Numerous calcified ova may be present in the lungs (Fig. 3), the liver (Fig. 4), sometimes with the nuclei of the inner embryo still visible, but without the slightest evidence of inflammatory reaction. The submucosa of the intestine may also contain large numbers of calcified or calcifying ova (Fig. 5) without significant inflammatory reaction. Even foreign body giant cells were lacking.

A similar calcification of ova is seen in cases of schistosomiasis due to *S. hematobium*. The urinary bladder may show numerous calcified or calcifying ova beneath the epithelium (Fig. 6). Most of these ova do not appear to be within blood vessels and yet there is no significant inflammatory reaction around them.

The foregoing illustrations and remarks concerning the non-reactive ova deposition in tissues infected by *S. japonicum* and *S. hematobium* should not be

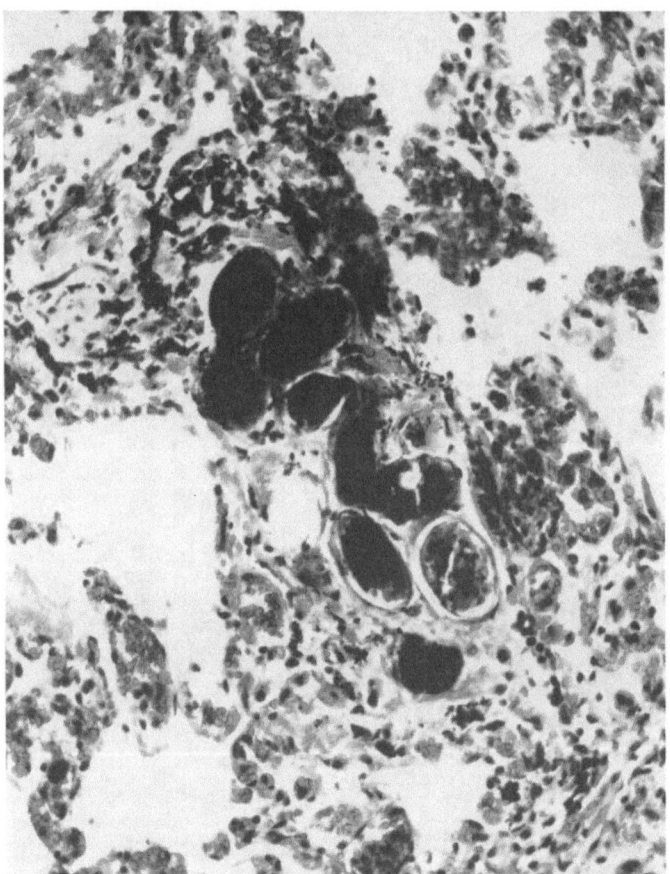

Fig. 3. Lung, showing ova of *S. japonicum*. H. & E. X 195. AFIP Neg. no. 65-4905

interpreted to mean that these parasitic eggs are incapable of illiciting an inflammatory reaction or producing granulomas. The ova of these parasites are the principle incitants of the disease just as are the ova of *S. mansoni*. There is an inflammatory infiltrate around calcified and calcifying ova (Fig. 7). The infiltrate consists of lymphocytes, some plasma cells, a few eosinophils and occasional multinucleated giant cells of foreign body type. Ova are also found in sections of brain, prostate, testis, urinary bladder, large intestine, small intestine, adrenal gland, liver, pancreas and lung. There is histologic evidence that the schistosome ova are widely distributed via blood vessels but that they are able to penetrate vascular walls and become deposited in groups within extravascular tissue (Fig. 8). These ova are surrounded by few if any inflammatory cells. The histologic evidence suggests that many of the ova of *S. hematobium* and *S. japonicum* may be sealed with mineral deposits which coat the surfaces of the ova. It seems possible that such a coating might prevent leakage of antigenic material through the shells into the surrounding tissue. Otherwise it is difficult to explain the lack of inflammatory response to so many ova. The possible anti-inflammatory role of mineralization is

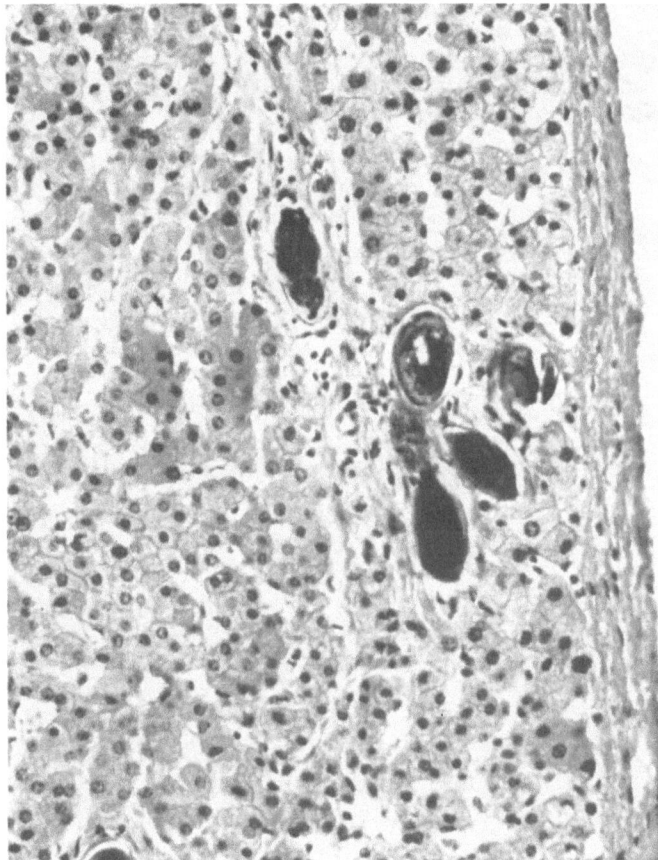

Fig. 4. Liver, showing ova of *S. japonicum*. H. & E. X 195. AFIP Neg. no. 65-4906

also suggested by the observation that those ova contained in well-developed discrete granulomas usually exhibit much less mineralization.

Reactions associated with allergy

In patients who are hypersensitive, discrete granulomas with epithelioid cell formation and allergic features such as eosinophil infiltration and central"fibrinoid" necrosis may be produced by ova of *S. mansoni, S. japonicum,* and *S. hematobium* (Fig. 9). Other diseases may be present. For example in the case illustrated in Fig. 9 the patient had *S. japonicum* infection. The liver showed many granuloma with ova and "fibrinoid" necrosis in the center. Surrounding the central necrotic area is a row of pallisaded epithelioid cells. Numerous eosinophils were observed in the peripheral portion of the granuloma. Many discrete granulomas were found throughout the liver. There was also in- volvement of lung, mesenteric lymph nodes, large intestine and rectum. In addition, how- ever, there was severe amebic colitis and proctitis. The patient had a left arm

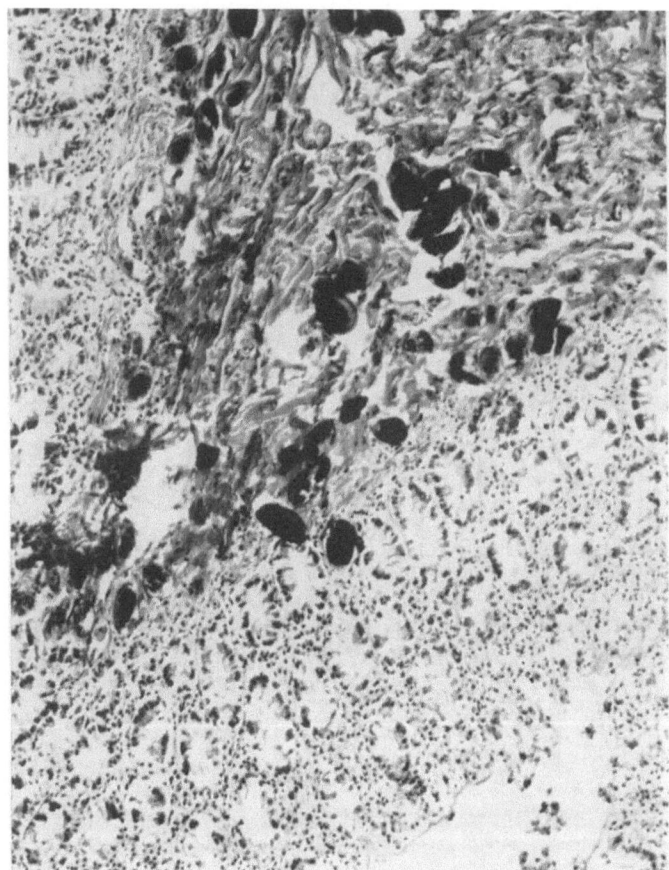

Fig. 5. Intestine, showing ova of *S. japonicum*. H. & E. X 84. AFIP Neg. no. 65-4907

amputation and had been treated with penicillin every 4 hours. Although he may have been sensitized only by the *Schistosoma japonicum*, there was ample opportunity for other factors to play a role. The influence of associated disease, malnutrition, repeated schistosomal infection and other factors on the extent and quality of lesions is poorly understood but probably accounts for the great variation in the clinical and pathological picture in schistosomiasis.

Hematin pigment

The nutritional requirements of the schistosomes in the human host are supplied by blood and their intravascular location is apparently necessary for their survival. Histological evidence supports this view. As previously stated, viable worms are frequently found within blood vessels in tissue sections. Around these there is no observable inflammatory reaction. Within the schistosome altered blood pigment can be found in the intestinal tract, appearing as brown granular pigment. The excretion of this hematin pigment by the schistosome into the circulating blood of the host is evidenced histologically by the presence of similar

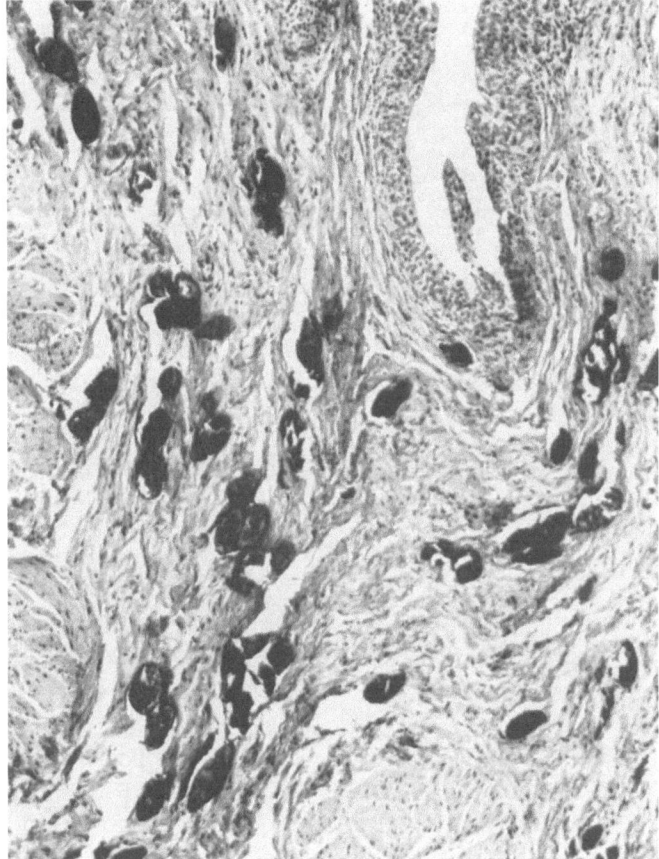

Fig. 6. Urinary bladder, showing ova of *S. hematobium*. H. & E. X 63. AFIP Neg. no. 65-4908

pigment granules in the Kupffer cells of the liver and within phagocytic cells in the spleen. It is probably similar to if not identical with malarial pigment and stains negatively with iron stains. Its presence in histologic sections should cause one to consider the possibility of schistosomiasis or malaria, from which it may not be differentiated by itself. In cases where the malaria is still active, one may find similar pigment within erythrocytes, providing a clue as to the source of the pigment. The pigment must be differentiated from formalin pigment which is somewhat lighter brown and not typically found within erythrocytes or phagocytic cells.

Species differentiation in histological sections

The histological differentiation of the three common types of human schistosomiasis can usually be made without much difficulty. As has already been stated,
the ova of *S. japonicum* and *S. hematobium* are usually very numerous, show a
marked tendency to calcify, and frequently are present within extravascular tissue

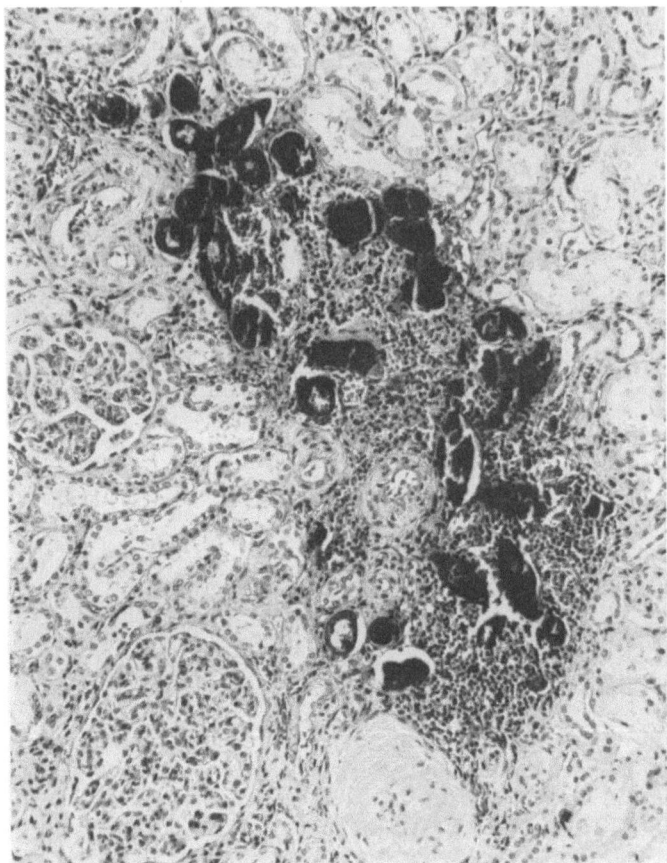

Fig. 7. Kidney, *S. hematobium* infection. H. & E. X 100. AFIP Neg. no. 65-4909

in groups without significant surrounding inflammation. The distribution of large
numbers of ova of *S. hematobium* in the genitourinary tract provides a clue aiding
in differentiation from *S. japonicum*. In addition the ova of *S. hematobium* appear
longer and less rounded than those of *S. japonicum*, and they have a prominent
terminal spine. The ova of *S. mansoni* have much less of a tendency to calcify, al most
always are associated with some tissue reaction, and have a long sharp and
prominent lateral spine. With regard to the spine points it is important to realize that
ova of *S. mansoni* which are so positioned that the spine upward or downward may
appear to have a terminal spine [10]. In any case for histologic diagnosis it may be
necessary to examine many ova under high power in order to determine the species.

Distorted or fragmented ova may sometimes give an erroneous impression of the true structure.

The histologic differentiation of the adult worms is somewhat more difficult. If good sections of viable worms are present, examination of the cuticle will be of particular aid in differentiation. The male cuticle of *S. hematobium* is finely tuberculated, that of *S. mansoni* is grossly tuberculated, and that of *S. japonicum*

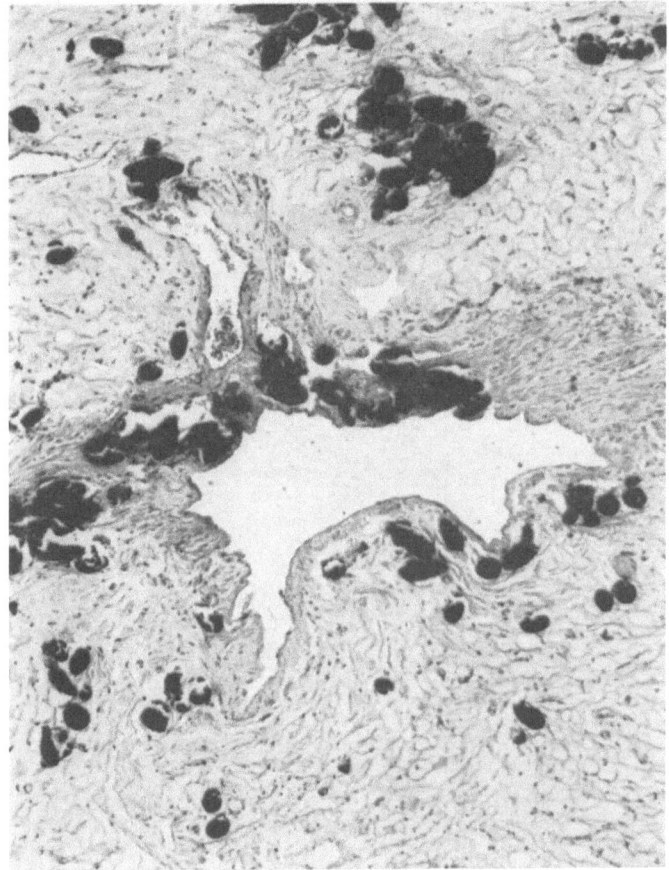

Fig. 8. *S. hematobium* ova in pelvic connective tissue. H. & E. X 63. AFIP Neg. no. 65-4910

is nontubercular. Other structural features which may be of aid in differentiating these adults are shown in the following table (from Chatterjee [2]):

Table 1. *Species differentiation in histological sections*

Organ	S. hematobium	S. mansoni	S. japonicum
Male testis	4—5; in groups	8—9; in a zigzag row	6—7; in single file
Female ovary	Posterior to middle of body	Anterior to middle of body	Middle of body
Uterus	20—30 ova	1—3 (usually 1)	50 or more ova

Many of the investigations concerned with schistosomiasis have had to do with the changes in the liver produced particularly by *S. mansoni* and *S. japonicum*. Some authors have suggested that the most important factor in producing disease of the liver is the presence of dying or dead worms in the small intrahepatic portal radicles [8]. It is true the "hepatic shift" of worms, especially following treatment may result in abscesses and large areas of necrosis within the hepatic parenchyma.

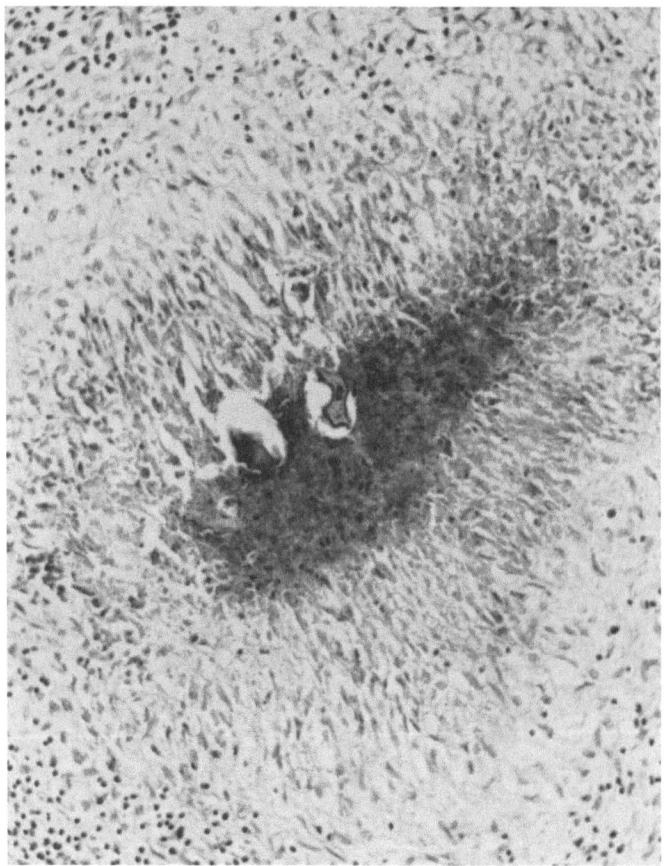

Fig. 9. Liver, granuloma caused by ova of *S. japonicum*. H. & E. X 145. AFIP Neg. no. 65-4911

It is possible that toxic products from dying worms may circulate to different parts of the liver and produce necrotizing or allergic effects. In general, however, it appears that most of the lesions in the liver directly traceable to schistosomiasis are caused by ova which, after extrusion from the female, become swept by the portal circulation into the liver. If the number of eggs is large, numerous granulomas are produced particularly in relation to the portal radicals. In time, severe portal fibrosis (Symmers' pipestem fibrosis) results, and in some cases, obstruction of the portal circulation produces portal hypertension.

Although a great deal is now known about the histopathology of schistosomiasis, there is still much to learn. The variations of the disease in different human hosts under certain environmental conditions when exposed to a certain species of cercariae "x" number of times poses complex problems which require further investigations of the experimental and natural disease.

Conclusion

The histopathology of schistosomiasis is concerned with morphologic phenomena associated with alterations of the parasite (particularly its ova) and the host. The imperfection of the host-parasite relationship together with the influence of various associated factors results in a certain degree of parasite mortality. The host becomes sensitive to the presence in its tissues of toxic and foreign material and responds by production of an inflammatory defensive reaction, sometimes appearing as suppurative foci but more often seen as chronic granulomatous lesions with more or less evidence of hypersensitivity. In infections with *S. japonicum* and *S. hematobium*, many ova appear to mineralize and fail to provoke an inflammatory reaction. The histologic evidence suggests that this mineralization may tend to prevent the expected host-parasite interaction. A review of histologic sections of many cases of human schistosomiasis and the accumulated literature suggest that, in general, the host-parasite interaction particularly occurs when the parasite is poorly adapted to its anatomic situation in the host and becomes devitalized. A well adapted parasite in a suitable anatomic position within the host provokes little if any inflammatory reaction. If this were not so, the infection could not become well established.

References

[1] CAMERON, G. R., and N. C. GANGULY: An experimental study of the pathogenesis and reversibility of schistosomal hepatic fibrosis. J. Path. Bact. **87**, 217—237 (1964).

[2] CHATTERJEE, K. D.: Parasitology, Calcutta, Sree Saraswaty Press Ltd. 1962.

[3] DIAZ-RIVERA, R. S., F. RAMOS-MORALES, E. KOPPISCH, M. R. GARCIA-PALMIERI, A. A. CINTRON-RIVERA, E. J. MARCHAND, O. GONZALEZ, and M. V. TORREGROSA: Acute Manson's schistosomiasis. Amer. J. Med. **21**, 918—943 (1956).

[4] FAUST, E. C., and H. E. MELENEY: Studies on schistosomiasis japonica. Amer. J. Hyg., Monograph Series No. 3, 1—325 (1924).

[5] ISHAK, K. G., and P. C. LeGOLVAN: Cardiopulmonary schistosomiasis, Pathology and pathogenesis. J. Méd. Liban. **10**, 347—365 (1957).

[6] MARCHAND, E. J., R. A. MARCIAL-ROJAS, R. RODRIGUEZ, G. POLANCO, and R. S. DIAZ-RIVERA: The pulmonary obstruction syndrome in Schistosoma mansoni pulmonary endarteritis. Arch. Intern. Med. **100**, 965—980 (1957).

[7] MARCIAL-ROJAS, R. A.: Protozoal and helminthic diseases. In: Pathology. W. A. D. ANDERSON, (Ed.) St. Louis, Mo.: C. V. Mosby 1966.

[8] MENEZES, H.: Embolizacao experimental dos ramos intra-hepaticos da Veia Porta de Coelhos, por exemplares adultos de Schistosoma mansoni. Rev. Inst. Med. Trop. S. Paulo **5**, 70—74 (1963).

[9] OGILVIE, B. M.: Reagin-like antibodies in animals immune to helminth parasites. Nature **204**, 91—92 (1964).

[10] PLAUT, A., and H. VOGEL: The differentiation of Schistosoma hematobium and Schistosoma mansoni according to the position of the spine. Arch. Path. **6**, 871 (1928).

Ecology and the Pathology of Bilharzia

R. Elsdon-Dew* and S. B. Bhagwandeen**

Of recent years there has been much controversy about the importance of bilharzia as a debilitating, killing disease. On the one hand, there are the schools centred in Egypt and South America, who consider that the condition is all important; on the other hand, there are large tracts of country infected with the *Schistosomes, mansoni* and *haematobium*, in which the manifestations of bilharzial disease are but slight by comparison with the distribution of the parasites. The third well-known form of bilharzia, due to *Schistosoma japonicum*, is in a slightly different position for here there cannot be much doubt as to the disease-producing potential of some strains of this particular parasite.

The concept that the more host-specific a parasite, the higher the probability of balance between host and parasite is certainly reflected in the relationship between the schistosomes and man. Though *Schistosoma haematobium* is most blatant, making itself manifest by flying a red flag, it is possibly responsible for less sequelae than are either of the other two schistosomes. *Schistosoma japonicum*, with the widest host-spectrum and therefore not so dependent on man for the maintenance of its species is least in equilibrium.

One must at this point revert to the general concept of host-parasite relationships. The evolution of such associations must have started in the very beginnings of time. Where such associations occur, host and parasite species have evolved together, almost as a single unit. The environment has selected those host-parasite relationships best adapted one to the other. Thus it is that, in the more highly-specialised parasites, equilibrium with the host is the rule. Theobald Smith, a prophet to whom honour has been given but to whom little attention has been paid, might be called the father of this concept. It is only when the development of pathogenesis increases probability of species survival of the parasite that the parasite may act to the detriment of the host species. Here one may quote tuberculosis as an example where pathogenesis by increasing dissemination increases ths chances of survival of the parasitic species. Amongst the parasites, larval forme such as hydatid may act in this way by making the victim more accessible to the predator host of the adult. For the most however it does a parasitic species little good to destroy its host species.

The extremely complicated life-cycle of the schistosomes cannot have arisen overnight and is an indication of the length of the evolutionary process. Thus we must expect that where schistosomiasis is still in a primitive relationship, equilibrium will be the rule, and disease manifestations small. However, the schistosome-man association evolved under primitive conditions and changes in the external

---

* Amoebiasis Research Unit, Durban, South Africa.

** Department of Pathology, University of Natal. Durban, South Africa.

environment may have changed the host-parasite relationship. Under primitive conditions the odds against the survival of a parasitic species are enormous — to counter this the parasite takes many bets in the lottery of life. In the schistosomes the multiplication within the intermediate host increases the probability of transmission many thousand-fold, a probability further enhanced by the host-seeking propensities of the infective phase. When man lived a pastoral life, his contacts with water were relatively few, and the parasites' chances of posterity small, but when man took to agriculture and above all to irrigation such contacts with the parasite became considerably more frequent and more prolonged.

So the odds against survival of the bilharzia species decreased. Where, before, the chances of finding a home for the children were but small, and one success in a million adequate, now there were pastures new and plenty. Where the bus service provided by the snail had been poor and erratic, man, by his lavish provision of water, not only provided more buses, but shortened the route to readily available apartment houses.

Small wonder then that a population explosion occurred. Small wonder that homes were overcrowded to the detriment of the buildings. Small wonder that eggs were laid, not in their proper place, but in every nook and cranny irrespective of their chances of survival or of the respect due to an hospitable host.

Thus the host-parasite equilibrium was upset. No doubt, given time, Nature would restore the balance, most probably by reduction of the numbers of the host-species through disease. This would indeed be poetic justice, as man, having disturbed the natural ecology for his own ends, is the guilty party. Having turned a gentle neighbour into a dangerous enemy, he must now destroy that neighbour or suffer the consequences.

The picture of varied ecology is to be seen in Southern Africa, and the contrast between the primitive disease picture and its changed counterpart is well illustrated by the manifestations of Schistosoma haematobium. Here, within a relatively short geographical distance, we have such extremes of pathognomy that it is difficult to conceive that the same parasite is responsible.

The writings of PRATES [10] from Lourenco Marques would certainly indicate that, in that area, Schistosoma haematobium is a formidable pathogen. We recall a visit to the necropsy rooms of the Miguel Bombarda hospital, where, for our edification, Dr. Prates' group had laid out the bladders of 100 consecutive necropsies. The demonstration was fabulous, in that within those 100 specimens one could find all manifestations of bilharzia ranging from the simple sandy patch to carcinoma. Over 80% of the bladders were visibly affected in one way or another. There must be few places where such a demonstration would have been possible.

The contrary picture is seen in Durban, a mere 250 air miles away, on the same coast. Here the appearance of such manifestations in the necropsy rooms is rare, and one would have to go through hundreds of bladders to find a single example.

To determine the incidence of such manifestations one of us reviewed, in 1958, [4] the post-mortem reports of the King Edward VIII Hospital in Durban, and, of some 5,000 cases at risk, that is to say over the age of five, there were but 8 cases in which, even remotely, bilharzia could have contributed to the death. That this concept was not due to lack of infection was suggested by survey [5] of the children of some of the local schools. A single urine examination carried out on

16*

peri-urban children revealed at age of approximately 15, schistosome eggs in something over 60% — a figure which implied that the infection rate would be of the order of 100% in this particular zone and yet, there was this apparently strange lack of manifestation at post-mortem.

To what might this differing manifestation be due? Why is it that in Lourenco Marques, *Schistosomiasis haematobium* is a formidable disease but in Durban as judged by the necropsy records it is by comparison unimportant? That this might be due to a difference in the race of the human population can be discounted immediately, as there has been considerable interchange between the African tribes in the area. This movement would also tend to disperse the Schistosome so that we may, at any rate initially, discount the possible difference in schistosome species. I would remind you that very shortly after Bilharz described the schistosome in Egypt, *Schistosoma capense* was described in the Eastern Cape Province of South Africa. The difference in name was probably based on the apparent difference in pathogenicity, the very difference we are now discussing.

Are there differences in the diets of the two people? The Zulu people do not, because of a tabu, eat fish, whereas the peoples of Moçambique do. This fish provides protein which is lacking to the Zulu people who were dependent on a cattle culture. The military tradition of these people caused them to despise agriculture, an attitude which not only led to the importation of Indians to work the Sugarcane fields, but no doubt restricted the Zulu contact with water, and their exposure to the schistosomes.

Differences in terrain may also play a part. The area around Lourenço Marques is an alluvial plain with meandering placid rivers. In most of Natal, the mountains are closer to the sea, and the turbulent, fast-flowing rivers are in deep valleys, making the water less accessible, and restricting the distribution of vector snails.

It would thus seem that the stage is set to give the peoples of Moçambique a much higher probability of infection than those of Natal. Nevertheless, the infection rate in coastal Natal is obviously already high, and we must therefore consider differences in individual load as being a factor determining the degree of pathogenesis. There is no easy method of determining load. To get some concept, tissue digestion of necropsy material was undertaken, and this somewhat rough and ready method has revealed that in Natal there are some fantastic loads even in the absence of pathognomy. [2]

Table. *Digestion for Schistosome ova in 200 necropsies*

Parasite	Bladder	Rectum	Liver	Lung
S. haematobium	65	54	28	28
S. mansoni	—	5	—	—
S. mattheei	9	5	1	2
Ova per gram				
Over 10^5	3	—	—	—
10^4—10^5	16	2	—	—
10^3—10^4	14	4	—	—
10^2—10^3	10	18	2	—
10—10^2	16	15	17	19
Under 10		6	10	9
Negative	135	145	171	172
All positive	32.5%	27.0%	14.%%	14.0%

Table 1 shows the findings from two hundred necropsies on cases over the age of two. This reveals that though pathology may not be apparent, ova can be found in the bladder in about a third of the cases, in the rectum, in about a quarter; in the liver and lung in about one eighth. This is no mean infection rate. In 23 cases there were over a thousand eggs per gram of bladder; in 19 cases, over 10 eggs per gram of liver; and in 19, over 10 eggs per gram of lung. It is apparent that more work must be done to allow breakdown into age and race groups, but it is equally apparent that heavy loads of S. haematobium are not uncommon in Durban. This leads to a question as yet unanswerable. − What constitutes a heavy load?

The apparent low incidence of pathology in the earlier necropsy series in Natal may have been misleading, in that the age-group of the patients dying in our hospitals is much higher than that in Lourenço Marques. It may well be that the older age group who now provides our necropsy material, were not in their youth exposed to Schistosoma haematobium to the same degree as are the youngsters of to-day who showed the extremely high incidence-rate referred to. This high incidence-rate is paralleled by the incidence of bilharzial pathology in the living.

The surgeons [3] will tell you of numerous cases of stricture of the ureter, of numerous cases with sandy patches in the bladder, and of malignant changes. On the other hand the non-oriented necrologist seeing an older age group is not impressed by the story. Is it that the majority of cases of bilharzia in Natal burn themselves out leaving little in the way of sequelae? Not only do the eggs disappear, but the tissue response too resolves. Is the failure of such resolution in Lourenço Marques, merely a result of overloading of the defences? By what mechanism does this operate?

In these days of revived interest in the immune response it is fascinating to speculate whether this is not the factor determining whether or not pathognomy results. The report by HSU and HSU [6] of protection afforded by non-pathogenic strains of S. japonicum brings the issue right into the present field. If, perchance, massive load results in immunological paralysis, this may well modify the tissue response.

The reported finding of circulating antigen in urine by OKABE and TANAKA [7] and by SHERIF [11] rather suggested that some such mechanism might be operative, but attempts to demonstrate such antigens, both by the techniques of the original authors, and by more refined, more sensitive techniques have uniformly failed in various laboratories, including our own.

The pattern of infection too may well modify the immune response. It might be that the Moçambique babies are exposed to infection so early in life that an immune tolerance is developed. We know nothing of the possibility of a sensitisation phenomenon. Does sensitisation change the histological picture? Are we perhaps by treating persons whom we cannot protect from reinfection not doing them a dis-service by interfering with some premunity? One can speculate almost ad infinitum.

Thus far the remarks have been concerned with S. haematobium, the commoner species in our part of Africa. But what of S. mansoni? The incidence of this parasite in Natal is low, and the disease subclinical. In the earlier review of 5,000 necropsies no cases of pipe-stem cirrhosis were noted, an observation which caused little surprise in view of the fact that the few cases discovered by clinical laboratory examination usually showed so few eggs that concentration was necessary for their detection. Dysentery due to *S. mansoni* is rare in the area. Nevertheless, the eggs are to be found, and the vector snails not uncommon in the lower reaches of our rivers.

Reappraisal of liver material from further cases revealed three cases of pipe-stem cirrhosis, in two of which *S. mansoni* eggs were found, and in the other, with *S. haematobium*, the condition was localised to the left lobe [1]. During further clinico-pathological study [2], a series of children presenting at the bilharzia clinic are being examined by rectal snip and ova of *S. mansoni* discovered in addition to those of *S. haematobium*. Cases are now being admitted to hospital for further study. Liver biopsy has so far been performed on eighteen cases, with results that can only be termed startling. Of these 14 had shown both *S. haematobium* and *S. mansoni* on rectal snip and 2 had *S. haematobium* only. All showed liver pathognomy. Four showed granulomata only, 2 showed eosinophilia and pigment, but 14 showed granulomata and eggs. The surprising feature was the number of eggs. In one needle biopsy specimen, weighing something of the order of 15 milligrams, 12 eggs were found. This means 800 eggs per gram, and, if the specimen be representative, implies a million eggs in the liver. It is difficult to conceive that such a load can leave no mark. The cases examined were a selected group in that it was the red flag of urinary bilharzia which brought them to hospital, and the fact that rectal snips had revealed an unsuspected *S. mansoni* infection. Nevertheless, this preliminary observation is alarming.

It will be noted in the digestion series that ova of *S. mattheei* were discovered in 17 cases. Infection with this bovine schistosome is by no means uncommon in South Africa, as has been shown by PITCHFORD [8] who has reported a rate of 25% in the Komatipoort area of the Eastern Transvaal. Such infection is not surprising in a people with a cattle culture. However, infections seem to be associated with those of *S. haematobium*. In Pitchford's series 100% of the subjects had this parasite, and "pure" cases of *S. mattheei* were not encountered in that series. Indeed, PITCHFORD [9] has suggested that these two species may hybridize. In our digestions too, no "pure" cases of *S. mattheei* infection were encountered and thus no speculation as to the activities of this fluke can be made. In cattle its depredations are usually considered unimportant, but are now under study at Onderstepoort, our Veterinary Research Institute. Whether this apparently less host-specific schistosome will, in an unusual host, behave as badly as do other parasites in such situations remains to be elucidated.

Too little work has been done on the mechanisms of the disease. Whilst there can be little doubt that the heavier loads resulting from greater exposure will cause greater pathognomy, this is not, by any means, the whole story. When one considers the way in which even large numbers of misplaced eggs can be disposed of, leaving little trace, one cannot but marvel at the reparative powers of the body. On the other hand we have seen that these can fail, but why do they fail?

It is certainly obvious that, despite the enormous volume of literature on Schistosomiasis, Bilharziasis or Bilharzia, the field is still wide open. We would plead for more attention to the host-parasite relationship at all levels and from all angles. We would stress the necessity for study of the factors determining the nature of the tissue response to varying levels of infection.

Acknowledgements

The authors would like to thank Prof. J. WAINWRIGHT, of the Department of Pathology, and Dr. S. ADNAMS, Superintendant of King Edward VIII Hospital, Durban, for advice and facilities. The Amoebiasis Research Unit is sponsored by the S. A. Council for Scientific and Industrial Research, the University of Natal, the Natal Provincial Administration, and the United States Public Health Service (Grant Al-p1592), and the junior author, Dr. S. B. BHAGWANDEEN would like to acknowledge a grant from Roche Products (Pty.) Ltd. (Grant 72—73).

References

[1] BHAGWANDEEN, S. B.: Bilharzial cirrhosis of the liver. Med. Proc. **10**, 199—206 (1964).

[2] — In preparation.

[3] CHAPMAN, D. S.: Personal communication.

[4] ELSDON-DEW, R.: The host parasite relationship in bilharzia. S. Afr. J. Sci. **54**, 43—44 (1958).

[5] FREEDMAN, L., and R. ELSDON-DEW: A note on the incidence of bilharzia in Durban Bantu children. S. Afr. Med. J. **32**, 311 (1958).

[6] HSU, H. F., and S. Y. LI HSU: The infectivity of four geographic strains of schistosoma japonicum in the rhesus monkey. J. Parasit. **46**, 228 (1960).

[7] OKABE, K., and T. TANAKA: A new urine precipitin reaction for schistosomiasis japonica; a preliminary report. Kurume Med. J. **5**, 45—52 (1958).

[8] PITCHFORD, R. J.: Cattle schistosomiasis in man in Eastern Transvaal. Trans. Toy. Soc. Trop. Med. Hyg. **53**, 285—290 (1959).

[9] — Observation on a possible hybrid between the two schistosomes, S. haematobium and S. mattheei. Trans. Roy. Soc. Trop. Med. Hyg. **55**, 44—51 (1961).

[10] PRATES, M.: Bilharzia in man. Leech **27**, 17—18 (1958).

[11] SHERIF, A. F.: Schistosomal metabolic products in the diagnosis of billharziasis. In: CIBA Foundation Symposium. Bilharziasis. WOLSTENHOLME, G. E. W., and M. O'CONNOR. (Eds.) London: Churchill 1962.

Experimental Bilharzia

J. H. S. GEAR*

With 8 figures

"Experiment is the beginning of knowledge." Nowhere has the truth of this motto been more evident than in the study of bilharzia. Indeed, in no other disease have its experimental studies been more rewarding. These have revealed the intermediate hosts of the parasites, their life cycles in the definitive hosts, the pathogenesis and pathology of the disease and the effect and value of drugs and, more recently, the biochemical and immunological reactions to the infection.

The first requirement for the experimental study of bilharzia is a susceptible laboratory animal. In nature, many species have been found infected with *Schistosoma japonica*, several with *Schistosoma mansoni*, and few with *Schistosoma haematobium*. Many of the commonly used laboratory animals are also susceptible to these infections and much valuable work has been done using white mice, guinea-pigs, rabbits and rhesus monkeys.

However, many remaining problems require elucidation and for the study of some of the aspects, the common laboratory animals are not altogether satisfactory. It appeared worthwhile, therefore, to determine the suitability of various South African veldt rodents and also the common South African vervet monkey for their use as experimental animals for the study of bilharzia.

A study of bilharzia in these experimental animals has been carried out by the Bilharzial Research Unit of the South African Institute for Medical Research for the past 15 years. The members of this team have inculeded Dr. B. DE MEILLON, Dr. H. LURIE, Dr. I. BERSOHN, Dr. B. WOLSTENHOLME, Miss H. HOWALDT, Miss B. TAPLIN and Miss G. LISTER. This report will describe briefly some of the findings.

Experimental bilharzia in South African veld rodents

In these studies the following animals have been tested in many different experiments for their susceptibility to the three species of *Schistosoma* — *S. mansoni, S. haematobium* and S. *mattheei*.

Multimammate mouse *(Praomys (Mastomys) natalensis)*
Pouched mouse *(Saccostomus campestris)*
Nile rat *(Arvicanthus niloticus)*.
African bush rat *(Aethomys chrysophilus)*.
Highveld gerbil *(Tatera brantsi)*.
White-tailed rat *(Mystromys albicaudatus)*.
White mouse *(Mus musculus)*.

All of these animals proved susceptible to *Schistosoma mansoni* infection and *Praomys (Mastomys) natalensis* has proved particularly valuable. It has been

---

* South African Institute for Medical Research, Johannesburg, South Africa.

used extensively, not only in our Institute but in many other institutions in other countries for investigation of many different aspects of bilharzia.

In a study sponsored by the World Health Organization, these veldt rodents have also been tested for their susceptibility to *Schistosoma haematobium* infection. All proved susceptible [3] They have also been shown to be susceptible to *Schistosoma mattheei*.

The most suitable as laboratory animals were *Mastomys natalensis*, *Saccostomus campestris*, *Arvicanthus niloticus* and *Mystromys albicaudatus*.

The multimammate mouse, *Praomys (Mastomys) natalensis* is one of the commonest and most widespread rodents in Africa. It is hardy and breeds prolifically under laboratory conditions but tends to bite its handlers. Some old established laboratory strains are docile and are easily handled.

The pouched mouse, *Saccostomus campestris*, occurs from the Cape to north of the Equator in East Africa. It is not a common species but is widely distributed, inhabiting sub-tropical savannah bush country. It is nocturnal. Pouched mice are small rodents weighing up to 90 g and need no special diet. They are easily handled except during the mating season when they become vicious and readily bite; the female, when pregnant, is liable to kill the male if the pair is kept together. They are relatively easy to breed, having about four litters in a year during the restricted breeding season between September and March (southern summer). They live in underground burrows, often in association with gerbils *(Tatera)* and tend to avoid water. They have not been found naturally infected with any schistosome. In the laboratory they are highly susceptible to *S. mansoni*, *S. mattheei*, *S. haematobium* and *S. rodhaini*.

The Nile rat, *Arvicanthus niloticus* occurs north of the Zambesi and is widely distributed in Central, West, North and East Africa. It is particularly numerous in cultivated areas. It is mainly nocturnal and breeds freely in the laboratory provided potatoes are given. It is relatively easy to handle and weighs up to about 150 g. The stock used in our laboratory have been bred from a nucleus established at the Virus Research Institute, Entebbe, Uganda. This species does not occur in Africa south of the Zambesi. It is highly susceptible in the laboratory to *S. mansoni*, *S. mattheei*, *S. haematobium* and *S. rodhaini*, but has not been found naturally infected although it does not avoid water.

The white-tailed rat or South African hamster, *Mystromys albicaudatus*, is the only member of the sub-family Cricetinae in Sub-Saharan Africa and is restricted to the South East of Southern Africa. It has been bred in the laboratory since 1940 and has been extensively used as an experimental animal. In the laboratory it is long-lived and may reach the age of six years. It breeds readily and may produce over 20 litters in its lifetime. It is thoroughly adapted to laboratory conditions and is now easy to handle. It weighs up to 180 g, needs no special care or diet and is susceptible to *S. mansoni*, *S. haematobium* and *S. mattheei*. In the field it avoids water and does not occur in the endemic bilharzia areas.

Our studies of bilharzia in these experimental animals have had the following purposes: to trace the course taken by the schistosomules in their migration from the site of infection to the portal system of veins where they mature and lay eggs; to study the pathogenesis and pathological lesions produced by the infection in the course of this migration; to correlate the development of pathological lesions with immunological and biochemical findings; to assess the value of serological tests in diagnosis; to determine the value of live vaccines in conferring protection against infection and to work out the limitations of this method of protection; and finally to test the value and toxicity of new drugs for the treatment of this disease.

Migration of schistosomules. Many attempts have been made to trace the migration of the schistosomules from the point of penetration of the skin by the cercariae to the mature worms in the tributaries and branches of the portal veins. Recently Stirewalt [6] in particular has studied the adhesion of the cercariae to the skin and the role of the secretions of the acinotubular glands in facilitating their penetration and passage through the skin to the deeper layers of the dermis where they enter lymphatic vessels.

In our studies, as in those of others, the schistosomules have been traced in their passage through the skin to the regional lymph glands to the lungs and finally their appearance in the portal veins in the liver has been noted. The reactions to this invasion have been observed.

In the skin, a mild inflammatory infiltration of cells, mostly polymorphonuclear leucocytes is evoked in the dermis. In animals sensitized by previous exposure the reaction is more severe and includes numerous polymorphonuclear leucocytes, eosinophilic leucocytes and round cells with some oedema. Little reaction results from the presence of the schistosomules in the lymph glands in primary infections. In the lungs the schistosomules appear to make their way to the periphery of the lobules and many come to lodge adjacent the visceral pleura. Perhaps they actively penetrate it and the diaphragm and the capsule of the liver to enter the portal veins. It is generally presumed that they return to the heart and from there are distributed via the general circulation and a few fortunate worms finally reach the portal veins. However, often over 50% of cercariae give rise to mature worms and this haphazard route appears unlikely. Further studies are necessary to elucidate the path by which the schistosomules travel from the lung to the liver.

Pathogenesis and pathology. In the portal veins of the liver the worms rapidly mature and soon produce eggs. In *S. mansoni* infections, eggs are found sometimes within five weeks, often within six weeks, and regularly within eight after exposure to cercariae. In *S. haematobium* infections, it takes about twice as long before eggs are first detected. In both infections a subacute to chronic progressive often fatal disease ensues. It is characterized by bilharzial lesions in the liver and intestine, often in the lungs and pancreas, sometimes in the spleen and rarely in the bladder. The characteristic lesion, the bilharzial tubercle, consists of a central multinucleate giant cell formed around an egg or the remnants of an egg, surrounded by a zone of polymorphonuclear and eosinophil leucocytes and a peripheral zone of monocytes, lymphocytes and plasma cells and in time by fibroblasts which form a capsule of fibrous tissue.

Numerous eggs and large egg nests are often found displacing lobules of the pancreas and in the submucosa of the intestine sometimes with loss of the overlying epithelium.

These lesions are clearly related to the presence of eggs in the tissues. Live worms appear not to be associated with an inflammatory reaction in their immediate neighbourhood. Their cuticles are free from adhering leucocytes, platelets and red cells. However, they excrete pigment granules, presumably haematin which is first seen in the phagocytic cells of the portal tracts, and then in the Kupffer cells lining the sinusoids and then widely distributed in reticulo-endothelial cells notably in the spleen and occasionally in distal lymph nodes.

The presence of live worms is also primarily concerned in inducing a state of hypersensitivity in their host manifest by some eosinophil leucocytes in the portal tracts and the eosinophilia in the blood. Their presence also stimulates the state of hyperreactivity manifest in the active germinal centres in the spleen and lymph nodes. The state of immunity induced by prolonged infection is also related to the presence of live worms.

Dead worms stimulate a marked reaction in their vicinity. There is great thickening of the intima and a marked perivascular cell collection. The body of the worm is invaded particularly by polymorphonuclear leucocytes and then by other phagocytic cells. In time the worm is dissolved completely and all signs of its presence obliterated except for strands of fibrous tissue.

The relative role of eggs and of worms and their other products in the pathogenesis of the lesions of bilharzia has long been a vexed question. It is clear that experimental studies offer an opportunity of analyzing the contributions made by each of the components to the stimulation of the reactions to bilharzial infection.

Role of nutrition. The role of nutrition in determining the progress of infection has also received attention. Somewhat contrary to expected findings, malnourished animals supported infections less well than those receiving adequate diets[2].

Effects of drug treatment. Several schistosomocidal drugs have been tested in these rodents. These results will not be considered in detail. It has been shown, however, that treatment with many of those currently used is highly effective and it is possible to study in detail the subsequent resolution of the lesions. In time the only sign to be seen of once florid lesions is a few firm onion skin fibrous nodules in the portal tracts. The lesions formed in the vicinity of dead worms appear to be completely resolved.

Malignant change. After three or more years a proportion of the Mastomys infected with *S. mansoni* have developed primary cancer of the liver. The significance of this finding has not yet been assessed. Its occurrence suggests lines of study of carcinogenesis in bilharzia.

Epidemiological and ecological studies. Dr. PITCHFORD [5] has used Mastomys extensively in epidemiological studies to determine the patterns of infection in different areas at different seasons. It has been shown that the incidence of infection of *S. mansoni* acquired by immersion in water has two peaks; one in late spring and the other in autumn. Few infections are acquired in winter. These studies could with advantage be applied to other regions and using other experimental animals, to other species of schistosome.

Bilharzia in monkeys

It may rightly be argued that the disease in rodents differs in many of its features from that seen in man. In this respect monkeys present a picture more comparable with that in human bilharzial infections.

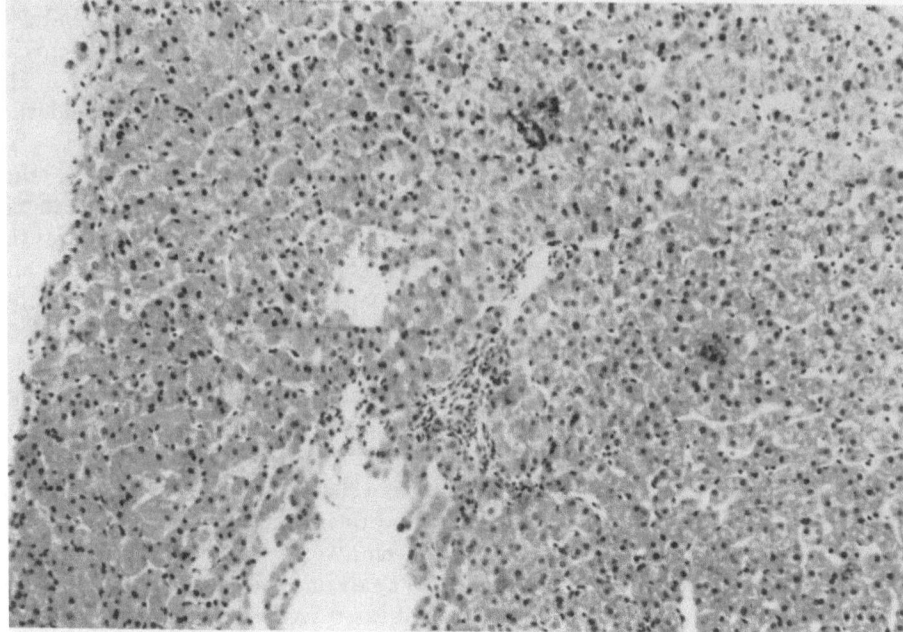

Fig. 1. Monkey 5/59. 26 weeks after first treatment. Liver biopsy. Some portal tracts show fibrosis, others a mild cellular infiltration but no evidence of bilharzia

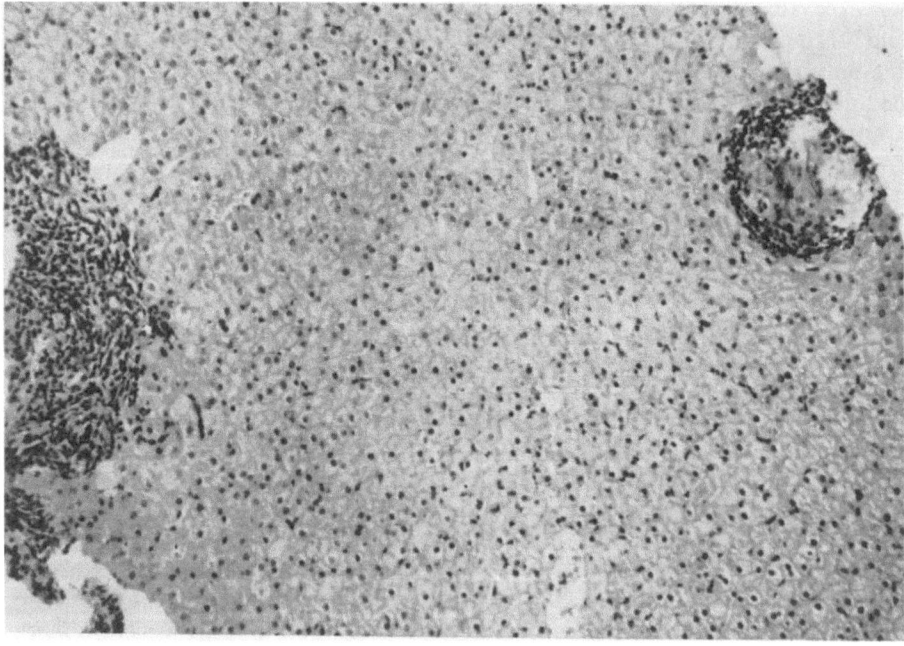

Fig. 2. Monkey 5/59, 52 weeks after first re-infection. Liver biopsy. Portal tracts show bilharzial tubercles and heavy cellular infiltration

Macacus monkeys have been used in the study of S. *japonicum* and S. *mansoni* infections. The latter tend to spontaneous cure after about one year. RICHIE and his co-workers have reported that in *Cercopithecus sabaeus* infected with a single dose of 100 cercariae, egg production continued for at least $3^1/_2$ years. Various aspects of S. *mansoni*, S. *mattheei* and S. *haematobium* infections have been investigated by our Unit. From our studies too it is clear that the course of infection in vervet monkeys, *Cercopithecus aethiops* more closely simulates that seen in man.

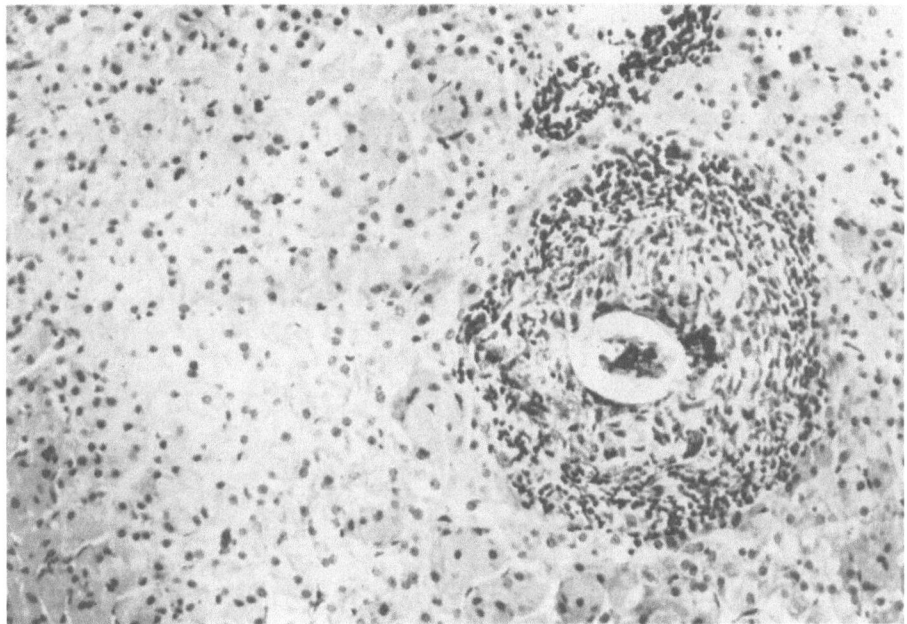

Fig. 3. Monkey 5/59, 53 weeks after second re-infection. Liver biopsy. Portal tract shows bilharzial tubercle with central multinucleated giant cells containing remnants of ovum and surrounded by endothelial cells, polymorphonuclear cells and numerous eosinophil leucocytes and round cells and few scattered pigment cells. Kupffer cells contain yellow pigment

Attention will be called briefly to a few of the findings in particular to the correlation of the pathological, biochemical and immunological events.

In a series of infected and control monkeys, liver biopsy specimens were taken at weekly, then monthly and then three monthly intervals. At the same time blood was taken for biochemical and serological tests.

The results obtained in two of these monkeys are given in the accompanying photographs (Fig. 1—8) to illustrate the salient features of these infections.

Pathologically, as seen in liver biopsy, the first evidence of infection appearing one to two weeks after infection was a mild inflammatory cell infiltration of the portal tracts associated with some parenchymal cell damage and degeneration Fig. 1—5. Biochemically this was associated with a transient positive reaction in the cephalin cholesterol test and an increase in the serum glutamic oxaloacetic transaminase (SGOT) level. The latter increased still further when the stage of egg laying began. Eggs were first detected in the portal tracts from 5—8 weeks after infection. The appearance of eggs was followed by the formation of bilharzial tubercles.

This coincided with biochemical changes involving alteration of the protein pattern with a marked increase in the globulin level due mainly to a rise in the gamma globulin content. The albumin level showed a significant decrease. Certain of these biochemical changes suggest parenchymal liver cell damage while others reflect stimulation of the reticulo-endothelial system [1].

Several monkeys have now been followed for nearly five years. The pathological changes include "pipe stem" fibrosis of the portal tracts; the biochemical changes including very high gamma globulin levels which suggest liver cirrhosis.

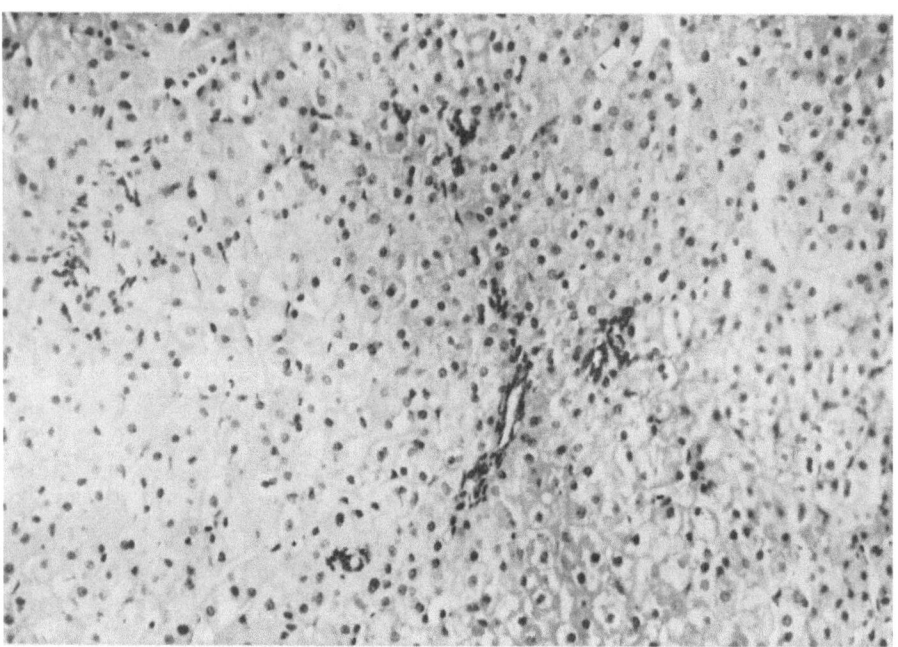

Fig. 4. Monkey 5/59, 13 weeks after third treatment. Liver biopsy. Portal tract shows slight increase in cells including few polymorphonuclear and eosinophil leucocytes and round cells and an occasional cell loaded with brown pigment. No worms or eggs. Kupffer cells contain no pigment

Other monkeys treated with Miracil D given in a dose of 100 mg/kg of body weight as a 2% aqueous solution by stomach tube on each of five consecutive days have been cured. The lesions in the liver have resolved and the pattern returned to normal. The biochemical pattern including the albumin globulin ratio, the level of gamma globulin and the zinc sulphate turbidity has also returned to normal.

When these monkeys were reinfected the same pathological (Fig. 6—8) and biochemical changes recurred and after cure again the pattern returned to normal.

The immunological response is also of interest. The complement fixation test gave positive results often three weeks after infection and usually one month after infection. Blood eosinophilia was usually apparent somewhat later from five weeks onwards.

Ova may be found in the faeces as early as six weeks but usually not until eight weeks have elapsed.

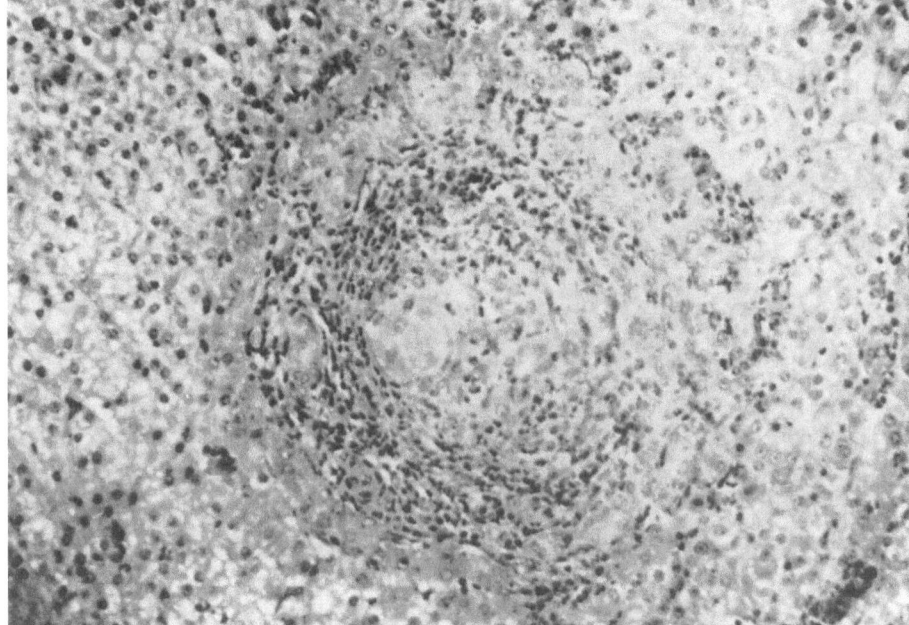

Fig. 5. Monkey 11/59, 29 weeks after infection. Liver biopsy. Portal tract shows marked infiltration of neutrophil and eosinophil leucocytes and lymphoid cells and a bilharzial tubercle with a central multinucleated giant cell and surrounding poly morphonuclear and eosinophil leucocytes, round cells and few pigment cells. Kupffer cells contain pigment

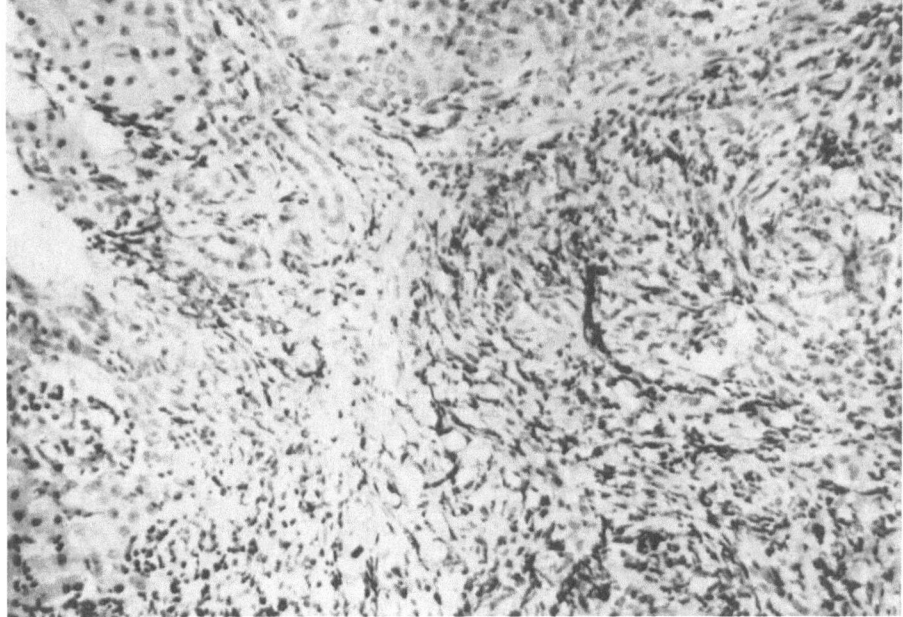

Fig. 6. Monkey 11/59, 10 weeks after re-infection; 40 weeks after infection. Liver biopsy. Portal tracts show infiltration of inflammatory cells and fibrosis. Kupffer cells contain large amounts of brown pigment

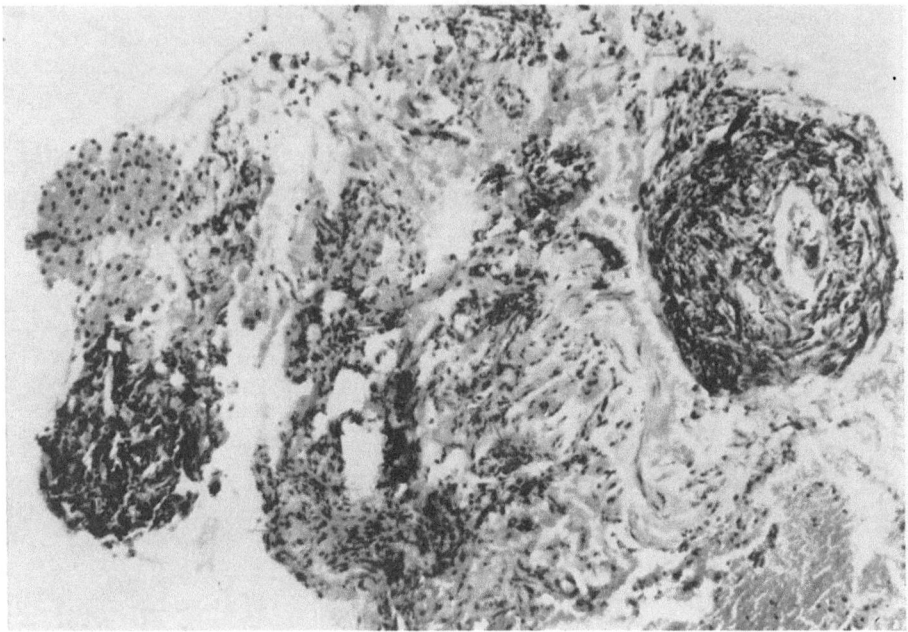

Fig. 7. Monkey 11/59, 51 weeks after re-infection; 81 weeks after infection. Liver biopsy. Portal tract shows heavy infiltration of cells and definite fibrosis and a bilharzial tubercle with central ovum

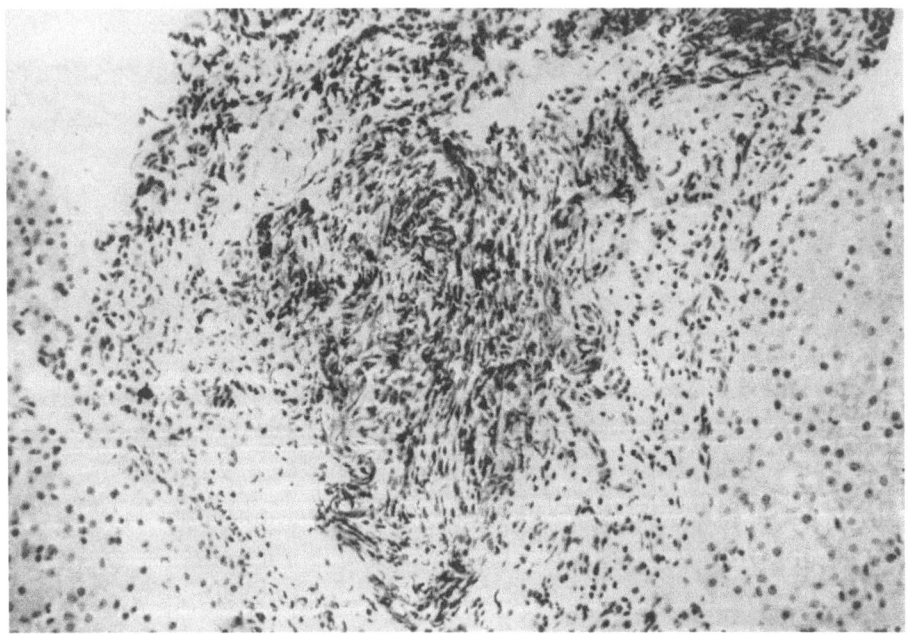

Fig. 8. Monkey 11/59, 173 weeks after re-infection; 203 weeks after infection. Liver biopsy. Portal tracts show marked infiltration of inflammatory cells, mostly round cells including lymphocytes, plasma cells and mononuclears and histocytes and fibroblasts and considerable fibrosis. Polymorphonuclear and eosinophil leucocytes are also present. No worms or ova detected

Diagnosis of bilharzia. These findings are relevant in considering the diagnosis of bilharzia for this sequence of events has a parallel in human infections. In the latter, as in the monkey, the first tests to give positive results are the biochemical tests. Rises in the transaminase levels and then a positive cephalin cholesterol reaction are found before the immunological tests give positive results. However, as they are not specific tests, they do not have specific diagnostic value. Of the specific diagnostic tests the complement fixation test and, as shown more recently, the fluorescent antibody test are the first to give positive results. These are first obtained sometimes as early as the third week and usually within one month after infection. Eosinophilia in the blood while not of specific value is very suggestive of infection in those known to have been exposed to infection. However, in man as in monkeys it may not become apparent until the fifth or sixth week after infection. The fact that the immunological tests give a clear clue to the diagnosis is of practical importance as treatment may be commenced before the tissue damaging egg laying stage has commenced. Eggs are not excreted in most human infections, as in the vervet monkeys, until towards the end of the second month or during the third month after infection.

Immunization with "cercarial vaccines". Clinical experience has indicated that in hyperendemic areas, the proportion of individuals excreting eggs tends to diminish with increasing age after adolescence. This in itself suggests the development of a state of immunity.

Some years ago LURIE and DE MEILLON [3] showed that mice first exposed to a relatively small dose of cercariae were able to resist successfully a heavy dose which in normal mice caused a high mortality. Since then, many studies carried out in several other institutions as well as our own, have suggested that infection with irradiated cercariae confers some degree of immunity to subsequent challenge with normal cercariae. However, the stimulation artificially of immunity and the development and use and value of cercarial vaccines is a large and important subject and merits full consideration on its own.

Summary

Experimental studies have shown that the multimammate mouse *Praomys (Mastomys) natalensis*, the pouched mouse *Saccostomys campestris*, the Nile rat, *Arvicanthus niloticus*, the African bush rat *Aethomys chrysophilus*, the highveld gerbil *Tatera brantsi* and the white tailed rat *Mystromys albicaudatus* are susceptible to infection with *S. mansoni* and *S. haematobium*. Because of their adaptability the most suitable were *Mastomys*, *Saccostomus*, *Arvicanthus* and *Mystromys*, and animals of the two former species have been used extensively in the study of the pathogenesis and pathology of bilharzia.

Attempts have been made to determine the route taken by the schistosomules from the point of penetration of the skin to the portal veins of the liver. They have been traced through the skin, the regional lymph glands and lung. The route taken from the lungs to liver needs elucidation.

In the skin a mild inflammatory infiltration of cells including eosinophil leucocytes is evoked in the dermis. Little or no inflammatory reaction occurs in their immediate vicinity in the lymph glands or lung. In the liver, the earliest signs include slight infiltration of the portal tracts and some degeneration of the paren-chymal cells around the central veins. Later the cell infiltration becomes marked and includes numerous eosinophil leucocytes, and when eggs are produced, cha-racteristic bilharzial tubercles consisting of a central multinucleate giant cell containing an ovum or the remnants of an ovum, surrounded by eosinophil and polymorph leucocytes, lymphocytes and plasma cells, and later by fibroblasts are formed. Live worms have no cells adhering to them. Dead worms stimulate a marked cellular reaction mostly of polymorphonuclear leucocytes. Finally all traces of the worm are removed by phagocytes.

The evolution of the bilharzial lesions in the South African vervet monkey *Cercopithecus aethiops pygerythrus* have been studied and correlated with the blood count, blood biochemistry and serological findings. The earliest pathological change is an acute hepatitis associated with corresponding changes in the liver function tests. Later coinciding with the appearance of the bilharzial tubercles there is a marked change in the serum protein pattern with a reversal of the albumin/globulin ratio, due mainly to a considerable increase in gammaglobulin.

The bilharzial lesions disappear after treatment and the biochemical pattern returns to normal.

The complement fixation test first gives positive results about 3—4 weeks after infection and remains positive for many months after successful treatment. Eosinophilia in the blood is usually noted 4—6 weeks after infection.

Infection of experimental animals with irradiated cercariae may protect to some extent against subsequent infection with normal cercariae. Further study is necessary to determine the value and limitations of this method of immunization.

References

[1] BERSOHN, I., and H. I. LURIE: Experimental bilharziasis in animals. II. Correlation of biochemistry (Liver function tests) and histopathological changes in the liver in early bilharziasis. S. Afr. Med. J. 27, 950—954 (1953).

[2] DE MEILLON, B., and S. PATERSON: Experimental bilharziasis in animals. Effect of a low protein diet on bilharziasis in white mice. S. Afr. Med. J. 32, 1086—1088 (1958).

[3] GEAR, J. H. S., and R. J. G. PITCHFORD: The susceptibility of South African veld rodents to schistosome infections (In press).

[4] LURIE, H. I., and B. DE MEILLON: Experimental bilharziasis in laboratory animals. V. Immunity in mice produced by repeated small infections. S. Afr. Med. J. 31, 68—69, (1957).

[5] PITCHFORD, R. J.: Personal communication.

[6] STIREWALT, M. A., and F. J. KRUIDENIER: Activity of the acetabular secretory apparatus of cercariae of Schistosoma mansoni under experimental conditions. Exp. Parasit. 11, 191—211 (1961).

Immunodiagnosis in Schistosomiasis

ELVIO H. SADUN*

Introduction

Approximately 150 million people throughout the world are estimated to be presently infected with schistosomes. Although it is known that human infection with this trematode constitutes an important clinical and public health problem in Asia, Africa and South America and, to a lesser extent in the West Indies, reasonably accurate data on the prevalence and intensity of this infection are not often available. In many instances we do not even know whether the incidence of schistosomiasis in a given population group is increasing or decreasing and whether the areas affected are expanding or contracting. This lack of essential knowledge is largely due to the fact that an unequivocal diagnosis of schistosomiasis is difficult to obtain.

Since the clinical picture is not well defined and the organisms cannot always be detected by direct microscopic examination of the excreta, there is a great need for reliable laboratory procedures which could provide a basis for the rapid and accurate diagnosis of this infection. For these reasons, many investigators in recent years have attempted to develop immunological tests of value in individual diagnosis, in epidemiologic surveys, in determining the results of treatment and in establishing the efficacy of control.

A judgment of the relative merits of direct identification of the organisms and indirect immunodiagnosis in schistosomiasis is beyond the scope of this presentation.

However, it is necessary to emphasize that although recovery of schistosome eggs is proof of schistosomiasis, negative stool or urine examinations do not exclude infection. Actually, in early mild infections and in cases which have been therapeutically affected, the finding of eggs in the excreta is rather unusual. Furthermore, microscopic examination of the excreta is time consuming and somewhat "impersonal" unless the specimen is produced in the same place it is examined. It is not uncommon to find individuals who for esthetic reasons, because of religious and social interdiction, or because of constipation will either fail to submit samples for examinations or present as their own stools those produced by members of their families or collected in the nearest pit privy. As far as urine examinations are concerned, anyone who had experience in endemic regions is aware that babies usually do not urinate into bottles.

On the other hand, great danger exists in placing too much confidence in indirect immunological techniques. A positive reaction may simply indicate a previous exposure to infection or the presence of antibodies to substances anti-

* Department of Medical Zoology. Division of Communicable Disease and Immunology. Walter Reed Army Institute of Research. Walter Reed Army Medical Center. Washington, D.C.

17*

genically related to schistosomes. Furthermore, whereas the number of eggs recovered in excreta may have some relationship to the number of parasites present in the host, no immunological test so far devised for schistosomiasis has been shown to have a proven relationship to the intensity of infection, to the virulence of the organisms involved or to the immunological status of the host.

Critical reviews of various techniques have been published recently [23, 26, 42]. Therefore, rather than attempt to review critically or even present a complete list of the numerous tests which have been developed for the immunological diagnosis of schistosomiasis during the last 50 years, only those techniques with which the author and his collaborators have been involved in the last decade will be detailed here. This should not be misconstrued as an attempt to suggest that the tests discussed here are the best or the only valuable ones for the laboratory diagnosis of schistosomiasis.

1. Intradermal tests

A world wide program for the standardization and evaluation of the intradermal test for schistosomiasis is being actively pursued through the encouragement and coordination of the World Health Organization. This test has distinct advantages since it is relatively inexpensive, permits screening of large population groups in a relatively short time and provides immediate results. Since the skin reactions appear within 15–20 minutes after introduction of the antigen, the results can be read before the patients have been dismissed.

Although the intradermal test is a valuable aid in some epidemiologic investigations and public health practices, its clinical applications are very limited in schistosomiasis since great variations in sensitivity and specificity are often encountered. These variations may be due to differences in the character of the antigens employed, age or sex of patients, duration of active infection or site of injection. Furthermore, difficulties are often encountered in standardizing the antigens employed, in performing the test and in reading the results. A wide variety of antigens from different stages of the life cycle of the schistosomes have been used, but in general, extracts from adult worms provide more sensitive antigens than do those from cercariae or eggs. Moreover, it was reported that homologous intradermal tests in S. japonicum endemic areas give better results than in S. mansoni areas [49], that children, and in particular females under the age of puberty, give a lower percentage of reactions [19, 37] and that the scapular region near the neck is a more sensitive site for skin testing than the forearm [23, 24], Cross reactions were observed in areas endemic for Schistosoma bovis [46], and in patients with other trematode infections [49]. This indicates that in areas of the world where nonhuman mammalian schistosomiasis, clonorchiasis or paragonimiasis is prevalent a large proportion of false positive reactions might occur with this test.

2. Serological tests

In vitro tests employing serum from individuals with suspected schistosomiasis have been in existence for more than half a century since YOSHIMOTO [64] first described a complement fixation procedure. Since then great strides have taken place in the development of a variety of serological procedures.

a) Complement fixation test. For a number of years relatively crude extracts of cercariae or of adult worms were used as sources of antigen in the complement fixation test. Although encouraging results were obtained, numerous cross reactions were observed, particularly with sera from syphilitic patients. This difficulty was obviated by extracting the parasite with anhydrous ether prior to extracting in buffered saline [13]. Further attempts to purify the antigenic material [27, 41], 43, 49, 50, 51, 52, 55, 56] and improve the performance of the test itself [27] have produced a complement fixation test with a high degree of sensitivity and specificity (Table 1). Similar levels of sensitivity and specificity were obtained in the complement fixation test using antigens from different stages of the schistosome life cycle (both endogenous and exogenous). However, sera which gave frank positive reactions with one antigen were frequently non reactive with another. This suggests that the antigenic mixtures used may not react with the same antibodies and that the relative concentrations of these antibodies may vary significantly during the course of infection and in different individuals. This test permits the detection of infection before the worms reach maturity and produce eggs. In general, one can conclude that the complement fixation test is the most reliable procedure when performed under optimal conditions. However, this reaction requires complicated and highly delicate techniques which must be performed under the supervision of experienced and competent serologists. Furthermore, unless blood obtained by venipuncture is transported rapidly to the laboratory, a large percentage of specimens develop anticomplementary properties which make them unsuitable for testing.

b) Slide flocculation test. Since flocculation techniques appear to fulfill the need for simple serological tests, many attempts to develop them have been made. BRANDT and FINCH [10] described a simple flocculation test for the diagnosis of this trematode infection. However, attempts by several investigators to obtain satisfactory reproducible results with such flocculation tests were unsuccessful. Similarly, the results of a different flocculation test reported by WRIGHT et al.

Table 1. *Summary of representative results obtained recently with sera from Schistosomiasis patients*

Test	Source of Antigen	No. of Specimens	Positive	Doubtful	Negative	Reference
Complement fixation	Adult	540	507	23	10	ANDERSON et al., [8]
Complement fixation	Cercariae	544	505	16	23	ANDERSON et al., [8]
Complement fixation	Cer. excr. secr.	61	54	0	7	SLEEMAN et al., [56]
Slide flocculation	Cercariae	519	470	40	9	ANDERSON et al., [8]
Slide flocculation	Adult excr. secr.	48	36	3	9	SADUN et al., [44]
Slide flocculation	Eggs	37	31	0	6	SADUN et al., [44]
SPC (serum)	Cercariae	29	27	0	2	SADUN et al., [45]
SPC (plasma)	Cercariae	189	186	3	0	SADUN et al., [45]
Fluorescent antibody (serum)	Cercariae	107	80	18	9	SADUN et al.,]48]
Fluorescent antibody (dried blood)	Cercariae	152	140	5	7	SADUN et al., [47]
Fluorescent antibody (soluble antigen)	Adult	87	86	1	0	TOUSSAINT and ANDERSON, [61]

[63] on sera obtained from military personnel harboring S. japonicum proved to be extremely variable.

Recently, Anderson [3] described a simple and reliable slide flocculation test which utilizes lipid-free cercarial antigen coated onto cholesterol-lecithin crystals. The sensitivity of the antigen in this test was greatly increased by removing the antigen-cholesterol-lecithin complex from the salt solution in which it was prepared and by resuspending the complex in fresh salt solution. This test was evaluated on sera from individuals with proven S. mansoni infection. As indicated in Table 1, only a few of these gave false negative results [8]. The specificity of this procedure was also found to be excellent [19]. The main advantages of this test lie in its reliability, relative simplicity and economy. Another favorable aspect is that all the serologically reactive antibody for this test can be removed without any dilution by simple absorption with a calculated volume of washed, packed and essentially dry antigen-cholesterol-lecithin complex, [2]. This permits the standardization of antisera in terms of amounts of antibody nitrogen, thus introducing into the field of schistosomiasis some of the quantitative criteria which in the past existed only in the serology of some bacterial infections.

Recently antigenic extracts from schistosome eggs and water soluble secretions and excretions from adult worms have been coated onto cholesterol-lecithin crystals [44]. This permitted investigations into the probable existence and relative diagnostic value of stage specific antigens. The reactions obtained in the slide flocculation test with antigens from eggs, cercariae, and adult excretions and secretions (ES) were compared in artificially immunized and experimentally infected animals as well as in naturally infected humans to determine whether they stimulated or detected distinct humoral factors or whether they differed only in the relative proportions of common antigens. Furthermore, attempts were made to isolate and define some of the soluble antigenic fractions present in egg, cercaria and adult S. mansoni extracts to ascertain which are common to various stages; to characterize the antigenic fractions which are adsorbed onto cholesterol-lecithin crystals, and to compare results obtained with the slide flocculation test and immunoelectrophoresis before and after homologous and heterologous serum absorption.

Although flocculation tests with all 3 antigens gave consistently satisfactory results, the ES antigen seemed to confer to the test the greatest sensitivity and specificity. Homologous and heterologous absorptions revealed the presence of stage specific reacting fractions which stimulate distinct humoral factors.

In this connection it is of particular interest to notice that antibodies against adult ES extracts could be detected in monkeys more than 3 years following a single exposure to infection and more than a year after antibodies against egg and cercaria extracts were no longer detectable. The slide flocculation (SF) test using adult ES antigen might also be of value in early infections as demonstrated in the experimentally infected animals. Further studies should also be conducted to determine whether the SF test employing egg extracts might offer promise as a possible means of evaluating the results of chemotherapy, although negative results obtained so far along these lines with other serological tests for schistosomiasis do not justify great optimism. The demonstration of stage specific antibodies in schistosomiasis is also of great interest in the study of possible mechanisms of acquired immunity to this infection. A major drawback in the use of this test, as in most other serological tests, is the requirement for fresh serum.

c) Plasma card test. The need existed for a test which would utilize a few drops of blood collected by finger puncture instead of serum. This led to the development of a card test [45] using one drop of plasma obtained from a few drops of finger with the Brewer's collection slide [11]. This technique, which is referred to as the schistosomiasis plasma card test, makes use of the slide flocculation test antigen suspension. After centrifugation the antigen complex sediment is resuspended in a solution containing charcoal powder as a visualizing agent [40]. Tests are performed on plastic coated cards which may be filed for future reference after proper drying. This test was evaluated in endemic areas [45], and found to possess a satisfactory degree of sensitivity and specificity (Table 1). The practical advantages of this field screening test are obvious. It is rapid, economical and does not require any of the usual laboratory equipment. All materials employed are disposable and supplies and apparatus for performing a hundred tests are included in a kit which occupies less than one square foot of space and weighs less than one pound. In addition, the cards provide permanent records for future reference. The main drawbacks of this test are that some samples can be read only with some difficulty and that quantitative determinations of antibody titers are not readily available.

d) Fluorescent antibody test. A fluorescent antibody technique has been developed for the serodiagnosis of schistosomiasis [48]. When this indirect test, employing formalin fixed cercariae or miracidia of any of the human schistosomes as a source of antigen, was evaluated with sera from people in endemic areas, it appeared to be approximately as sensitive and specific as the complement fixation test and the slide flocculation test (Table 1). One of the great advantages of this test is that it is easily standardized. An early difficulty was the need for relatively freshly shed cercariae or miracidia, since their storage for a few days rendered them unsuitable for diagnostic work. This was due to internal staining which occurred in these stored organisms when exposed to fluorescein-tagged globulins regardless of whether they had been previously exposed to normal or immune serum specimens.

This technique was improved and rendered more practical by the introduction of rhodamine bovine albumin (RBA) as a counterstain [6]. The use of this fluorochrome gives the organisms a bright orange-red coloration which contrasts vividly with the greenish-yellow color of fluorescein when the specimens are viewed with ultraviolet light. This method obviates the need for maintaining a fresh supply of cercariae in the central diagnostic laboratory and permits satisfactory results even with cercariae which have been preserved in formalin for longer than a month, or frozen or lyophilized. Cercariae thus treated could be mailed and used for the test by distant serological laboratories.

A further improvement of this test was introduced when extracted fluids from minute quantities of dried blood smears on filter paper were used successfully in place of serum, thus obviating the need for venipuncture [7, 47]. In this way minute drops of finger blood obtained in an endemic area, smeared on filter paper, allowed to dry and mailed to a central laboratory can be extracted and used for the fluorescent antibody test. The combination of mailing dried blood specimens and of using preserved cercariae makse the fluorescent antibody test one of the simplest and most practical serologic methods for the diagnosis of schistosomiasis and bridges the usually conspicuous gap between endemic areas and central laboratories. This technique has been evaluated by several investigators in different parts of the world [14, 18, 21, 29, 38] with excellent results.

The principal advantages for the test performed on dried blood smears are: a) large collections of specimens may be obtained in endemic areas even from infants, since only one or two drops of blood are required; b) blood may be collected by puncture of finger, toe or heel with a minimum of apparatus; c) collection may be made by relatively untrained personnel without regard to sterility of the specimens; and d) dried blood smears may be placed in an envelope and mailed to a central laboratory where the tests can be performed with standardized reagents by adequately trained laboratory personnel. The main disadvantages of this test are: a) fluorescent microscopy equipment is rather expensive and not available to many laboratories; b) booklets of filter paper for blood collection are not commercially available at the present time; c) extensive cross reactions occur with non human schistosomes [46]; and d) unless batches of antiglobulin are carefully prepared and titrated, unsatisfactory results may be obtained [12].

A recent modification of the fluorescent antibody test for schistosomiasis was introduced by using soluble delipidized adult somatic extracts on an artificial matrix of cellulose acetate filter paper [60, 61]. A small cellulose acetate paper disc containing the antigen is used in each test. Following testing by the indirect FA procedure the results are read on a fluorometer fitted with a paper chromatogram door. The instrument is set at zero using a normal serum control disc and the specific fluorescence of the the test zera is determined. Findings obtained with homologous and heterologous antisera indicated that the method yields excellent results.

e) Other serologic procedures. Many other serological tests have been described for the laboratory diagnosis of schistosomiasis. Leading among those employing soluble antigens are the precipitin tests [33, 35, 59] the hemagglutination test [25], and the conglutination test [36]. Among the serological tests employing whole organisms, the most promising procedures are: the cercarienhuellen reaction [62], the cercarial agglutination test [30], the miracidial immobilization test [53], the circumoval precipitin test [31], and the phagocytic response test [34]. Some of these tests must still be regarded as research tools because of limited evaluation for routine diagnosis and because they may require living organisms not readily available to most laboratories.

Discussion

In spite of the great progress achieved in recent years, the immuno-diagnosis of schistosomiasis is still at a formative stage. Many serological tests have been developed and noteworthy advances have been made in the attempt to reduce cross reactions by purifying antigens through physical and chemical fractionation. Nonetheless, *in vitro* cross reactions between *S. mansoni* antigens and serum from patients with *Trichinella spiralis* infection have been shown in different tests from all stages of the schistosome life cycle. Fortunately, since the geographic distribution of the two diseases is fairly distinct this cross reaction does not represent a serious limitation in the practical application of schistosome serology, unless one is interested in detecting infections in troops or other persons not indigenous to an endemic schistosome area. Yet, the fact that such cross reaction occurs between two organisms which are so phyliogenetically separated is quite intriguing and demonstrates the complexity of helminth serology. Absorption studies to determine the relationship of the schistosome and *Trichinella* antigens [7] have shown that the cross reaction between *S. mansoni* and *T. spiralis* lacks reciprocity and that the homologous antigen fails to remove reactivity toward the heterologous antibody. In this connection, one must consider that we are in fact dealing with most complex mixtures, that the antigens used are from tissues which are made of different cells built up of many different molecules of functional antigen. Each functional antigen probably consists of a mosaic of small structural units each of which is a potentially specific immunologic determinant. Since only a few amino acids or sugars are involved in each determinant of immunological specificity, it is indeed remarkable that naturally complex materials such as helminths have specific properties at all and show a relative lack of common determinant [4].

In the serology of schistosomiasis there is still no test suitable for the detection of early infections and of chemotherapeutic cures. Therefore, the search for more sensitive and specific antigens to be derived from different stages of the life cycle of the parasite must continue.

Greater emphasis on evaluating excretory and secretory antigens from the various stages of the life cycle of schistosomes in different serological tests may resolve some of the unanswered questions on the subject. In this connection, the interesting results reported by SHERIF [54] using *S. haematobium* miracidial metabolic antigen in the intradermal and precipitin tests should be followed-up by other investigators. Promising results were obtained in preliminary experiments by using cercarial secretory and excretory antigens in the complement fixation test [56] and analogous products from the adult worms in the slide flocculation test [44].

Recent attempts at obtaining better definition of soluble antigens through agar-gel diffusion and immunoelectrophoresis should be mentioned [9, 22, 26, 44, 58].

Because of the complexity of crude extracts or partially purified materials used for the immunodiagnosis of schistosomiasis, our knowledge of the biochemistry of these antigens is still fragmentary. While improved physical and chemical methods have been applied in the fractionation and analysis of some schistosome antigenic components, the identity of the immunologically reactive fractions has not been clearly established. Polysaccharides have been demonstrated in complement fixing fractions [52] but have not been considered to be the only reactive component [39]. Recent investigations [16, 27, 41, 55, 57] suggest strongly that the basic antigenic components operating in the complement fixation test are lipoprotein. Qualitative chemical analyses of cercarial excretions and secretions revealed the presence of protein, carbohydrate and lipid [56]. These investigations were expanded by FIFE et al., [17]. Descending paper chromatography of hydrolyzed and unhydrolyzed exoantigen using a n-butanol: acetic acid: water solvent system revealed the presence of two reducing components. One of these showed a RF corresponding to that of glucose and/or galactose, whereas the other corresponded to that of glucosamine and/or galactosamine. It is noteworthy, however, that glucose could be reasonably excluded as an antigen constituent; hydrolysates of the antigen gave no reaction whatsoever in the highly specific enzyme test using glucose oxidase. On the basis of these findings, galactose therefore appeared to be the hexose present in the exoantigen. Further enzymatic tests indicate that galactose and possibly galactosamine are present. Paper chromatograms with a variety of solvent systems are being employed in efforts to more precisely define the amino sugar present in the product. Although some protein appears to be associated with the exoantigen, repeated attempts to detect amino acids by chromatographic methods thus far have been unsuccessful.

In contrast to the exoantigen, the major component of the cercarial antigen appeared to be protein rather than carbohydrate in nature. There was considerable phosphorus present, and acid hydrolysis effected no increase in detectable amino nitrogen. Thus, there were marked qualitative as well as quantitative differences between the somatic and exoantigens. Water extracts of adult and cercarial forms of S. mansoni were compared in terms of their protein, carbohydrate and lipid constituents and antigenic potential [26]. Obviously, there is great need for further basic biochemical studies of this trematode. Experiments might be undertaken to determine the sites of groupings required for antigen activity. This could be accomplished by studies on the products of partial hydrolysis, the blocking of groups or competitive reactions.

In addition to the application of more imaginative and sophisticated techniques for the isolation and definition of specific antigenic components to be used in serological tests, favorable results might be obtained by attempting to detect the presence of antigen in the host. This might be achieved by adaptations of the method described by Okabe and Tanaka [32] for the extraction of antigen from the urine of patients infected with S. japonicum. Other techniques, such as modifications of the respiratory test devised by Desowitz [15] may provide means of detecting and measuring concentrations of protective antibodies to schistosomes. This is particularly needed since all attempts to correlate antibody titers, intensity of infection and acquisition of immunity in schistosomiasis have failed [20].

Some advance in this direction might be provided by further investigations with the phagocytic response test described by Newsome [31]. This test involves the incubation of adult worms in the presence of serum and leukocytes taken from the animal to be tested. The flukes remain alive for several days in sera and cells from normal animals, but they become heavily covered with leukocytes and are killed in one or two days when exposed to sera and cells of highly immune animals.

Although good progress has been made in the immunodiagnosis of schistosomiasis, the intricacies of immunochemistry and serology in such complex organisms as schistosomes still constitute a challenge to parasitologists. It is doubtful that anyone will solve the entire problem with a bold stroke since each component will need separate tedious study, but therein lies both the lure and the opportunity for parasitologists, immunologists and biochemists with vision and courage.

References

[1] Anderson, R. I.: Current and potential value of immunodiagnostic tests employing a whole organism. Amer. J. Hyg. Monogr. Ser. 22, 97—109 (1963).
[2] — Relationship of antibody nitrogen to titer obtained in the cercarial antigen slide flocculation test for schistosomiasis. Exp. Parasit. 12, 434—440 (1962).

[3] ANDERSON, R. I.: Serologic diagnosis of Schistosoma mansoni infections. I. Development of a cercarial antigen slide flocculation test. Amer. J. Trop. Med. Hyg. 9, 299—303 (1960).

[4] — E. H. SADUN, and M. J. SCHOENBECHLER: Cross absorption studies performed with Schistosoma mansoni and Trichinella spiralis antigens in sera from patients with trichinosis. Exp. Parasit. 14, 323—329 (1963).

[5] — — Some recent advances in the diagnosis of schistosomiasis. Med. Ann. D. C. 31, 211—215 (1962).

[6] —, and J. S. WILLIAMS: Preserved cercariae in the fluorescent antibody (FA) test for schistosomiasis. Exp. Parasit. 11, 226—230 (1961).

[7] — — — A technique for the use of minute amounts of dried blood in the fluorescent antibody test for schistosomiasis. Exp. Parasit. 11, 111—116 (1961).

[8] —, and D. H. NAIMARK: Serologic diagnosis of Schistosoma mansoni infections. II. Sensitivity of intradermal and serologic tests on individuals with an unequivocal diagnosis of schistosomiasis. Amer. J. Trop. Med. Hyg. 9, 600—603 (1960).

[9] BIGUET, J., A. CAPRON et P. TRAN VAN KY: Les antigenes de Schistosoma mansoni. I. Etude electrophoretique et immunoelectrophoretique. Caracterisation des antigenes specifiques. Ann. Inst. Pasteur 103, 763—777 (1962).

[10] BRANDT, J. L., and E. P. FINCH: A simple flocculation slide test for the diagnosis of schistosomiasis. Amer. J. Clin. Path. 16, 141—152 (1946).

[11] BREWER, J. H., and A. HARRIS: Presented at Meeting of Maryland Branch. Amer. Soc. Microbiol., 1962.

[12] BUCK, A. A., E. H. SADUN, R. I. ANDERSON, and E. SHAFFA: Comparative studies of some immunologic screening tests for schistosomiasis in Ethiopia. Amer. J. Hyg. 80, 75—84 (1964).

[13] CHAFFEE, E. F., P. M. BAUMAN, and J. J. SHAPILO: Diagnosis of schistosomiasis by complement-fixation. Amer. J. Trop. Med. Hyg. 3, 905—913 (1954).

[14] CLARKE, V.: Personal communication, 1963.

[15] DESOWITZ, R. S.: Effect of antibody on the respiratory rate of Trypanosoma vivax. Nature 177, 132—133 (1956).

[16] ELIAKIM, M., and A. M. DAVIES: The complement-fixation test in bilharziasis. II. Preparation and preservation of antigens from Schistosoma mansoni worms extracted in Coca's solution. Parasitology 45, 189—194 (1955).

[17] FIFE, E. H., K. A. SLEEMAN, and J. I. BRUCE: Studies on the exoantigens of Schistosoma mansoni cercariae. (In Press).

[18] FOSTER, R.: Skin antigen tests and the fluorescent antibody technique in the diagnosis of schistosomiasis. (In Press).

[19] JACHOWSKI, L. A., and R. I. ANDERSON: Evaluation of some laboratory procedures in diagnosing infections with Schistosoma mansoni. Bull. Wld Hlth Org. 25, 675—693 (1961).

[20] — —, and E. H. SADUN: Serologic reactions to Schistosoma mansoni. I. Quantitative studies on experimentally infected monkeys (Macaca mulatta). Amer. J. Hyg. 77, 137—145 (1963).

[21] KAGAN, I. G.: Personal communication, 1963.

[22] —, and L. NORMAN: Analysis of helminth antigens (Echinococcus granulosus and Schistosoma mansoni) by agar gel methods. Ann. N. Y. Acad. Sci. 113, 130—153 (1963).

[23] — J. PELLEGRINO, and J. M. P. MEMORIA: Studies on the standardization of the intradermal test for the diagnosis of bilharziasis. Amer. J. Trop. Med. Hyg. 10, 200—207 (1961).

[24] — — A critical review of immunological methods for the diagnosis of bilharziasis. Bull. Wld Hlth Org. 25, 611—674 (1961).

[25] — Hemagglutination after immunization with schistosome antigens. Science 122, 376—377 (1955).

[26] KENT, J. F.: Current and potential value of immunodiagnostic tests employing soluble antigens. Amer. J. Hyg. Monogr. Ser. 22, 68—90 (1963).

[27] —, and E. H. FIFE, JR.: Precise standardization of reagents for complement fixation. Amer. J. Trop. Med. Hyg. 12, 103—116 (1963).

268   Elvio H. Sadun:

[28] Kent, N. H.: Comparative immunochemistry of larval and adult forms of Schistosoma mansoni. Ann. N. Y. Acad. Sci. 113, 100—113 (1963).
[29] Lewert, R. M.: Personal communication, 1963.
[30] Liu, C., and F. B. Bang: Agglutination of cercariae of Schistosoma mansoni by immune sera. Proc. Soc. Exp. Biol. 74, 68—72 (1950).
[31] Newsome, J.: Investigation of anti-schistosome opsonins in vivo. Trans. Roy. Soc. Trop. Med. Hyg. 58, 58—62 (1964).
[32] Okabe, K., and T. Tanaka: A new urine precipitin reaction for schistosomiasis japonica. Kurume Med. J. 5, 45—52 (1958).
[33] — Y. Koga, H. Shibue, and M. Matsuse: Immunological studies on schistosomiasis japonica. 3. Intradermal and precipitin tests for schistosomiasis japonica. Kurume Med. J. 1, 85—89 (1954).
[34] Oliver-Gonzalez, J.: Anti-egg precipitin in the serum of humans infected with Schistosoma mansoni. J. Infect. Dis. 95, 86—91 (1954).
[35] —, and C. K. Pratt: Skin and precipitin reactions to antigens from the cercariae and adults of Schistosoma mansoni. Puerto Rico J. Publ. Hlth 20, 242—256 (1944).
[36] Pautrizel, R.: Personal communication, 1963.
[37] Pellegrino, J.: The intradermal test in the diagnosis of bilharziasis. Bull. Wld Hlth Org. 18, 945—961 (1958).
[38] — Immunological methods for the diagnosis of schistosomiasis mansoni. In: Procedings Seventh Internat. Cong. Trop. Med. Malaria, Rio de Janeiro, 1, 21—23 (1963).
[39] — E. Paulini, J. M. P. Memoria, and D. G. Macedo: A reacao intradermica na esquistossomose com una fracao polissacaridea isolada de cercarias de Schistosoma mansoni. Malar. Doen. Trop. 8, 527—534 (1956).
[40] Portnoy, J., J. H. Brewer, and A. Harris: Rapid plasma reagin card test for syphilis and other treponematoses. Publ. Hlth Rep. 77, 645—652 (1962).
[41] Rieber, S., R. I. Anderson, and M. G. Radke: Serologic diagnosis of Schistosoma mansoni infections. III. Isolation and purification of antigen from adult S. mansoni for the complement fixation test. Amer. J. Trop. Med. Hyg. 10, 351—355 (1961).
[42] Sadun, E. H.: Trichinosis, hydatid disease, schistosomiasis and ascariasis. In: Immunological diseases. Sampter, W., and H. L. Alexander (Eds.). Boston: Little Brown and Co. 1965.
[43] — Recent advances in the diagnosis of the most prevalent human trematode infections in Asia. Abstracts of the Ninth Pacific Congress, Bangkok, Thailand, 1957.
[44] — M. J. Schoenbechler, and M. Bentz: Multiple antibody response in schistosoma mansoni infections. Amer. J. Trop. Med. Hyg. 14, 977—995 (1965).
[45] — R. I. Anderson, and M. J. Schoenbechler: A plasma card test for rapid serodiagnosis of schistosomiasis (SPC). Proc. Soc. Exp. Biol. 112, 280—283 (1963).
[46] —, and E. Biocca: Intradermal and fluorescent antibody tests on humans exposed to Schistosoma bovis cercariae from Sardinia. Bull. Wld Hlth Org. 27, 810—814 (1962).
[47] — R. I. Anderson, and J. S. Williams: Fluorescent antibody test for the laboratory diagnosis of schistosomiasis in humans by using dried blood smears on filter paper. Exp. Parasit. 11, 117—120 (1961).
[48] — J. S. Williams, and R. I. Anderson: Fluorescent antibody technic for serodiagnosis of schistosomiasis in humans. Proc. Soc. Exp. Biol. 105, 289—291 (1960).
[49] — S. S. Lin, and B. C. Walton: Studies on the host parasite relationships to Schistosoma japonicum: III. The use of purified antigens in the diagnosis of infections in human and experimental animals. Milit. Med. 124, 428—436 (1959).
[50] — A. A. Buck, and B. C. Walton: The use of purified antigens in the immunodiagnosis of paragonimiasis in humans and experimental animals. J. Parasit. 44 (Suppl.) (1958).
[51] Schneider, M. D., and M. G. Radke: Further observations on a complement fixing substance from Schistosoma mansoni. Proc. Med. Soc. (Washington) 24, 137—139 (1957).
[52] — —, and M. T. Coleman: Immunologically reactive substance from Schistosoma mansoni. Exp. Parasit. 4, 391—397 (1956).
[53] Senterfit, L. B.: Immobilization of Schistosoma mansoni miracidia by immune serum. Proc. Soc. Exp. Biol. 84, 5—7 (1953).

[54] SHERIF, A. F.: Schistosomal metabolic products in the diagnosis of bilharziasis. Ciba Fundation Symposium Bilharziasis, WOLSTENHOLME, G. E. W., and O'CONNOR, M. (Eds.). Boston: Little Brown and Co. 1962.

[55] SLEEMAN, H. K.: Isolation and study of a specific complement fixing antigen from adult Schistosoma mansoni. Amer. J. Trop. Med. Hyg. **9**, 11—17 (1960).

[56] — E. H. FIFE, and J. I. BRUCE: Isolation and characterization of serologically active components from secretory and excretory products of Schistosoma mansoni cercariae. J. Parasit. **19**, 36 (1963).

[57] — J. D. BURKE, and J. F. KENT: Physicochemical and serologic studies of Schistosoma mansoni antigens. Amer. J. Trop. Med. Hyg. **7**, 241 (1958).

[58] SMITHERS, R. S.: Gel-diffusion studies on Schistosoma mansoni. Trans. Roy. Soc. Trop. Med. Hyg. **54**, 8 (1960).

[59] TALIAFERRO, W. H., W. A. HOFFMAN, and D. H. COOK: A precipitin test in intestinal schistosomiasis (S. mansoni). J. Prev. Med. **2**, 395—414 (1928).

[60] TOUSSAINT, A. S.: Improvement of the soluble antigen fluorescent antibody procedure. Exp. Parasit. (in press).

[61] TOUSSAINT, A. J., and R. I. ANDERSON: A soluble antigen fluorescent antibody (SAFA) technic. Appl. Microbiol. **13**, 552—558 (1965).

[62] VOGEL, H., u. W. MINNING: Hüllenbildung bei Bilharzia-Cercariaen im Serum Bilharzia-infizierter Tiere und Menschen. Zbl. Bakt. **153**, 91—105 (1940).

[63] WRIGHT, W. H., J. BOZICEVICH, F. J. BRADY, and P. M. BAUMAN: The diagnosis of Schistosomiasis japonica. V. The diagnosis of Schistosomiasis japonica by means of serological tests. Amer. J. Hyg. **45**, 150—163 (1947).

[64] YOSHIMOTO, M.: Über die Komplement-Bindungsreaktion bei der Schistosomum-Krankheit in Japan. Z. Immun.-Forsch. **5**, 438—445 (1910).

Fluorescent Antibody Studies on the Immunopathology
of Schistosomiasis Mansoni

Donald V. Moore*

With 8 figurees

The first fluorescent antibody studies in schistosomiasis were concerned with the use of this procedure as a diagnostic aid and for the determination of antibody titer in experimental animals. Sadun and co-workers [10–13] using preserved miracidia and cercariae as antigens showed that the fluorescent antibody test is both sensitive and specific and is a practical survey procedure. This subject is discussed by Sadun elsewhere in this volume. Sadun and co-workers demonstrated that schistosomulae removed from the skin of infected animals showed specific immunofluorescence.

Andrade, Paronetto and Popper [2] were the first to use immunocytochemical methods to study the localization of schistosome antigens and gamma globulin in the tissues of the infected host. These investigators studied cryostat sections from albino mice experimentally infected with *Schistosoma mansoni*. Such sections were treated with fluorescein conjugated anti-mouse gamma globulin prepared in rabbits and with fluorescein conjugated gamma globulin from patients infected with *Schistosoma mansoni*. Using fluorescein conjugated anti-mouse gamma globulin they were able to demonstrate gamma globulin in the cells of the hepatic granulomas; littoral cells of hepatic sinusoids and in the red pulp of the spleen. As the age of the infection increased and the granulomas became more fibrotic, the gamma globulin-containing cells disappeared but some diffuse fluorescence was observed in the connective tissue. However, the gamma globulin-containing cells in the hepatic sinusoids and in the red pulp of the spleen increased in number as the age of the infection increased.

Andrade et al. [2] also provided good evidence for the immunologic nature of the tissue reaction seen in schistosomiasis. This was demonstrated by the removal of the fluorescent activity of the anti-mouse gamma globulin by treatment of the sections with an acid pH which split the gamma globulin from its combination with antigen in the tissue. When such sections were treated with anti-schistosome gamma globulin, fluorescent activity reappeared indicating that the schistosome antigen remained in the tissue. From this evidence these authors postulate that the necrosis around the schistosome eggs in the tissue of the host is due, at least in part, to an antigen-antibody complex rather than free antigen which has escaped from the egg shell into the surrounding tissue. They also presented evidence that splenic enlargement in schistosomiasis is due not only to portal hypertension but also to reticuloendothelial hyperplasia which has an immunologic basis.

---

* Department of Microbiology. The University of Texas Southwestern Medical School Dallas, Texas.

ANDRADE et al. [2] also showed that the schistosome egg shell is not antigenic but that structures in the miracidium within the egg exhibited specific immunofluorescence. In some miracidia within eggs in the liver they observed a fluorescent multilobulated mass suggestive of a penetration gland. They also described specific fluorescence of adult worms in the tissues.

In a study concerned with antigen sequestration and destruction in the schistosome pseudotubercle, von LICHTENBERG [5] observed that miracidia and worms in the tissues of the mammalian host showed specific immunofluorescence. In this study tissues from albino mice experimentally infected with S. mansoni were cut in a cryostat, treated with immune mouse serum, then stained with fluorescein-conjugated anti-mouse globulin. In addition to studying antigen in cercaria induced infections, tissues of mice receiving intravenous injections of purified S. mansoni eggs were examined and in vitro studies of the S. mansoni eggs were made.

The cuticle, intestinal lining and intestinal contents of schistosomula and worms exhibited the strongest fluorescence. Apical glands of stages in the skin and lungs also exhibited bright staining. The major site of antigen concentration in the miracidia appeared to be in the penetration glands. A homogeneous specific fluorescent precipitate coated the inside and outside of egg shells in the tissue. The egg shell exhibited a nonspecific orange fluorescence. When intact eggs were incubated in vitro with immune serum then treated with fluorescent tagged anti-mouse globulin, the circumoval precipitates showed a bright specific fluorescence but there was little staining of the miracidium within the intact egg. Free miracidia and those in eggs with broken shells showed intense specific staining. This relates the antigen seen in vivo to the circumoval precipitate seen in vitro. Parasite nuclei were negative.

In addition to the above described clear homogeneous fluorescence, a dust-like halo of small fluorescent granules was seen near the eggs in the center of the granulomas. Occasionally a diffuse fluorescent staining was seen in the necrotic centers of the granulomas. This was most intense in the well developed cellular granulomas. Late fibrotic nodules showed little or no fluorescence.

The use of animals receiving an intravenous injection of eggs by von Lichtenberg provided a convenient method of studying the fate of the antigen in the sensitized and non-sensitized host since the picture was not complicated by continuing egg production of female worms. Four stages of antigen disposal were observed after the intravenous injection of eggs: (1) dissemination of antigen prior to the host cell reaction (1—24 hours); (2) "antigen sequestration" in which antigen production continued as well as antigen uptake by host phagocytes (24 hours to 4 days) which was coincident with the accretion of a cell halo; (3) this was followed by antigen destruction ending with the disappearance of cellular deposits as the granuloma reached its peak (16—32 days); and (4) the complete disappearance of antigen from the miracidium and host cells which is coincidental with the healing phase of the granuloma (over 70 days). In animals presensitized by an intraperitoneal injection of eggs, the antigen disposal and host cell reaction were accelerated. von LICHTENBERG interpreted his findings as a result of a balance between antigen release by the eggs and the phagocytic-catabolic activity of the host cells [5].

Recently Magalhães, Krupp and Malek [6] studied the localization of antigen and the presence of antibody in the tissues of mice infected with *S. mansoni* as detected by the fluorescent antibody technique. In addition these authors studied the cellular reaction of the infected host and the relationship of this reaction to the antigenic stimulus. Circulating antibodies were detected by the cercarial fluorescent antibody test and the cercarienhüllen reaction. Antigen in the tissues of experimentally infected mice was detected by treating cryostat sections with fluorescein conjugated anti-*S. mansoni* serum from an infected nutria *(Myocaster coypus)* which had a high antibody titer. Antibody in the tissue sections was located by the use of fluorescein-conjugated anti-mouse gamma globulin. Sections of liver, lungs, spleen and lymph nodes were examined.

Circulating antibody was first detected 42 days after infection by the use of the cercarial fluorescent antibody test and at 47 days by the cercarienhüllen reaction indicating that the fluorescent test is more sensitive. Antigen deposition in the tissues of the mice was detected as early as 15 days after exposure to cercariae which was considerably earlier than the detection of circulating antibodies. This early stage antigen was localized in the endothelium of blood vessels and in the neutrophils, lymphocytes and histiocytes in the liver and lungs. Later in the prepatent period antigen was found in inflammatory cells infiltrating perivascular tissue in the liver and lungs. During the patent period the fluorescence of antigen deposits in the tissues was much brighter and a greater number of cells contained antigen than during the prepatent period. The egg substance at the center of granulomas and neutrophils at the periphery were positive for antigen. In the lung, antigen was concentrated in lymphocytes and monocytes infiltrating alveolar septa and perivascular spaces. In the spleen, a few neutrophils and macrophages in the follicles and many in the sinuses surrounding blood vessels were positive for antigen. The only antigen containing cells in the lymph nodes were neutrophils and histiocyctes.

Antibody was first observed during the prepatent period, 25 days after infection, by fluorescence in the inflammatory cells in perivascular spaces and in histiocytes in the parenchyma of the liver and lungs as well as inflammatory cells in interlobular spaces. A few lymphocytes in the spleen were positive for antibody at this time. During the patent period the same cells were positive for antibody and in addition some neutrophils in the periphery of liver granulomas showed fluorescence.

When mice were given repeated exposures to cercariae the same cells were positive for antibody but the intensity of the fluorescence was increased which is interpreted by the authors as indicating a rise in antibody production due to secondary antigenic stimuli. Magalhães et al. [6] also state that active phagocytosis and marked hyperplasia of the cells of the reticuloendothelial system and the fibrinoid necrosis in hepatic granulomas seen in hyper-stimulated animals indicates a hyper-immuno-allergic condition.

The purpose of studies conducted in our laboratory was to use the fluorescent antibody procedure to detect the presence of antigenic material in the host cells and to determine the morphologic location of major antigenic sites in the developing and mature schistosome in the mammalian phase of the life cycle.

Materials and Methods

The mammalian host used in this study was the golden hamster, which was exposed to *S. mansoni* (Puerto Rican strain) cercariae obtained from laboratory-reared and infected *Australorbis glabratus*. In order to obtain schistosomulae in the skin, hamsters were anaesthetized with pentobarbital sodium and the hair shaved from the abdomen. A plasticine ring 1.5 cm in diameter and 3–4 mm high was affixed to the shaved abdomen by a thin film of petrolatum. The ring was then filled with a heavy suspension of freshly shed cercariae. After an exposure period of 1–2 hours, the water was pipetted from the ring and the ring removed from the skin. The area of skin penetrated by cercariae was biopsied, placed on an appropriate sized piece of acetate membrane filter and fixed in cold 95% ethanol. Pieces of skin were removed at 45 minutes, 1 hour and 45 minutes, and 24 hours after exposure. Other hamsters were exposed by the shaved percutaneous method. The fur was clipped from the posterior third of the body and the animals placed in dechlorinated tap water at a depth of 2 inches for an hour to encourage the passing of feces and urine prior to exposure to cercariae. Hamsters were exposed by placing them in 400 ml beakers with 500 cercariae in dechlorinated tap water 2 cm deep. Lung tissue was removed at 7 days; liver tissue at 14 and 21 days and both liver and intestine tissue at 7 weeks after exposure. In the preliminary phase of this work, tissue sections were cut in a cryostat. Extensive fibrosis due to the heavy infection resulting from exposure to 500 cercariae caused considerable difficulty in obtaining good sections by this method. Later it was found that the paraffin sectioning method described by SAINTE-MARIE [14] eliminated most of the difficulties associated with the cutting of frozen sections. We found that the paraffin method produced excellent fluorescent preparations and that the histological structure of the host and worm tissue was well preserved and resulted in excellent hematoxylin-eosin preparations following study by fluorescent staining. Briefly this procedure consists of fixation in cold 95% ethanol with subsequent dehydration and clearing carried out at 4° C. Tissues are infiltrated and embedded in paraffin and the blocks stored at 4° C prior to cutting. Sections 6 μ thick are placed on clean slides without adhesive. After removal of paraffin with cold xylene and hydration in cold solutions the sections are stained with fluorescein conjugated globulin, washed, and mounted in buffered glycerol in the usual manner.

Rabbits were immunized with the acid-soluble protein fraction [7] of lyophilized cercariae and adult *S. mansoni* in complete Freund's adjuvant. Antisera titers were determined by the latex agglutination test [8]. Gamma globulin was separated from anticercarial, antiadult and normal rabbit sera by ammonium sulfate precipitation and conjugated with fluorescein isothiocyanate according to standard procedures. Conjugated globulins were absorbed with mouse liver powder before being used in the fluorescent antibody staining procedure.

After removal of paraffin from the sections and hydration, they were stained for 30 minutes with fluorescein conjugated globulins; washed in 3 changes of buffered saline and mounted in buffered glycerol. Fluorescent microscopy was done with an AO monocular microscope and a Leitz ultraviolet illuminator equipped with an Osram HBO 220 light source. The exciter filter was a Corning 5840 and the barrier filter a Wrattan 2B. Color photographs were made with High Speed

274   Donald V. Moore:

Ektachrome and Anscochrome 200. Black and white photographs were made with
Polaroid film Type 47. After the sections had been studied with ultraviolet light,
they were stained with hematoxylin and eosin and fields which had been photographed for fluorescence were photographed again with conventional white light.

Controls consisted of staining adjacent sections with conjugated normal rabbit
gamma globulin; treating other adjacent sections with unconjugated anticercarial
and antiadult globulin followed by staining with conjugated anticercarial or antiadult globulin as well as treatment of other adjacent sections with unconjugated
normal rabbit globulin followed by staining with conjugated anticercarial or antiadult globulin.

Results

All controls were satisfactory. When sections were stained with fluorscein
conjugated normal rabbit gamma globulin there was no immunofluorescence in the
tissue or schistosome material. Specific immunofluorescence was inhibited when
sections were treated first with unconjugated anticercarial or antiadult gamma globulin followed by staining with conjugated anticercarial or antiadult globulin. Prior
treatment of sections with unconjugated normal rabbit globulin followed by staining with either conjugated anticercarial or antiadult globulin did not inhibit the
specific fluorescence. Very little nonspecific autofluorescence was observed in skin,
lung, and intestine sections. Liver sections exhibited more nonspecific autofluorescence but for the most part this could easily be differentiated by the apple green
color of the specific immunofluorescence. If paraffin blocks were stored for longer
than 3 weeks at 4° C, the nonspecific autofluorescence increased to a point where it
became troublesome, especially in liver sections. Sainte-Marie [14] states
that paraffin blocks which have been stored for 2—3 months are satisfactory but
that autofluorescence does increase with storage. The length of time that such
paraffin blocks may be stored at 4° C before becoming unsatisfactory for fluorescent
antibody studies is dependent upon the type of study being conducted and the
immune system used.

One purpose of this study was to determine whether any difference in fluorescent
antibody reaction could be detected between conjugated antiadult and anticercarial gamma globulins. No difference in the specific immunofluorescence of these
two antibodies could be detected, thus in the remainder of this presentation no
differentiation will be made between anticercarial and antiadult globulin.

At 45 minutes after exposure the cercariae or schistosomulae were for the most
part just penetrating or were in the process of penetrating the skin. When the time
was extended to 1 hour and 45 minutes after exposure, more schistosomulae were
in the dermis and subcutaneous tissue. At 24 hours most of the schistosomulae were
in the subcutaneous tissue, some associated with hair follicles. There was evidence
of growth of the schistosomulae seen 24 hours after exposure in that they were
larger than those seen at earlier times and the syncytial cells (Figs. 3a and b) seemed
to have undergone some enlargement. Schistosomulae could readily be detected in
the sections by their bright specific immunofluorescence. Longitudinal, cross, and
tangential sections of schistosomulae were observed.

The cuticular complex comprising the body wall of the schistosomulae exhibited
the brightest specific fluorescence. Strands of fluorescent material, less bright than

the cuticular complex were present in the syncytial tissue (Figs. 1a and b). Nuclei of the syncytium of the schistosomulae were conspicuous by the absence of

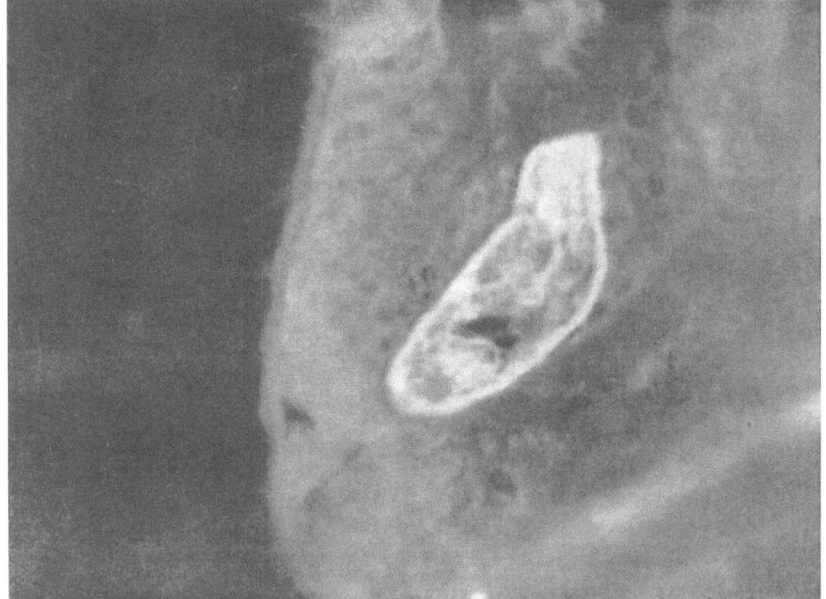

Fig. 1a. Schistosomula penetrating skin of hamster 45 minutes after exposure. Stained with fluorescein conjugated antiadult (*S. mansoni*) globulin, showing concentration of specific immunofluorescence in the cuticular complex

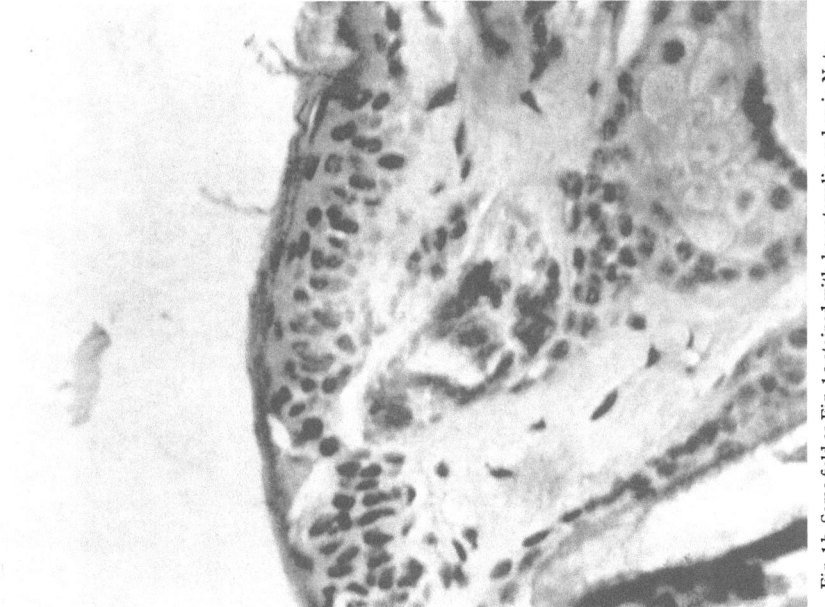

Fig. 1b. Same field as Fig. 1a stained with hematoxylin and eosin Note numerous syncytial nuclei of schistosomula which do not stain in the fluorescent preparation

fluorescence. In some sections of schistosomulae, bright fluorescent bands were seen inside the body. In one instance (Figs. 2a and b) this area was identified as part of the oral sucker complex. Some organisms possessed a thin fluorescent shell

18*

outside of and detached from the cuticula in places. Interpretation of this is difficult since it could represent the outermost layer of the cuticle which had

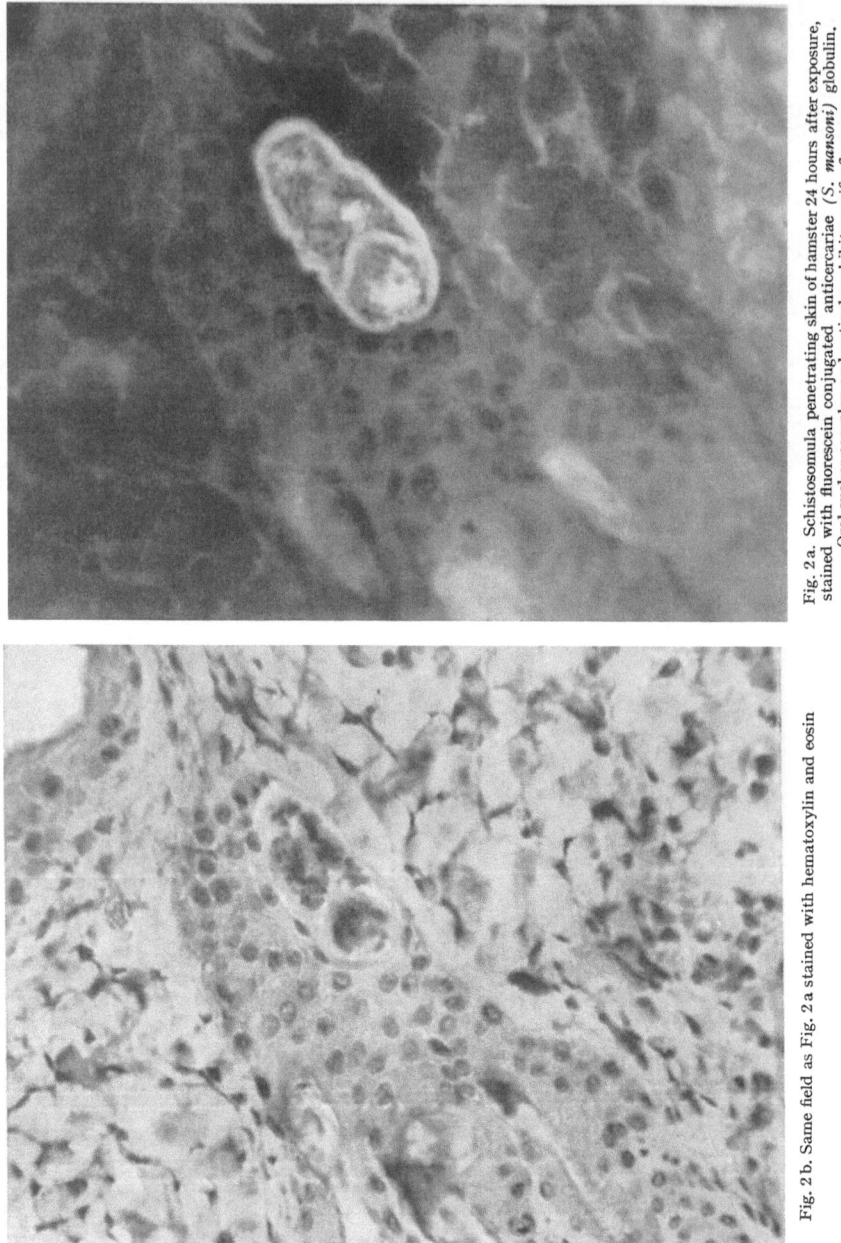

Fig. 2a. Schistosomula penetrating skin of hamster 24 hours after exposure, stained with fluorescein conjugated anticercariae (*S. mansoni*) globulin. Oral sucker complex and cuticule exhibit specific fluorescence

Fig. 2b. Same field as Fig. 2a stained with hematoxylin and eosin

become detached from the worm, or it could represent an accumulation of glandular secretions adhering to the outermost portion of the body of the penetrating schistosomula. No glands were identified as such in any of the sectioned schistosomulae studied. This is not an unexpected finding since the glandular secretions were undoubtedly utilized in the initial penetration of the host. The cells lining the

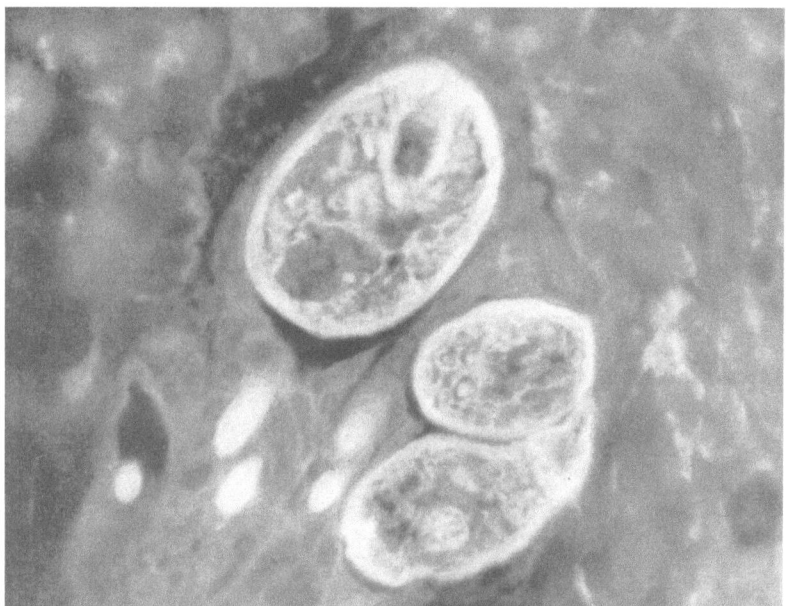

Fig. 3 a. Three schistosomulae in skin of hamster 24 hours after exposure, stained with fluorescein conjugated anticercaria globulin. These worms are associated with hair follicles and show evidence of growth and concentration of fluorescence in the cuticular complex

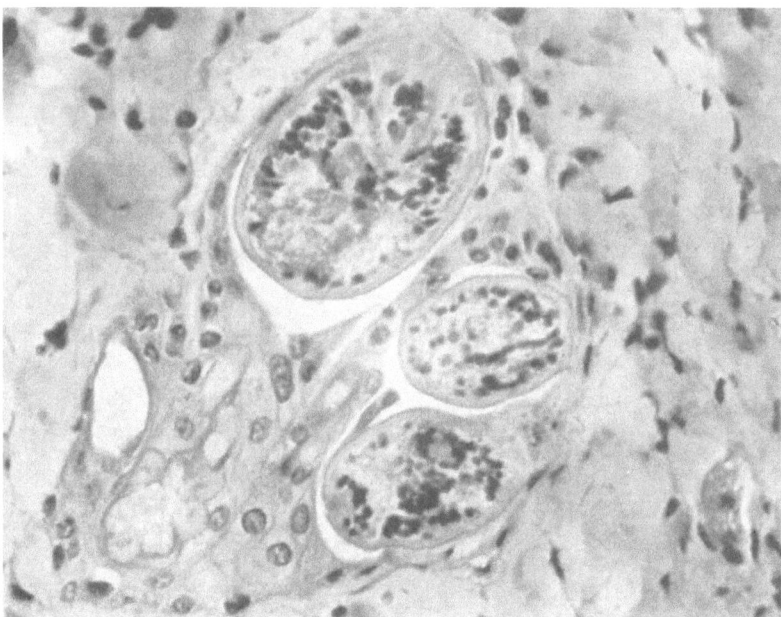

Fig. 3 b. Same field as Fig. 3 a stained with hematoxylin and eosin

digestive tract of the schistosomulae exhibited a bright fluorescence. In some sections discrete spots of less intense specific fluorescence were observed in the host cells ahead of and along the path of the penetrating schistosomulae (Fig. 7). This

18a Bilharziasis

was apparent in sections made 24 hours after exposure to cercariae. These undoubtedly represent uptake of parasite secretory- excretory or metabolic antigens by the cells of the host.

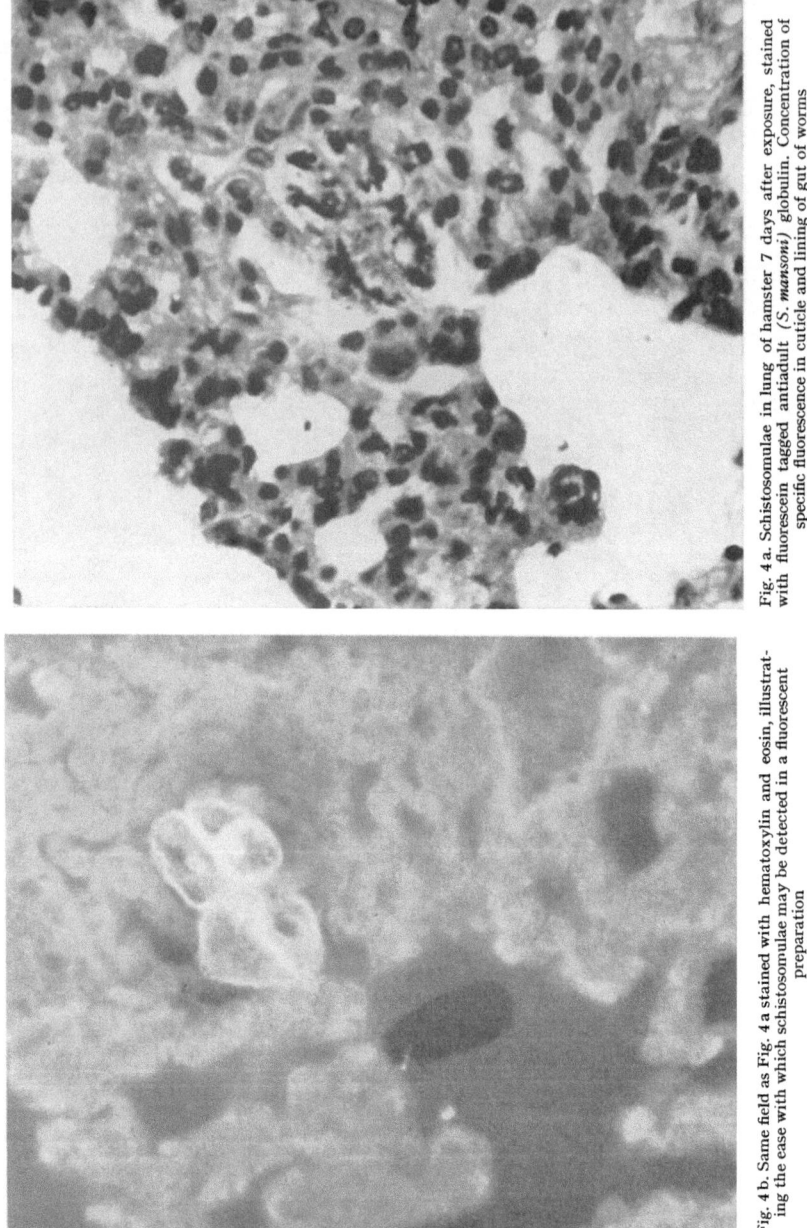

Fig. 4 a. Schistosomulae in lung of hamster 7 days after exposure, stained with fluorescein tagged antiadult (*S. mansoni*) globulin. Concentration of specific fluorescence in cuticle and lining of gut of worms

Fig. 4 b. Same field as Fig. 4 a stained with hematoxylin and eosin, illustrating the ease with which schistosomulae may be detected in a fluorescent preparation

According to the studies of YOLLES, MOORE and MELENEY [16] schistosomulae are migrating through the lung at 7 days after exposure. The detection of young worms migrating through the lung is greatly facilitated in sections stained with fluorescein-conjugated antischistosomal globulin. The cuticular complex and the cellular lining of the ceca of the young worms in the lung exhibited the brightest

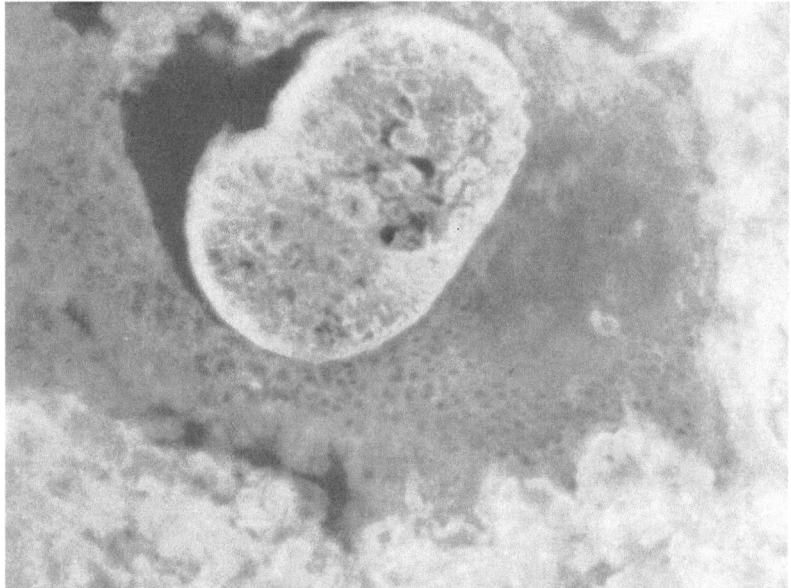

Fig. 5 a. Cross section of female S. *mansoni* in intrahepatic portal blood vessel of hamster 21 days after exposure, stained with fluorescein tagged antiadult globulin. Note concentration of specific fluorescence in cuticular complex and lining of intestinal cecum and strands of fluorescent material in the somatic syncytium of the worm

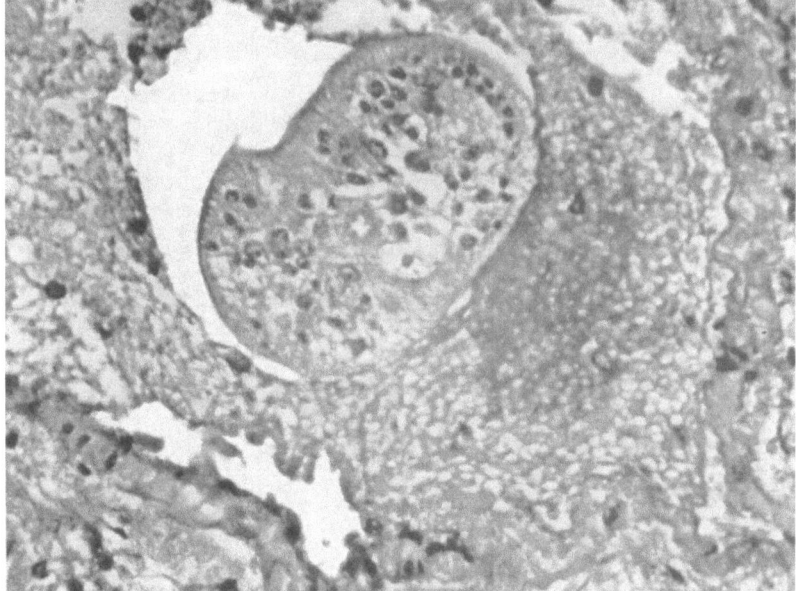

Fig. 5 b. Same field as Fig. 5 a stained with hematoxylin and eosin

fluorescence with strands of syncytial material staining less brilliantly (Figs. 4 a and b). Differentiation of organs has not begun in the 7-day-old schistosomula, thus there is little worm tissue to act as antigen. Schistosome antigen outside the worms was not detected in the lung sections studied.

At 14 and 21 days after exposure the developing worms have not attained sexual maturity, thus there are no eggs in the host tissue at this time. The predominant fluorescence was again the cuticle and the lining of the intestinal ceca of

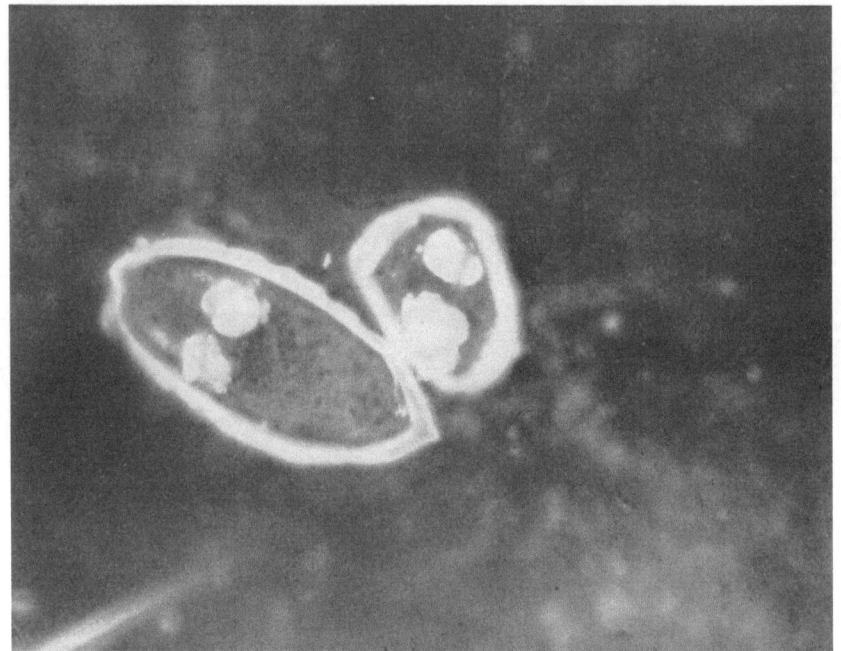

Fig. 6a. Two fully developed S. *mansoni* eggs in liver of hamster 7 weeks after exposure, stained with fluorescein conjugated anticercaria globulin. Note multilobulated cephalic penetration glands of miracidium and convoluted ducts in top egg showing bright specific immunofluorescence. Fainter specific fluorescence of body of miracidium. Egg shell has nonspecific orange fluorescence

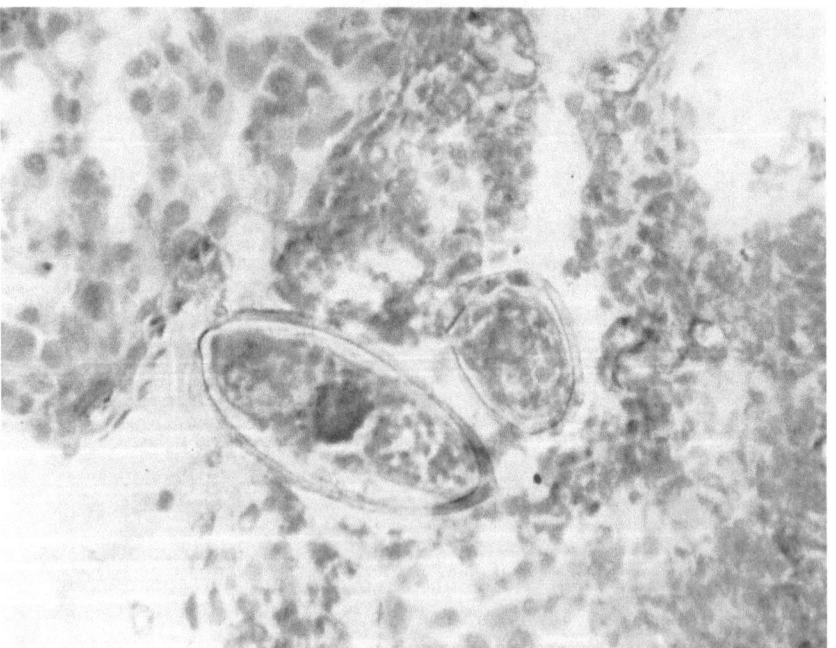

Fig. 6b. Same field as Fig. 6a stained with hematoxylin and eosin. Note nerve mass and syncytial nuclei which show no fluorescence in Fig. 6a

the developing worms. Occasional cells in the lining of blood vessels containing worms, near the location of the worms, showed areas of specific fluorescence. Cells in areas of perivascular infiltration also showed the presence of antigen.

When an *S. mansoni* infection has attained the age of 7 weeks in the hamster, the worms are sexually mature and have produced large numbers of eggs, many of which are in the host tissue. Sections of liver and intestine usually contained sections of worms as well as schistosome granulomas in varying stages of development.

Longitudinal, cross, and tangential sections through different portions of male and female worms were studied. As was seen in other stages of development, the cuticular complex and the lining of the intestinal ceca in the adult worms continued to exhibit the brightest fluorescence. Muscle fibers and cytoplasmic strands in the syncytial tissue of the worms also showed specific fluorescence (Figs. 5a and b). The cytoplasm of egg cells in the ovary exhibited specific fluorescence but not the nuclei. The delimiting membrane of the ovary and the wall of the oviduct (Fig. 8) also serve as a source of antigen as indicated by fluorescence. Syncytial nuclei were conspicuous by the absence of fluorescence. In some instances the vitelline glands

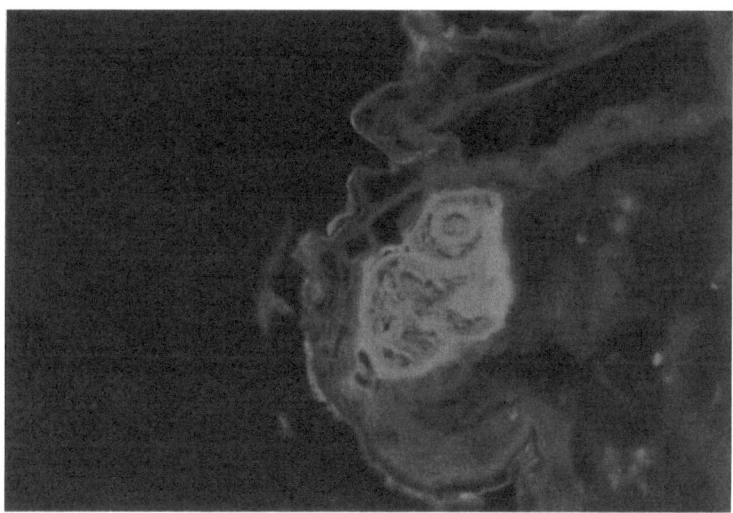

Fig. 7. Schistosomulae in skin of hamster 24 hours after exposure, stained with fluorescein conjugated antiadult *(S. mansoni)* globulin. In addition to specific fluorescence of cuticle and syncytial strands, this section shows some particles of specific fluorescence in the host tissue ahead of the penetrating worms

of the female showed a nonspecific white fluorescence. Hematin in the intestinal ceca always fluoresced red. This is in contrast to the findings of von LICHTENBERG [5], who reported that the intestinal contents of adult worms showed bright specific fluorescence.

The shell material of eggs in the tissue shows a nonspecific orange fluorescence which is in agreement with the findings of other investigators. Miracidia within the egg in the tissue sections exhibit a specific fluorescence in the cuticle and a fainter fluorescence in strands of the syncytial material. The most outstanding and by far the brightest specific immunofluorescence was observed in the cephalic penetration glands of the miracidium. When a miracidium is sectioned in the proper plane, the lobulate form of the glands and the convoluted ducts leading from the glands to the external openings on either side of the oral opening can be clearly seen (Figs. 6a and b). The nerve center and the syncytial nuclei of the miracidium are conspicuous by their lack of fluorescence. No fluorescence was seen in the primitive gut, which is thought to have a secretory function. If this structure does have such a function, no antibody to the secretions was present in the antiserum used in this study.

The perivascular infiltrations in liver and intestine associated with the presence of adult worms showed a few cells containing some antigen, as indicated by fluorescence. Most of the granulomas observed were devoid of fluorescent material. In a

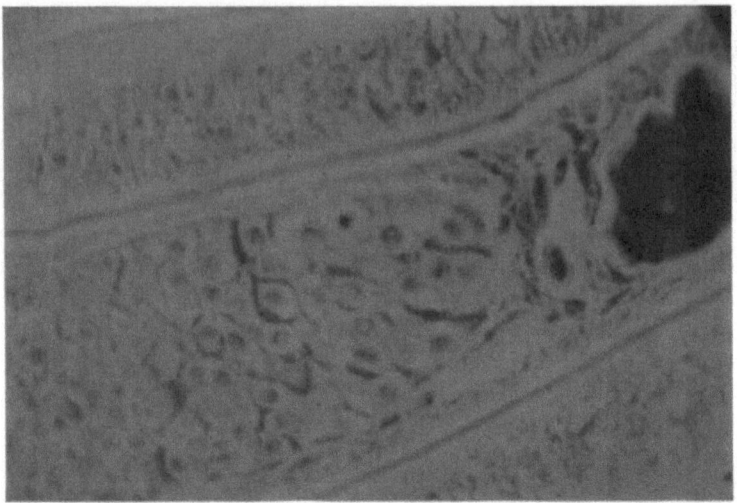

Fig. 8. Section of male and female in copula in section of hamster intestine 7 weeks after exposure. Note concentration of specific fluorescence in cuticle, intestinal ceca lining, and lining of oviduct of female worm. Other areas showing fluorescence are muscle fibers, strands of syncytial tissue, and cytoplasm of ovarian cells

number of sections the granulomas were conspicuous as dark areas even when liver sections showed autofluorescence of the parenchymal cells. These granulomas undoubtedly represent older stages in which the antigen had been destroyed, as has been demonstrated by the work of VON LICHTENBERG [5].

Discussion

The fluorescent antibody technique, in addition to being an efficient and practical diagnostic aid in schistosomiasis as discussed by SADUN in this volume, provides a procedure whereby the complex problems of immunogenesis and immunopathology in schistosomiasis may be studied and results compared with other experimental procedures used in studying the same or similar problems.

KAGAN [3] and LEVINE and KAGAN [4] performed experiments to determine the role of metabolic or secretory-excretory antigens in acquired resistance in schistosomiasis. These authors were able to demonstrate a partial resistance in mice as a result of immunization with metabolic antigens of S. mansoni in Freund's adjuvant. With the aid of the fluorescent antibody technique such antigens may be located in the tissues of the mammalian host. SADUN, ANDERSON and WILLIAMS [12] showed that when cercariae were fixed in acetic acid and subjected to staining with fluorescent antibody there was bright fluorescent staining of the postacetabular glands. The secretions of these glands assist the cercariae in the penetration of the skin of the final host. Droplets of stainable schistosome antigen were described by VON LICHTENBERG [5] close to and along the tract of the schistosomulae in the skin. Similar material was seen diffusing into nearby lymphatics. In addition, VON LICHTENBERG described a bright fluorescence in the central part of a schistosomula in the skin. This area was interpreted as being an apical gland. The droplets of stainable material near the penetrating schistosomulae were not discernible 24 hours after exposure. Similar observations were made in the present study except that we observed such stainable material in the host cells in the vicinity of penetrating schistosomulae 24 hours after exposure. Since we used hamsters and VON LICHTENBERG used mice, this difference in observations may be due to a difference in host response to schistosome metabolic antigens.

In reviewing studies on acquired resistance following vaccination in schistoso-miasis, STIREWALT [15] concluded that adult worm tissue provides a more effective antigen for the development of resistance to reinfection than cercarial tissue. If such is the case, then one may conclude from fluorescent antibody studies that the major sources of antigen in adult worm tissue are the cuticular complex and the lining of the alimentary canal. Since both areas are metabolically active, one might assume that metabolic antigens are important in the production of resistance and that antigens seen in the endothelial cells of portal and pulmonary vessels and antigens in the inflammatory cells infiltrating perivascular spaces as described by MAGALHÃES [6] may be metabolic antigens.

Circumoval precipitates were first described by OLIVER-GONZALEZ [9]. The formation of such precipitates on the shells of schistosome eggs in immune sera are thought to be the result of the leakage of secretory-excretory antigens of the miracidium through the shell. These circumoval precipitates show specific immuno-fluorescence as demonstrated by VON LICHTENBERG [5]. All papers dealing with the immunofluorescence of schistosome material in the tissues of the mamma-lian host have reported the bright specific fluorescence of the cephalic penetration glands of the miracidium, indicating that these glands represent the major antigen localization in this stage of the schistosome life cycle. Thus, there seems to be a definite relationship between the antigen which produces circumoval precipitates when combined with antibody and the cephalic glands of the miracidium. VON LICHTENBERG [5] reported that when living miracidia hatched from eggs were injected into mice, typical pseudotubercules are not produced but that pseudotubercles could be produced by the injection of eggs containing living miracidia or even the injection of autoclaved eggs. It was shown that the fluores-cence associated with the pseudotubercles produced by autoclaved eggs was less intense than that seen in pseudotubercles resulting from the injection of eggs containing living miracidia. It is postulated by VON LICHTENBERG [5] that the egg shell may have an adjuvant-like activity resulting in the slow release of antigen from the miracidium into the surrounding tissue. The work of ANDRADE et al. [2] indicates that some of the pathology in schistosomiasis is due, at least in part, to an antigen-antibody complex rather than free antigen. These findings illustrate the complexity of the problem of immunopathology in schistosomiasis.

As has been shown, the fluorescent antibody technique has a definite use in studies of this type but there are a number of shortcomings. The procedure is not sufficiently specific to detect differences in stage specific antigens which may be present. In this study we were unable to detect any difference in the reactivity of anticercaria and antiadult conjugated globulins since both stained schistosomulae, adult worms, and miracidia with equal intensity. This is due in part to the fact that the acid-soluble protein fraction of cercariae and adult worms used for the production of antisera is essentially a crude antigen. This points up the need for methods resulting in better fractionation and purification of antigens.

Summary

Gamma globulin from rabbits immunized with an acid-soluble protein fraction (Melcher's antigen) of cercariae and adult worms of *S. mansoni* were conjugated with fluorescein isothiocyanate and used in direct and indirect fluorescent antibody procedures to study the immunopathology of *S. mansoni* infections in hamsters. Sections were prepared from the tissues of animals following a primary exposure to cercariae. Skin sections taken at 45 minutes, 1 hour and 45 minutes, and 24 hours after exposure were studied. Lung tissue was examined at 7 days, liver tissue at 14 and 21 days, and liver and intestine at 7 weeks after exposure.

All developmental stages of *S. mansoni* exhibit a bright specific fluorescence in the cuticular complex and the lining of the intestinal ceca, indicating that these areas of the worm provide the major source of antigen which can be demonstrated in cells of the host tissue. The cytoplasm of the syncytial tissue and the muscle fibers also serve as a source of antigen but exhibit a less intense fluorescent staining. Nuclei of syncytial tissue and other organs of the worm show no fluorescence, indicating that they are not a source of schistosome antigen. In the miracidia within the egg in the tissue of the host, the cephalic penetration glands and their ducts exhibit an intense specific immunofluorescence, indicating a major source of antigen in this stage. The relationship of the schistosome antigens exhibited by fluorescent antibody studies to acquired resistance and to secretory-excretory or metabolic antigens is discussed.

Schistosome antigens from schistosomulae were demonstrated in host tissue during the penetration of the skin. Other locations of schistosome antigens in the host tissue were in cells lining blood vessels and in perivascular infiltrations associated with the presence of adult or developing worms. Older pseudotubercles were conspicuous by their lack of specific fluorescence. In this study no difference in the staining reaction of conjugated anticercarial and antiadult globulin could be detected. The status of studies on fluorescent antibody in the mammalian host of *S. mansoni* is discussed and reviewed.

References

[1] ANDERSON, R., E. H. SADUN, and J. WILLIAMS: Preserved cercariae in the fluorescent antibody test for schistosomiasis. Exp. Parasit. 11, 226—230 (1961).
[2] ANDRADE, Z. A., F. PARONETTO, and F. POPPER: Immunocytochemical studies in schistosomiasis. Amer. J. Path. 39, 589—597 (1961).

[3] KAGAN, I. G.: Contributions to the immunology and serology of schistosomiasis. Rice Inst. Pamphlet 45, 151—183 (1958).

[4] LEVINE, D. M., and I. G. KAGAN: Studies on the immunology of schistosomiasis and passive transfer. J. Parasit. 46, 787—792 (1960).

[5] LICHTENBERG, F. VON: Studies on granuloma formation. III. Antigen sequestration and destruction in the schistosome pseudotubercle. Amer. J. Path. 45, 75—94 (1964).

[6] MAGALHÃES FILHO, A., I. M. KRUPP, and E. A. MALEK: Localization of antigen and presence of antibody in tissues of mice infected with Schistosoma mansoni, as indicated by fluorescent antibody technics. Amer. J. Trop. Med. Hyg. 14, 84—99 (1965).

[7] MELCHER, L. R.: An antigenic analysis of Trichinella spiralis. J. Infect. Dis. 73, 31—40 (1943).

[8] MOORE, D. V.: Detection of schistosome antibodies by latex agglutination. J. Parasit. 50, 23 (1964).

[9] OLIVER-GONZALEZ, J.: Anti-egg precipitins in the serum of humans infected with Schistosoma mansoni. J. Infect. Dis. 95, 86—91 (1954).

[10] SADUN, E. H., J. S. WILLIAMS, and R. I. ANDERSON: Fluorescent antibody technic for serodiagnosis of schistosomiasis in humans. Proc. Soc. Exp. Biol. 105, 289—291 (1960).

[11] — R. I. ANDERSON, and J. S. WILLIAMS: Fluorescent antibody test for the laboratory diagnosis of schistosomiasis in humans using dried blood smears on filter paper. Exp. Parasit. 11, 117—120 (1961).

[12] — — — The nature of fluorescent antibody reactions in infections and artificial immunizations with Schistosoma mansoni. Bull. Wld Hlth Org. 27, 151—159 (1962).

[13] — Seminar on immunity to parasitic helminths. VII. Fluorescent antibody technique for helminth infections. Exp. Parasit. 13, 72—82 (1963).

[14] SAINTE-MARIE, G.: A paraffin embedding technique for studies employing immunofluorescence. J. Histochem. Cytochem. 10, 250—256 (1961).

[15] STIREWALT, M. A.: Seminar on immunity to parasitic helminths. IV. Schistosome infections. Exp. Parasit. 13, 18—44 (1963).

[16] YOLLES, T. K., D. V. MOORE, and H. E. MELENEY: Post-cercarial development of Schistosoma mansoni in the rabbit and hamster after intraperitoneal and percutaneous infection. J. Parasit. 35, 276—294 (1949).

Mechanisms of Schistosome Immunity

F. v. Lichtenberg*

With 8 figures

In 1953, Vogel and Minning [50] published their well-documented study of acquired resistance to *S. japonicum* in *Macaca mulatta*, following long-term infection. Since then, immunity has been produced in macaques with the cattle adapted Taiwan strain of *S. japonicum* [7, 34], and with gamma-radiated cercariae of the human-pathogenic strains of *S. japonicum* and *S. mansoni* [6, 33]. Recent results indicate that a high degree of resistance can be attained by repeated infection of macaques with "attenuated" schistosomes, but the applicability of these findings to human vaccination is not clear. The present status of this research has been ably summarized by Sadun [30]. Both practical and biological considerations demand that research be directed toward the underlying mechanisms of schistosome immunity. Progress in this field, however, has been slow.

Within the wide experimental host spectrum which has been studied with laboratory strains of *S. mansoni*, acquired resistance was best shown in the partly susceptible macaque. This host develops longterm infection, followed by resistance to challenge, and eventually by self-cure [14, 23, 27, 50]. Immunity is less clearcut in the more highly susceptible mouse [26, 30, 47], and in the less susceptible rat or rabbit [19, 30]. Currently, data on other species, particularly on primates, are being actively collected in several laboratories. The position of man within this host spectrum is thought to lie toward the highly susceptible side [25].

In the long-term infected macaque which we shall take as a model, immunity is eventually suppressive, but established worms are less affected than schistosomula introduced with a new challenge, and the total extermination of adult parasites may require many months, whereas the peak mortality of new schistosomula occurs within their first 60—80 days [27]. The results of the challenge must be interpreted in the light of the fact that each host species, independently of the immune state, can be characterized by a "normal loss" of schistosomula which occurs between the time of penetration and the establishment of the worms; this loss is always substantial, and its size depends on many factors, but it is statistically definable. The primary criterion of schistosome immunity is the reduction of the number of worms attaining maturity to a level significantly lower than the expected mean. All other criteria, such as disturbances of parasite sex ratio, growth, egg production, or position of worms in the host vessels, are auxiliary. Current sampling methods are not sufficiently precise to construct mortality curves for schistosomula, but marked differences are invariably found as regards the retention sites in the host organism, and the degrees of growth impairment of

* Department of Pathology, Peter Bent Brigham Hospital, Harvard Medical School Boston, Massachusetts. — This work was supported by a grant from the Institute of Allergy and Infectious Diseases, National Institutes of Health (No. AI-2631) and by a contract with the U.S. Army Medical Research and Development Command (No. DA-49-193-MD-2253).

different individual worms. In trying to represent this distribution, one visualizes an imaginary bell-shaped curve, elongated on its far side, as the likeliest abstract model of the observed death pattern. This makes allowance for the frequent survival of residual worms for an indefinite period, although in some monkeys worm suppression is total [14, 23]. This idealized model should be kept in mind when lesser degrees of immunity are examined and when histopathological findings are to be interpreted.

While there are impressive quantitative and histopathological differences between schistosome immunity and bacterial immunity, it is not clear which can be attributed to the biology of the parasite, and which — if any — represent unique forms of host reaction. The status of worms as biological individuals, their complex physiology, and their ability to compensate for damage [14] may have a far-reaching influence in the total picture of schistosome immunity. Regardless of the reasons, in schistosomiasis there is a slowing of the manifestations of the immune process to the pace of a delayed action movie, which can thus be studied profitably for features which might escape attention in other infections.

Although schistosome worms and eggs share a variety of antigens, including those concerned with immunofluorescence [9, 11], single or repeated injections of purified eggs fail to protect mice or monkeys from cercarial challenge [17, 40]. Cercariae have species, as well as stage-specific antigens [4, 11], but the relationship of such antigens to immunity is not clear. In contrast to the findings in *D. viviparus* [10], infection with radiated cercariae produces a feebler immunity than infection with normal cercariae [33]. SMITHERS found a modest but definite immune effect when monkeys were challenged only three weeks after primary infection [42], but long-term infection is vastly more effective. Conversely, in a single successful experiment of this kind, transplantation of adult worms into the portal vein later resulted in immunity [41]. These findings suggest that all mammalian stages of the worm are immunogenic rather than any specific developmental stage alone.

Thus far, worm extracts and homogenates have been effective only in the rat, but have failed to produce immunity in many other species [30], and live organisms have generally been required. If this is due to methodological difficulties, one may hope that — as in transplant antigens — cell-free immunogenic preparations will eventually be obtained by improving fractionation methods. Some workers are proceeding with differential antigen-centrifugation techniques [43], while others are following leads derived from worm physiology. Current thinking favors "metabolic" rather than "structural" antigens [4]. We recently failed to detect antigen in the dialyzate of a protein-free culture medium, in which axenic adult worms had been incubated for 6 to 8 days [20]. More information about this increasingly competitive area of research can be found in the papers of SADUN [30] and SMITHERS et al. [43]. Little work has been done on species specificity, other than the studies of the HSÜS [7] and of SWANSON and WILLIAMS [46] on *S. japonicum* strains; it has been shown that *S. mansoni* modified subsequent *S. douthitti* infection, but not vice versa [8]. Very likely, other cattle and rodent schistosomes will soon be similarly tested.

Diffusion of cercarial enzymes [12] and of immunofluorescent antigen [13] takes place in the host skin soon after penetration, but the pathway taken by immune stimuli, or the changes in immunologically competent cells have not been studied systematically. Although Vogel tells of the virtual abolishment of immunity in a pregnant macaque [49], suppression of the immune response by drugs or gamma radiation has not been reported. Studies on the effect of splenectomy are currently being carried out [31]. Production of tolerance has been attempted unsuccessfully in the opposum [32].

Reports on passive transmission of schistosome immunity with hyperimmune serum are conflicting. After many failures, success has been claimed in mice *(S. japonicum)* and in rats *(S. mansoni)* [30]. The absence of reports regarding passive transfer by immune cells or cell-fractions is surprising, but if such attempts have been made they have not been published. The problem of the transmission of immunity is thus left in a state of uncertainty. Nevertheless, it has become quite plain, that in contrast to immunity against Nippostrongylus [35], Dictyocaulus [10] and Ascaridia [29], precipitating antibodies are not important, and that the supposed smothering of young worms by circumferential precipitates does not occur in schistosomiasis. This will become even clearer when we turn to the effector stage of immunity.

Most of the information on this point has come from histopathological and correlated immunofluorescent studies of the crucial organs in the migration of *S. mansoni*, i.e., skin, lung, liver and gut, in conjunction with worm-recovery and other parasitological data. One such study, in collaboration with Ritchie [14] was a comparison of cercarial transit in non-immune and in long-term infected, immune *Macaca mulatta*. A similar study [28] is now being undertaken in *Cercopithecus sabaius* (the St. Kitts Green-face Monkey). Studies were also carried out, with Sadun and Bruce, in a series of wild animals, with variable degrees of insusceptibility toward *S. mansoni* [19], and in mice exposed to gamma-radiated cercariae at different radiation levels [16]. An unpublished study with Sadun and Bruce brought together, as representative examples, monkeys and mice immunized with gamma-radiated cercariae (immune hosts); muskrats with primary infection (naturally insusceptible host), and their various controls, all challenged with normal cercariae [18]. Finally, and likewise still unpublished [15], a series of immunofluorescent studies was carried out on schistosomula and young worms in neonatal and adult mice nad rats and in challenged long-term infected *M. mulatta* and *C. sabaius*.

In order to extract useful information from this plethora of data, one must recall the principle, mentioned above, that mortality of schistosomula will be spread over a wide range of time and migration sites, and that the timing and location of their peak mortality will be a function of the severity of damage to the worms. This was found to be true not only in immunity but also when worm damage was due to other causes. Both in mice exposed to cercariae radiated with increasing gamma-dosages, and in wild animal hosts arranged in order of decreasing susceptibility, which were infected with normal cercariae, there were shifts in the timing and site of the peak mortality of schistosomula. With increasing gamma-dosage and/or insusceptibility, the site of maximal worm retention passed from the liver to the lung and, ultimately to the skin. As the shift toward the earlier migration sites occurred, the scatter of retained organisms became lesser, and the peak of retention better defined; simultaneously, the pathology associated with the schistosomula became more localized so that, at high levels of radiation and/or host insusceptibility, organ damage was confined to fewer areas. The susceptible host (mouse or macaque) receiving normal cercariae in moderate numbers and for the first time is somewhat of a problem, since most of the schistosomula dying as a result of "normal loss" cannot be located, even by exhaustive serial sectioning. Migrating cercariae in these hosts lack significant tissue reaction (Fig. 1); a few organisms, presumably retained and dying, are found in the lung during the 2nd and 3rd week of infection in sharply defined, granulomatous foci. The same

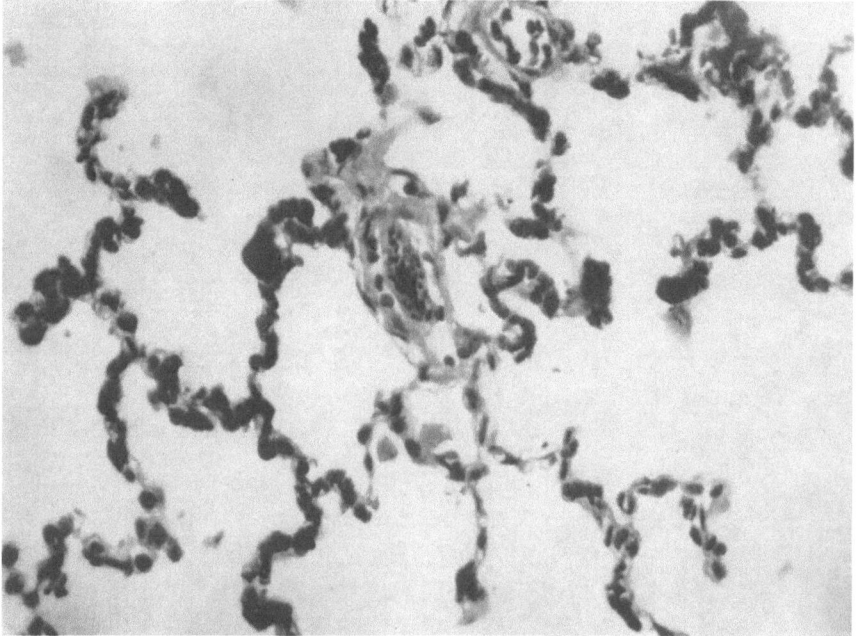

Fig. 1. 8th-day schistosomulum in mouse lung (primary infection, susceptible host). H & E stained, X 240. Note absence of significant host reaction

granulomatous reaction is seen around schistosomula after gamma-radiation and in the organs of the insusceptible hosts (Fig. 2). Some diffuse inflammation may also be present, particularly in the skin, but in the lung this is generally mild, and, with a few exceptions, it is proportional to the number of worms retained there. While these histological studies are less satisfactory quantitatively than the corresponding worm-recovery data, both are mutually consistent. The observation that gamma-radiation and natural insusceptibility have essentially identical effects suggests that the mechanism of retention and death in natural insusceptibility is the inability of worms to feed and grow, as is thought to be the case in "atreptic immunity" [16, 19].

As might be expected, in the immune host similar shifts of worm retention sites are also found. To make this as graphic as possible, one might say that the effect of immunity in the average long-term infected macaque is similar to the effect of 3000 to 4000 rep gamma administered to cercariae of *S. mansoni* before infection of a fully susceptible mouse. In both cases, skin retention will be slightly increased if at all, lung retention will be dominant, and a small number of worms will arrive in the portal radicles where all but a very few will have died by the end of two months. Since this is the maximal degree of immunity to *S. mansoni* which can be produced experimentally thus far, some of the extreme patterns of natural insusceptibility will not occur in the immunized animal, and most immunity patterns will be characterized by lung retention, and reduced portal recovery or accelerated mortality of young adults. To complete this picture, evidence of slowed migration has been found in some of the host types discussed here. The claim has

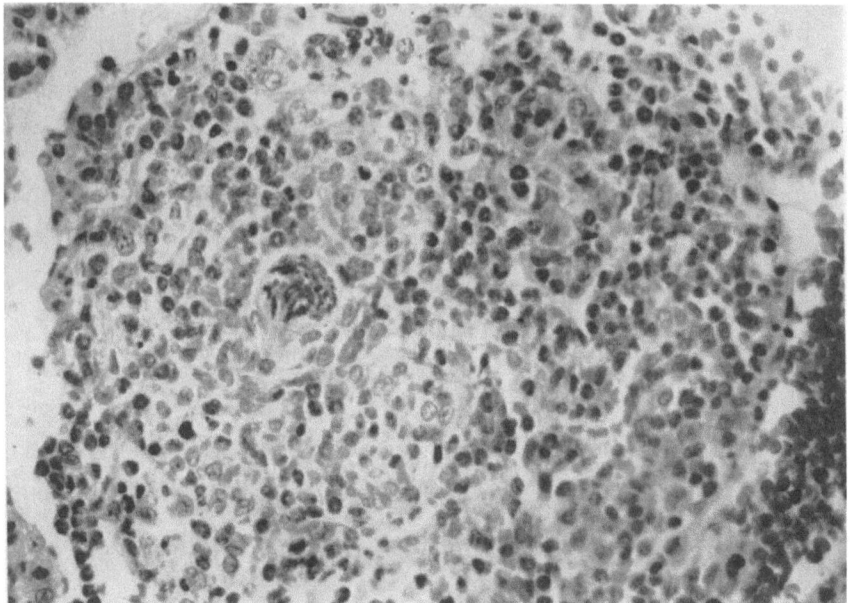

Fig. 2. 8th-day schistosomulum in lung of muskrat (partially insusceptible host, primary infection). H & E stained, X 240. Host reaction is granulomatous

been made [47] and contested [26, 30], that in the mouse this, rather than increased worm mortality may be the only immune effect. While our work was not concerned with migration velocity, slowing of migration would fit very nicely into the pattern, since slowing is likely to occur prior to total immobilization and death of the worms.

Other workers have likewise observed similarities between the challenged, immune host, and hosts bearing metabolically impaired parasites [5], but there is one striking difference in the immune host which has not been sufficiently emphasized, and this is the enhancement of the host cellular reaction. This feature is best observed in lung sections obtained 6 to 10 days after challenge, where one sees characteristic exudative foci, the "tuft-like foci", (Fig. 3) oriented initially along the capillary branches of arterioles; later there is consolidation, and formation of pneumonic foci which eventually resolve. Schistosomula lacking foci are seen to cause leukocyte clumping and endothelial swelling; more such foci are seen than can be accounted for by the number of schistosomula, and — at the height of the reaction — there is considerable scattered inflammatory activity in the macaque lung. When one confronts lung sections from immune and non-immune macaques, these differences are quite dramatic, but further confrontations were undertaken to insure that we were dealing with an integral phenomenon of schistosome immunity and not with a limited experimental situation [18]. Initially, confirmation was obtained in an enlarged series that tuft-like foci did not occur in naturally insusceptible hosts, such as the muskrat, nor after gamma radiation of cercariae in mice. Next, it was shown that such foci were not a species-specific feature of the macaque, since they were found, although lesser in number and smaller in size, in

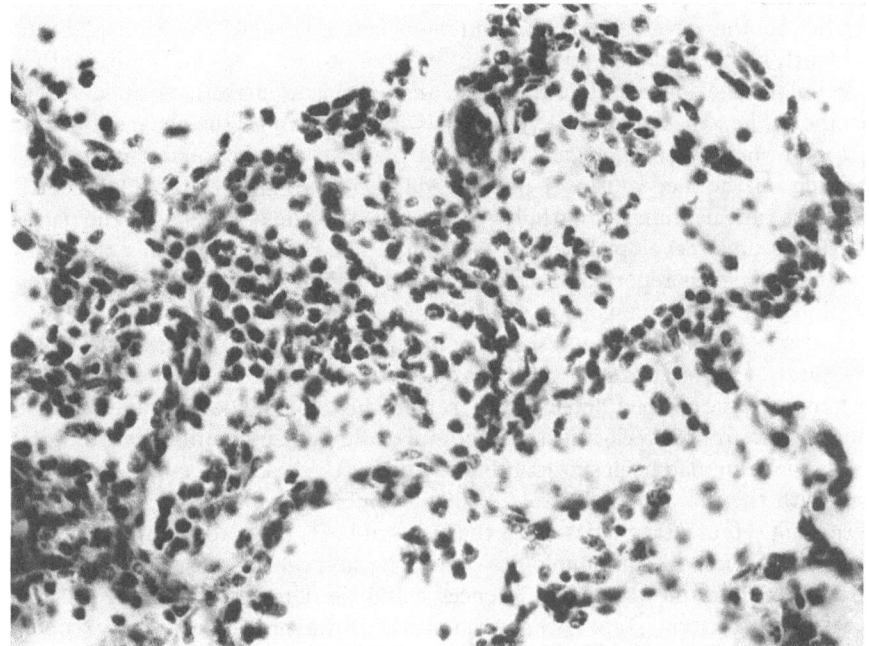

Fig. 3. 6th-day schistosomulum in lung of Macaca mulatta monkey (host previously immunized by long-term infection, and schallenged). H & E stained, X 240. Note exudative host cell response forming "tuft-like focus"

mice immunized with radiated cercariae and challenged. Further, it was demonstrated that the size and number of foci were related to the degree of immunity (as determined by worm-recovery data): foci were largest and most numerous in long-term infected macaques, fewer and smaller in macaques infected with radiated cercariae, and fewest in immunized mice, when compared at closely similar dates after challenge. Finally, and somewhat surprisingly, foci appeared to be related to immunity rather than to re-infection as such, since they were not found in the challenged long-term infected *C. sabaius*, which had received multiple doses of normal cercariae, without developing detectable evidence of acquired resistance.

We therefore concluded that schistosome immunity is characterized by two constant features:

A. Metabolic impairment of worms which — in common with other forms of damage — expresses itself in shortening of life span, shift in the retention peak of schistosomula, and disturbances of worm-migration and development, and

B. Accelerated and enhanced host cell response to migrating worms which is

19*

probably systemic, and is prominently expressed by the formation of exudative foci during the lung stage of worm migration.

Having attained these conclusions after considerable labor, we must acknowledge that they return us, essentially, to our point of departure, since these two phenomena are precisely the two classical ingredients of any immune response to infection, but our work was at least useful in giving us better insight into the modus operandi of the immune process under the particular conditions of bilharzial infection, and we can now eliminate the myth that schistosome immunity is a radical departure from other immune responses. This recognition is somewhat parallel to the development of immunological theory in the transplant field. Evidently, little is gained by studying immune processes in the traditional terms of cellular-versus-humoral factors. What is needed, instead, is an analysis of specificity, i.e., the features of the agent which determine the choice of a specific weapon from the immunological arsenal of the host; even more urgent, perhaps, is research on the mechanism of parasite damage and suppression. Both of these problems turn us from the pathology of the host to the pathology of the parasite, a hitherto underdeveloped field of endeavor. The remainder of this chapter will present a progress report on recent studies in this field, ending with a listing of possible effector mechanisms in schistosome immunity.

Initially, an immunofluorescent technique was used in a search for immune precipitates and/or changes in the antigen of schistosomula in immune hosts wich might have escaped detection by routine histology. The technique, based on immune sera from 8-week-infected mice and on fluorescein-conjugated-rabbit-anti-mouse-globulin, had been successful in studying schistosome egg-antigen, and was used with the prescribed controls. Schistosomula were located in serial cryostat sections of representative tissues of the series of hosts cited above, which varied in regard to species, age, immunological reactivity and cell response to schistosomula [15]. No significant staining differences could be detected in these hosts when corresponding worm stages were compared. However, these negative findings should not be overestimated, since technical factors cannot be ruled out, and the location of antibody was not studied.

An intriguing finding in this research, was weakened staining of the cuticle and entire soma of schistosomula in the interval between penetration and the hepatic stages, particularly in the lung 7 to 14 days after exposure, found in all the host species (Figs. 4, 5). Our initial interpretation, that this might reflect a change in antigenic composition of the cuticle, has not been borne out by fine-structural studies, and we now believe that, during this stage of maximal locomotion, and limited organ development "de-immunofluorescence" reflects the thinness of the cuticle, and the dissipation of earlier worm-products, e.g., acetabular gland secretions. In the young adults, which occupy portal radicles after the 3rd week, immunofluorescent staining is intense, and is brightest in the cuticle, cells closely underlying the cuticle, the gut lining, testes and vitellaria. Similar results were recently reported by Moore, using a different technique; he did not observe antigen-diffusion in the host skin, however [22].

Immunofluorescence failing to provide a short cut for interpreting the effector mechanisms of immunity, a more exacting approach was now called for, and the resources of molecular biology had to be mobilized. Here, we were able to start from the vantagepoint of knowledge on the metabolism and enzyme biochemistry of the schistosomes, which had been carefully accumulated by Bueding [1, 2], Senft [36, 37] and others, the axenic culture studies directed by Weller [3, 39],

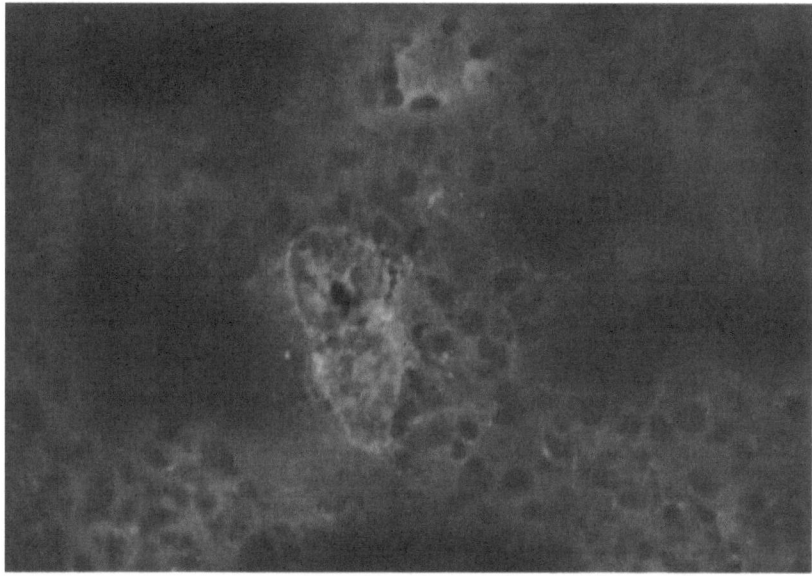

Fig. 4. 14-day schistosomulum in mouse lung, primary infection. Stained by the indirect immuno-fluorescent technique. X 400. Blackish pigment present in cecum. Note faintness and incompleteness of cuticular staining, partial dissipation of stainable antigen

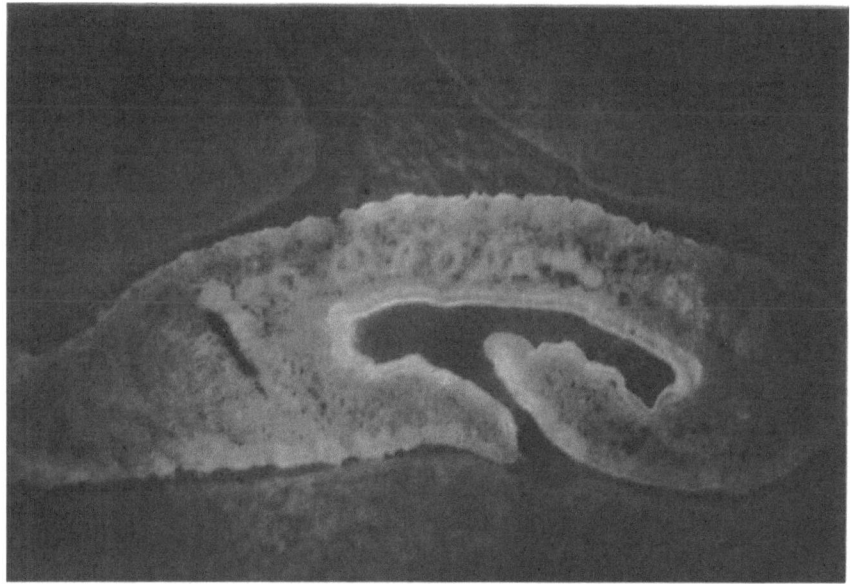

Fig. 5. 28-day young adult male schistosome, in mouse liver, primary infection. Indirect immunofluorescent technique, X 120. Note strong and complete staining of cuticle and subcuticular cells. Portal radicale and adjacent liver tissue essentially negative

19 a Bilharziasis

and the studies of Stirewalt, on the early metamorphosis and development of schistosomula [45]. Since studies on *in vivo* mobility and fine structure of worms were incomplete [38], we chose to concentrate on these latter features. First, the normal baseline had to be defined. Samples of normal cercariae, lung-stage schistosomula, and adult worms of *S. mansoni* were collected, and compared, with emphasis on the cuticle. Worms were fixed in osmium, and epon-embedded for electron microscopy. In addition, cryostat- and paraffin sections, and "thick" epon

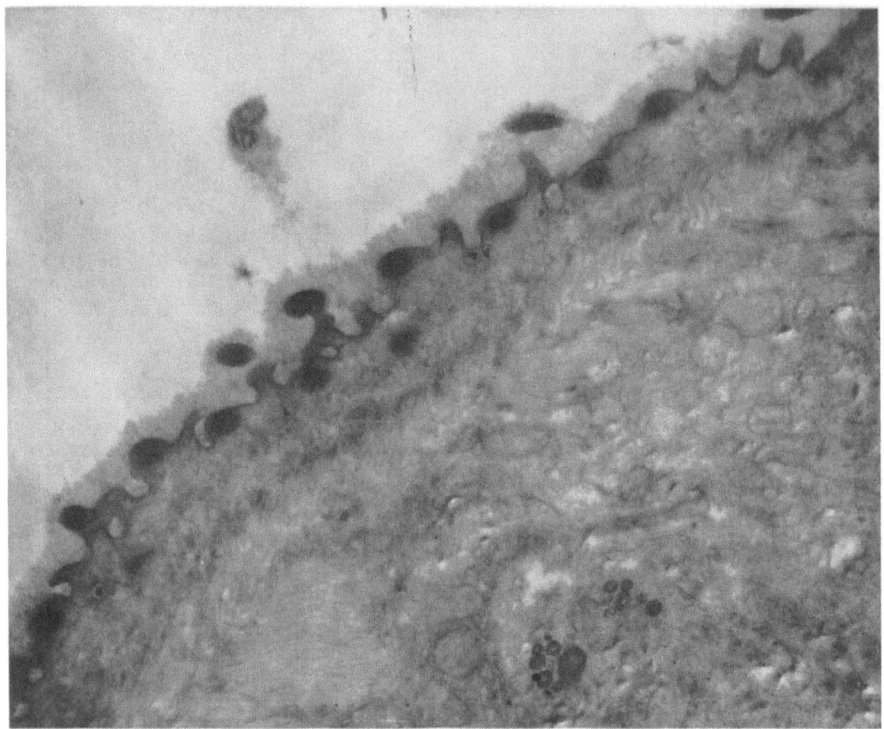

Fig. 6. Cercarial integument, electron micrograph; features shown include Cercarienhulle, setae, and basement membrane. Upper left shows cross-section of a cilium

sections of adult worms were stained with a battery of light microscope stains. These unpublished studies were done in collaboration with Drs. J. H. Smith and E. S. Reynolds [21].

The integument of cercariae, schistosomula and of adult worms is cytoplasmic in nature; it contains membranous profiles and vacuoles, as well as mitochondria. To date, no nuclear structures have been identified. There is, however, continuity with cytoplasmic elements in the parasite soma, situated between muscle fibers.

In cercariae, a finely fibrillary layer (Cercarienhülle) covers the cytoplasmic structure. The integument is relatively thin and uniform and has few organelles and setae. There is a well-defined, straight basement membrane (Fig. 6). In schistosomula, complexity is greater, the integument somewhat thicker, and it lacks an amorphous covering. There is considerable vacuole formation and large indentations are seen. A unit membrane has been discerned in the outer boundary of this cuticle, and a finely granular, homogeneous basement membrane underlies the integument, and is thickened at the points of apparent muscle attachment. Regionally, development of setae can be demonstrated (Fig. 7). The adult membrane shows the greatest complexity. A striking feature is the formation of dorsal tubercles in the male of *S. mansoni*. These appear to be herniations of cytoplasm of cells which resemble or are identical with the varieties found in the worm soma,

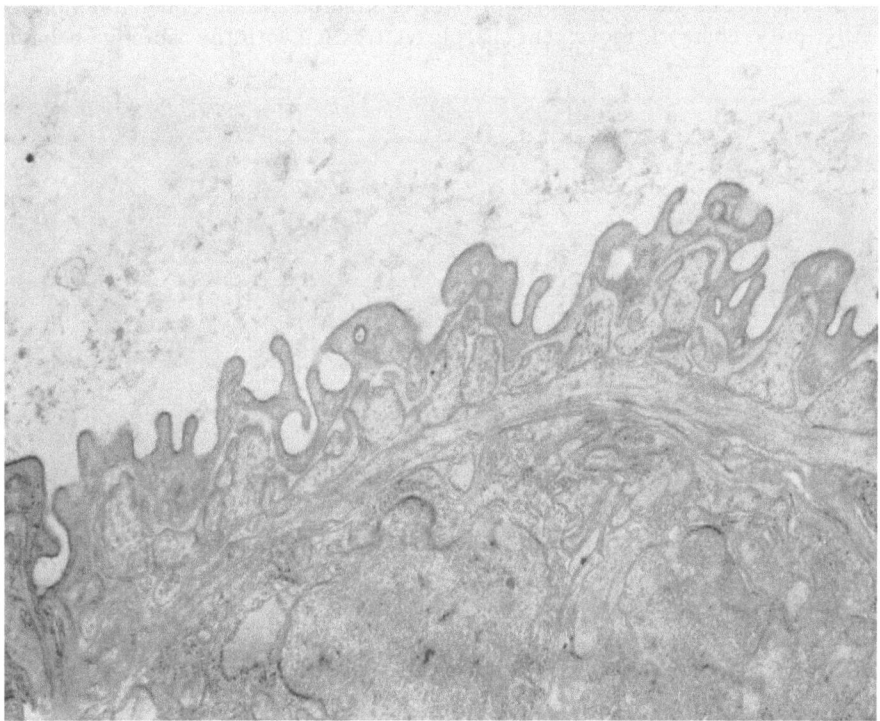

Fig. 7. Integument of schistosomulum, electron micrograph; absence of fibrillary covering, thick integument with marked vacuolar activity; complex basement membrane

through a hiatus in the dorsal circular muscle. At the margins of the tubercles, there is an intense elaboration of cystenae which are continuous with the plasma boundary adjacent to the basement membrane. The cells in the adult tubercle are, in part, vacuolated and lipid containing, while others are finely granular, and metachromatic or positive for PAS. The bubbling activity of the adult cuticle is very intense. Some of its inclusions are osmiophilic, and it would be of considerable interest to determine the direction of transport in this structure.

Staining with toluidine blue at various pHs shows that at pH 3, practically all worm structures are negative, indicating absence of chondroitin-sulphuric acids A and C. At pH 4, there are several structures deeply stained, including the vitelline glands. This presumably indicates presence of hyaluronate or of RNA. PAS stain differentiates the setae of the cuticle, and the basement membrane, as well as certain cells in the tubercles. The most intense PAS positivity is found in the vitelline glands.

In collecting lung-stage schistosomula, additional information was abtained about their *in vivo* behavior, and their structural organization compared with cercariae and adults. These forms were collected from the lung of heavily infected adult Swiss white mice, 160—168 hours after exposure, using a simple technique derived from previous work [3]. A few young and neonatal rats were also studied.

Schistosomula move actively for over 30 minutes, while under illumination, with a quick, energetic movement sharply contrasting with the "stately" behavior

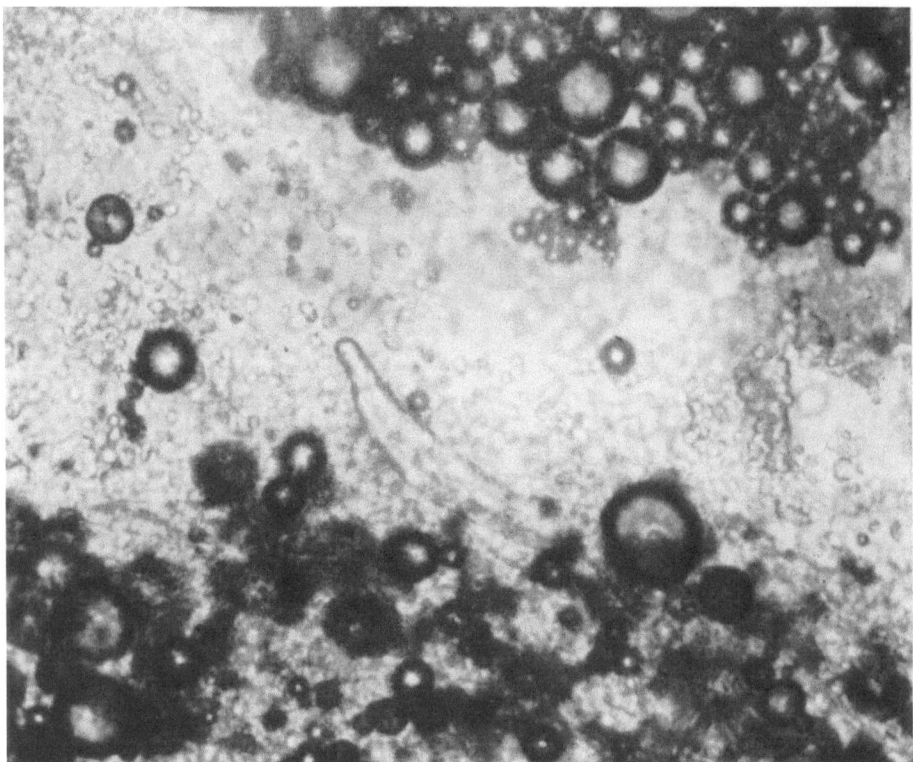

Fig. 8. Actively motile schistosomulum, 7th day, mouse lung, seen in compression preparation; shows oral end protruding between alveolar air bubbles

of the adult worm. From a resting position of flexion, the worm quickly elongates and extends dorsally, often with a sigmoid repeating movement which gradually displaces it. Muscular contraction bands are seen, most conspicuously at the poles, both of which undergo frequent changes in shape. The cecal ampullae move up- and downward and the entire worm cytoplasm seems to be in flux. Return to the resting position is somewhat slower (Fig. 8).

The number of schistosomula varied greatly, with a maximum of 11 organisms per lung. Comparison with stained and serially sectioned preparations showed that this still represented only 30 to 50% of schistosomula demonstrable by histology. No motile organisms were found in either primarily infected or challenged baby rats, although schistosomula were demonstrated histologically. There was considerable variation in size, shape and cecal content at the 7-day lung stage suggesting individual variations in development. Measurements varied between 212 micra in contracted worms and 392 micra in extended worms, with a width of 28 to 15 micra (average size of cercarial body without tail: 190–70 micra). Sexual dimorphism could not be ascertained at the 7-day lung stage!

Mounts of whole. stained schistosomula (tol. blue) show an oral depression or slit versus a conical caudal pole, the integument is thin, villous, pale and not metachromatic; a developing acetabulum is sometimes seen near the oral pole. Thus far, no vitellariae or other sexual apparatus have been visualized. A central esophagus runs through at least $2/_3$ of the worm, ending in a distinctly bifurcated cecal anlage which may contain red cells and/or debris. On thick section, muscular contractions give a scalloped appearance to the schistosomulum, and most of its soma was seen to consist of myocytes, which contain axial bundles of myofibrils lacking cross-striations or other substructures. The gut is composed of dark staining epithelial cells rich in ribosomes and organelles, whose cell boundaries have not yet been located, and which bear, on their inner surface, numerous terminally clubbed plicae, similar to but less numerous than those of the adult worms (Fig. 7). The protonephridial canaliculi show flame cells. With the exception of the – as yet unidentified – sexual elements, the schistosomulum is in many ways similar to the adult worm, but its organization is different from the cercaria.

These current studies are the first stage of a long-term effort, whose next stage should be the correlation of structural and physiological properties of normal worms, and whose final stage – the pathobiology of immunity – cannot yet be clearly envisaged. However, since research is unrewarding in the absence of a guiding set of hypotheses, I would like to return briefly to possible effector-mechanisms in schistosome immunity:

Host attack is likely to be multi-pronged, and, likewise, worm defense is apt to be complex. Two worm-surfaces are mainly exposed to potential damage: the integument and the gut. The latter is accessible only to plasma entering with the blood meal, the former both to plasma and to cells. Since energy requirements of worms (at least in adults) can be met by cuticular transport for relatively prolonged periods [3, 39], damage to the gut (by host antibodies, or "anti-enzymes") would have a delayed effect, and might express itself by maturation delay, sexual impairment, and dwarfing, all prominent features in schistosome immunity. While the relative importance of hematophagia and intestinal metabolism in the schistosomes is not yet known, recent data indicate that the gut has a specific enzyme for splitting amino acid chains off the heme molecule [37, 48]. In earlier studies of the immune macaque [14] the appearance of amorphous eosinophilic aggregates in the ceca of lung-stage schistosomula was disregarded as an inconstant feature, but this is certainly suggestive of damage to the gut. As to the integument, sensitization of host cells to the surface-bound antigens of schistosomula could result in complement-independent enhancement of the adhesiveness of host endothelia and leukocytes, termed "immune adherence" by SOULSBY [44]. Schistosome-infected baboon sera carry an opsonin which induces this phenomenon in vitro, but its relationship with immunity is unclear, and the factor was not detectable in

macaques [24]*. In the presence of immune adherence, the migration of schistosomula through capillary beds would become a contest of their endurance and, the
slower migration, the likelier the arrival of further sensitized cells homing in on
their target. This could explain the formation of tuft-like foci seen by histological
study. Occupation of worm integument by adhesive host cells might facilitate
transmittal of cell- or plasma-bound antibody, or "anti-enzyme" capable of
inhibiting membrane movement and regeneration of the cuticle, which is required
for active transport; and this, in turn, would eventually lead to energy starvation
and death. Evèn prior to total immobilization, the schistosomula would find
themselves cornered by host-cell-predators ready for phagocytic removal of their
disintegrating carcass.

What has been said about potential host mechanisms also applies, mutatis
mutandis, to the potential defenses of the parasite. Young worms would enter the
contest with variable endowments of vigor, and ability to resist. Choice of migratory
routes may also be important.

It is, of course, possible that a single one of the above factors, or another factor,
not yet envisaged, should be by far the most decisive mechanism in schistosome
immunity, but this is not likely, if biological analogy holds true. It will take time
and effort to develop the methods and carry out the experimentation necessary to
únravel this mystery. However, if this can be achieved, it will certainly represent
a milestone of immunology.

References

[1] BUEDING, E.: Metabolism of parasite helminths. Physiol. Rev. 29, 195—218 (1949).
[2] — Mechanisms of action of schistosomicidal agents. J. Pharmacol. Exp. Ther. 11, 385—392 (1959).
[3] CHEEVER, A. W., and T. H. WELLER: Observations on the growth and nutritional requirements of Schistosoma mansoni in vitro. Amer. J. Hyg. 68, 322—339 (1958).
[4] FIFE, E. H., and J. T. BRUCE: Studies on the exoantigens of Schistosoma mansoni cercariae. Presented to 13th Annual Meeting Amer. Soc. Trop. Med. Hyg. Nov. 7, New York, 1964
[5] HSU, H. F., J. R. DAVIS, S. Y. LI HSU, and J. W. OSBORNE: Histopathology in albino mice and Rhesus monkeys infected with irradiated cercariae of Schistosoma japonicum. Z. Tropenmed. Parasit. 14, 240—261 (1963).
[6] — S. Y. LI HSU, and J. W. OSBORNE: Immunization against Schistosoma japonicum in Rhesus monkeys produced by irradiated cercariae. Nature 194, 98—99 (1962).
[7] HSU, S. Y. LI, and H. F. HSU: A new approach to immunization against Schistosoma japonicum. Science 133, 766 (1961).
[8] HUNTER, G. W. III., and C. J. WEINMANN: Studies on schistosomiasis XVI. Non-reciprocal acquired resistance between Schistosoma mansoni and Schistosomatium douthitti. J. Parasit. 46, 5 (Section 2, Suppl.), 34 (1960).
[9] JAIMES, S., and F. v. LICHTENBERG: Host response to eggs of Schistosoma mansoni IV. Fluorescent antibody titers in mice infected with normal cercariae. gamma-radiated cercariae and with purified eggs. Amer. J. Trop. Med. Hyg. Under review.
[10] JARRET, W. F. H., F. W. JENNINGS, W. T. M. McINTYRE, W. MULLIGAN, and G. M. URQUHART: Immunological studies on Dictiocaulus viviparus infection. Immunity produced by the administration of irradiated larvae. Immunology 3, 145—151 (1960).

* Since this manuscript was completed, several authors have emphasized possible role of
reagin antibodies, demonstrable by passive cutaneous anaphylaxis, in schistosome immunity.
This constitutes another promising approach, and is in harmony with the observed cellular
phenomena described in this essay.

[11] KENT, N. H.: Comparative immunochemistry of larval and adult forms of Schistosoma mansoni. Ann. N. Y. Acad. Sci. 113, 100—113 (1963).

[12] LEWERT, R. M., and C. L. LEE: Studies on the passage of helminth larvae through host tissues I. Histochemical studies on the extracellular changes caused by penetrating larvae. II. Enzymatic activity of larvae in vitro and in vivo. J. Infect. Dis. 95, 13—51 (1954).

[13] LICHTENBERG, F. v.: Studies on Granuloma Formation III. Antigen-sequestration and destruction in the schistosome pseudotubercle. Amer. J. Path. 65, 75—94 (1964).

[14] —, and L. S. RITCHIE: Cellular resistance to schistosoma of Schistosoma mansoni in Macaca mulatta monkeys following prolonged infections. Amer. J. Trop. Med. Hyg. 10, 859—869 (1961).

[15 — —, and E. S. REYNOLDS: Immunoflourescent and fine structural studies on schisto-somula. Paper presented to 13th Annual Congress, Amer. Soc. Trop. Med. Hyg., New York, Nov. 7, 1964.

[16] —, and E. H. SADUN: The parasite migration and host reaction in mice exposed to irradiated cercariae of Schistosoma mansoni. Exp. Parasit. 13, 256—265 (1963).

[17] — —, and J. T. BRUCE: Host response to eggs of Schistosoma mansoni. III. The role of eggs in resistance. J. Infect. Dis. 113, 113—122 (1963).

[18] — — — Pulmonary tissue reactions in natural insusceptibility, in acquired resistance and in artificial immunization against. S. mansoni. Amer. J. Trop. Med. Hyg. In preparation (1965).

[19] — — — Tissue responses and mechanisms of resistance in Schistosomiasis mansoni in abnormal hosts. Amer. J. Trop. Med. Hyg. 11, 347—356 (1962).

[20] —, and A. W. SENFT: Unpublished. Abstract obtainable through U.S. Army R & D Command. A.F.E.B. Report, March 1, 1965.

[21] — J. H. SMITH, and E. S. REYNIOLDS: Unpublished. Abstract obtainable through the U.S. Army R & D Command. A.F.E.B. Report, March 1, 1965.

[22] MOORE, D. V.: Studies on the immunopathology of Schistosomiasis mansoni using the fluorescent antibody procedure. Paper presented to 13th Annual Meeting. Amer. Soc. Trop. Med. Hyg., New York, Nov. 7, 1964.

[23] NAJMARK, D. H., A. S. BENENSON, J. OLIVER-GONZALEZ, D. B. McMULLEN, and L. S. RITCHIE: Studies on schistosomiasis in primates: Observations on acquired resistance (Progress Report). Amer. J. Trop. Med. Hyg. 9, 430—435 (1960).

[24] NEWSOME, J.: Immune opsonins in schistosoma infestations. Nature 195, 1175—1179 (1962).

[25] — Problems of fluke immunity with special reference to schistosomiasis. Trans. Roy. Soc. Trop. Med. Hyg. 50, 258—274 (1956).

[26] RADKE, M. S., and E. H. SADUN: Resistance produced in mice by exposure to irradiated Schistosoma mansoni cercariae. Exp. Parasit. 13, 134—142 (1963).

[27] RITCHIE, L. S., W. B. KNIGHT, D. B. McMULLEN, and F. v. LICHTENBERG: The influence of infection intensity of S. mansoni on resistance against existing and subsequent infections in Macaca mulatta monkeys. Amer. J. Trop. Med. Hyg. Under review.

[28] — and F. v. LICHTENBERG: The pathobiology and immunology of Schistosoma mansoni infection in the green monkeys. In preparation.

[29] SADUN, E. H.: The antibody basis of immunity in chickens to the nematode, Ascadiagalli. Amer. J. Hyg. 49, 101—116 (1949).

[30] — Immunization in schistosomiasis by previous exposure to homologous and heterologous and heterologous cercariae, by inoculation of preparations from schistosomes and by exposure to irradiated cercariae. Ann. N. Y. Acad. Sci. 113, 418—439 (1963).

[31] — Personal communication.

[32] — Personal communication.

[33] — J. T. BRUCE, and P. B. MACOMBER: Parasitologic, pathologic and serologic reactions to Schistosoma mansoni in monkeys exposed to irradiated cercariae. Amer. J. Trop. Med. Hyg. 13, 548—557 (1964).

[34] — A. YAMAKI, S. S. LIN, and J. C. BURKE: Studies on the host-parasite relationships to Schistosoma japonicum. VI. Acquired resistance in mice and monkeys infected with the Formosan and Japanese strains. J. Parasit. 47, 891—897 (1961).

[35] Sarles, M. P., and W. H. Taliaferro: The local points of defense and the passive transfer of acquired immunity to Nippostrongylus muris in rats. J. Infect. Dis. **59**, 207—220 (1936).

[36] Senft, A. W.: Observations on amino acid metabolism of Schistosoma mansoni in a chemically defined medium. Ann. N. Y. Acad. Sci. **113**, 272—288 (1963).

[37] — Recent developments in understanding of amino acid and protein metabolism in vitro by Schistosoma mansoni. Abstract, Int. Cong. Parasitology, Rome, July, 1964.

[38] — D. E. Philpott, and A. H. Pelofsky: Electron microscope observations of the integument, flame cells and gut of Schistosoma mansoni. J. Parasit. **47**, 217—229 (1961).

[39] —, and T. H. Weller: Growth and regeneration of Schistosoma mansoni in vitro. Proc. Soc. Exp. Biol. **93**, 16—19 (1956).

[40] Smithers, S. R.: Stimulation of acquired resistance to Schistosoma mansoni in monkeys: Role of eggs and worms. Exp. Parasit. **12**, 263—273 (1962).

[41] — Discussion of paper by E. H. Sadun. In: Proceedings Seventh International Congress of Tropical Medicine and Malaria, Rio de Janeiro, **2**, 31—32, 1963.

[42] — Personal communications, 1964.

[43] — R. J. M. Wilson, and D. B. Brodyn: Morphological, biochemical and antigenic characteristics of subcellular fractions of adult Schistosoma mansoni. In: Proceedings, Seventh International Congress of Tropical Medicine and Malaria, Rio de Janeiro **2**, 97 1963.

[44] Soulsby, E. J. L.: The nature and origin of the functional antigens in helminth infections. Ann. N. Y. Acad. Sci. **113**, 492—509 (1963).

[45] Stirewalt, M. A.: Cercaria vs. schistosomule (Schistosoma mansoni), absence of the pericercarial envelope in vivo; and the early physiological and histological metamorphosis of the parasite. Exp. Parasit. **13**, 395—406 (1963).

[46] Swanson, V. L., and J. E. Williams: Pathology of Schistosoma japonicum in the Taiwanese monkey (Macaca cyclopis) I. Comparison of Formosan and Japanese strains. Amer. J. Trop. Med. Hyg. **12**, 748—752 (1963).

[47] Szumlewicz, A. P., and L. F. Oliver: Schistosoma mansoni: Development of challenge infections in mice exposed to irradiated cercariae. Science **140**, 411—413 (1963).

[48] Timms, A. R.: Schistosome enzymes, pp. 41—49. In: Host influence on parasite physiology. L. A. Stauber (Ed.) New Brunswick, N. J.: Rutgers University Press 1960.

[49] Vogel, H.: Acquired resistance to schistosoma infection in experimental animals. Mimeographed Abstract. W.H.O. African Conference on Bilharziasis, Brazzaville, 1956.

[50] —, and W. Minning: Über die erworbene Resistenz von Macacus rhesus gegenüber Schistosoma japonicum. Z. f. Tropenmed. Parasit. **4**, 418—505 (1953).

The Measurement of Schistosome Populations

David J. Bradley*

With 3 figures

I. Introduction

The study of bilharziasis has now reached the stage where some attempt to be systematic is essential: the data available are too numerous to be comprehended individually. The position has also been reached where much is known about every aspect of the disease and its transmission, but different parts have been studied in different places and circumstances, and it is often impossible to interpret one set of results without local information on another part of the life cycle, which may be lacking. Recently the need for full study of schistosome population dynamics has become clear, but in most places one particular stage has been studied in great detail — cercariae in water, or eggs in excreta for example — rather than as part of a complete analysis. It appears then that there is a need for review of the available techniques for measuring schistosome populations at each stage of the life cycle. The course of such a review has shown that a few broad general principles and methods underlie the mass of technical detail concerned, and an attempt has been made to give these prominence here.

The basis of any complete study of schistosome population dynamics is a census at each state in the life cycle, perhaps with further subdivision of the longer stages into age-groups. For most of the stages the habitat is the host, and a host census is the first step towards parasite census. There are vertebrate and molluscan hosts, and fresh water is the habitat of the free-living stages. Fortunately an adequate summary of snail host census techniques is now available [46], and there are numerous books on general limnology. The sampling of human populations, though often very difficult in bilharzial field work, has also been adequately covered in standard works on human demography and preventive medicine. It will be assumed that Mrs. Beeton's principle of "first catch your host" has been observed and census within the micro-habitat — vertebrate, water or mollusc—only is considered here. The stages and their habitats are listed in Table 1 and are considered serially.

Methods of clinical diagnosis and prevalence survey are not dealt with, nor are indirect methods suggesting heavy or light parasite loads. They are omitted as the clinician and population ecologist have different aims, though less separate than either sometimes believes, and too many unsatisfactory methods have resulted from confusion of aims. Indirect methods, immunological or chemical, may eventually become good substitutes for census techniques but at present they are not, and need much further comparison with parasite counts before they can be used in this way.

* Department of Microbiology, University of East Africa. — Makerere College Medical School. P.O. Box 2072, Kampala, Uganda.

Table 1. *The stages of the schistosome life cycle and their habitats*

Section of Chapter	Stage in Schistosome life cycle	Microhabitat	
A.	excreted eggs	excreta	free
	excreted eggs	snail habitat	
B.	miracidia	water bodies	
C.	miracidia	snails	
	mother sporocysts	snails	
	daughter sporocysts	snails	molluscan host
	cercariae		
D.	cercariae	emerging from snails	
	cercariae	water bodies	free
E.	cercariae	vertebrate surface	
	cercariae	vertebrate skin layers	
F.	schistosomules	vertebrate organs	vertebrate host
	adult worms	vertebrate organs	
G	eggs	vertebrate tissues	

Complete coverage of the literature was impossible with the available library facilities, and the papers quoted have been selected from a far greater number describing variants of technique. Since the problems of sample size in relation to accuracy of results merely involve general statistical considerations, they have been largely omitted; they are reviewed in a bilharzial context in the paper by Uemura (WHO mimeographed document) and in part by WHO [126].

Certain basic procedures recur in the enumeration methods for many stages of the life cycle, and although the extent of this convergence will not be apparent till later in the chapter, these basic techniques are discussed first to avoid repetition.

II. Apparatus and basic procedures*

1. Filtration

The use of filtration to replace sedimentation as a means of extracting schistosomes from volumes of turbid fluid has increased in recent years, and is just emerging from the experimental stage to becoming a reliable routine procedure. A variety of apparatus, filters, and stains is available, covering a great range of costs as well as applications. An attempt has been made to be selective and to suggest commercially available equipment where possible.

Apparatus. Although ordinary conical filter papers may be used for extracting cercariae from small volumes of water, all really useful methods employ a flat Büchner-type funnel. Pressure filtration can be used [98, 99], but tends to damage the schistosomes. Unaided filtering is too slow, and therefore suction is applied. This may be provided from an ordinary filter pump which is adequate for egg counts on urine [18], or by various types of manual stirrup pump with reversed valves. These are usable in the field. So is a 50 ml syringe with one-way valves fitted. For laboratory procedures and particularly in the presence of much debris, as in stool egg counting, an electric vacuum pump is best. Under no circumstances should a liquid trap near the pump be omitted. With poor suction the capacity of filtration systems is limited by the time it takes to filter the sample. With an adequate vacuum source it is limited by the thickness of debris deposited on the paper. This

---

* For the addresses of firms to which reference is made in the text see page 327.

will depend on the density of particles in the suspending medium and their size in relation to the filter. Other things being equal, however, the sensitivity of any procedure is proportional to the area of filter membrane. For very large volumes, as in the measurement of cercarial populations in natural waters, an 18.5 cm filter diameter, area about 250 cm², is used [101] in a plastic Büchner funnel. For stool egg counting BELL [7] used a 7 cm diameter paper (32 cm²) and for work with urines I have used areas from 2 cm² to 10 cm². The complete range of possible requirements is covered by four types of apparatus, and for most purposes only one or two are needed for all stages of the life cycle. The four suggested types are:

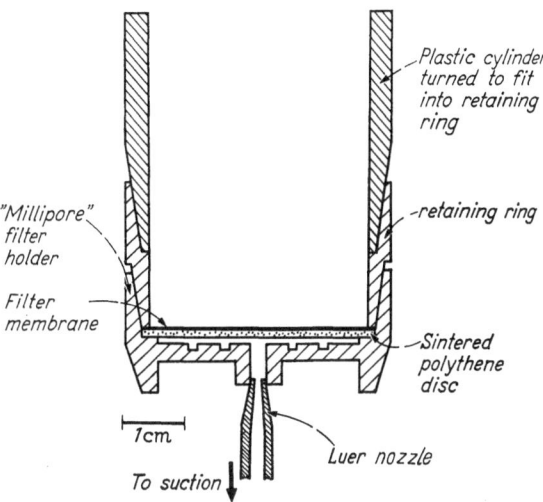

Fig. 1. Section of portable filter holder made largely from commercially available parts; after BRADLEY [20]

A. A 6 cm² rectangular filter holder commercially obtainable (Millipore XX20.017.00) and having the advantage of taking a rectangular filter suitable for mounting on a traditional 3″ by 1″ glass slide. It is suitable for urine studies in particular, and for organ digest work, but is too small for stool counts in S. mansoni as the capacity of one filter is approximately 20 mg of stool only. Filter membranes and papers can be readily cut by the user to fit this holder.

B. A 10 cm² circular filter holder. This may also be obtained commercially, in either of two forms. The bench one (e.g. Millipore XX10.047.00) resembles the preceding model except for having a circular filtering area, of diameter 35 mm. It is intended to hold membranes of 47 mm diameter. This leaves a large margin for labelling but, unfortunately, is not a standard size for filter *papers*. However, a 42.5 mm paper can be used. The alternative form is a disposable plastic holder (Millipore M000037AO) as used in field urine studies [19] but with an open top and used in a non-disposable manner, with a filter support of sintered polythene (Fison's Scientific, V/3/030). The top may be extended with plastic tubing, and the apparatus is shown in Fig. 1. The suction orifice then fits a standard Luer nozzle for connection to a syringe or other vacuum source. Provided that the retaining ring for the filter is adequately pressed down, the seal is good and these have the advantage of being cheap and portable for field use. For laboratory work the more conventional holder is preferable.

C. A filter holder for 7 cm diameter papers does not appear to be commerically available and is best made from clear plastic ("Perspex" or "Lucite"), glued together with a solution of plastic shavings in chloroform. The removable cylinder can be of 7 cm external diameter plastic tubing, or of glass with the edges ground flat, or of stainless steel, depending on materials available. Alternatively a tripartite

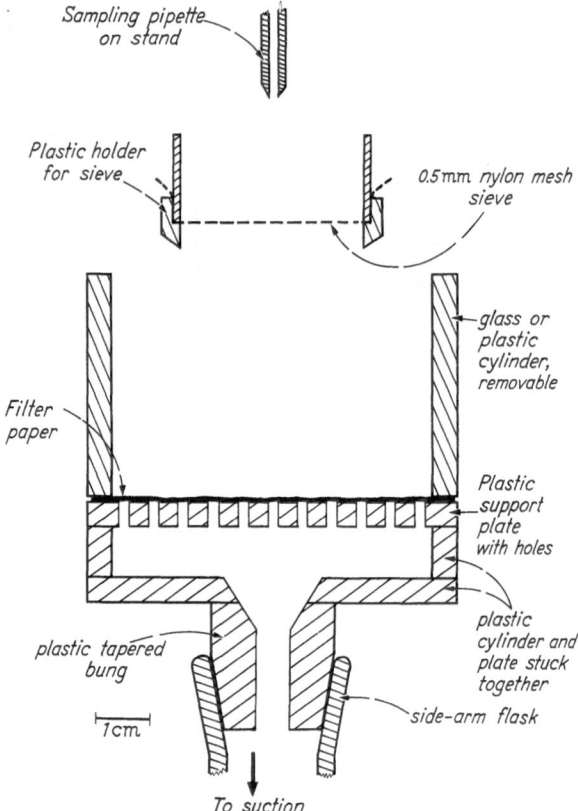

Fig. 2. Section of filter holder for stool egg counts; after BELL [1, 8]

porcelain Büchner funnel of Hartley tape (e.g. Griffin and George S26-845 type 15) may be used, but the perforated plate rarely has enough holes in and may be replaced by a suitably drilled sheet of ground plastic. The home-made variety is illustrated in Fig. 2.

D. For large, 250 cm², filtering surfaces a plastic funnel may be improvised [101] or porcelain ones may be bought, free-standing (e.g. Thomas 5592K size 5) or to fit into a jar (e.g. Griffin and George S26-845 type 40), though the latter type, due to its wide flange, needs a 24 cm diameter paper.

In general, filter holders of types A and C will cover all usual needs except cercariometry, and will not provide difficulties in obtaining suitably sized papers and membranes.

Filter membranes. The choice lies between paper, cellulose ester and netting membranes. The first two are alternatives for many purposes. Cellulose ester membranes have a smoother surface, more accurately standardised pore sizes, and can be rendered transparent in appropriate media. They are exceedingly expensive and not, therefore, feasible for large scale use. Papers, whilst having a rougher surface and remaining opaque, or at best translucent, are cheap, robust and can be obtained in a great variety of sizes, porosities and tensile strengths. They expand when moist and therefore should always be damped before the top of a filtering apparatus is clamped into them. A mention should be made of glass fibre filters (e.g. Whatman GF/A) in passing: they are very retentive and yet fast-filtering and become transparent in xylene or balsam. They are resistant to almost all stains and solvents. They provide a regular but undulating surface and their main defects are excessive thickness and low wet strength. Whilst they are of value for work with *Trichuris* and *Ascaris* and are less costly than cellulose ester, their use in bilharzial studies is confined to special investigations.

For the retention of schistosomes at almost any stage in their life cycle, papers are used unless there are additional exacting requirements, for which cellulose ester membranes are suitable. Miracidia are hard to preserve by any filtration method, but are best on ester membrane. In the latter case the most coarse grade made is usually best, with holes 5–10 microns in diameter. These retain the helminths and yet allow a fairly rapid filtration rate. The Van der Waals forces created within these membranes tend to retain also smaller particles than the pore size so they clog rather rapidly. BROWNE and THOMAS [21] have utilised cellulose ester membrane (Millipore SS) for depositing eggs from hepatic digests. When papers are used there is a wide range of suitable ones. S and S 404 [101] is certainly adequate for cercarial and egg retention [102]. Whatman No. 1 [18, 65] is also adequate. BELL [7] used Whatman 541. This has great wet strength, is fairly thin, and is translucent when wet, through the pores are rather large. Whatman 3 MM gives a smoother surface and 3 MMH is strong as well. These two papers are quite thick and therefore stand handling well but are relatively opaque to light. A variety of other papers has been tried but without advantages over those already mentioned. The writer has not had the opportunity of using S and S 404. Where the Whatman range is that most readily available 3 MMH is ideal except for very turbid suspensions (stools and sewage) where 541 is less readily clogged. No. 1 is always available and may be used where the others are not to hand.

Netting or sieve materials are useful for retaining adult worms in perfusion washings, and for extracting large particles from suspension before using filter paper for the helminths, as in BELL's [7] apparatus. Wire gauze and phosphor-bronze screens have been widely used for these purposes and are sometimes necessary, but in most census procedures they can usefully be replaced by nylon mesh sifting cloth. This is available in a wide range of rigidly standardised meshes and is inexpensive enough to be discarded when badly clogged. It is easily obtainable with mesh apertures down to 61 microns (e.g. from Henry Simon, Stockport) and is now available down to 25 μ aperture. This will retain most schistosome eggs but is not a practicable method for census work with them. These nylon cloths can conveniently be held between two retaining rings from "Millipore" disposable filter holders. Bolting cloths of silk are readily obtainable but the uneven shape of the pores and projecting silk filaments make them inferior to nylon for selective sieving.

Staining procedures. Since the various filter membranes available are not transparent it is difficult, though not impossible, to see the unstained schistosomes at most stages and some form of colouring is needed. Many different methods have been put forward. That preferred by ROWAN [98, 101], BELL [7], and the writer [16, 20] uses saturated or else 2% aqueous ninhydrin followed by gentle heating. Protein matter turns blue. Certain simple precautions need to be observed. Several killing and fixing agents tend to interfere with the reaction. In particular strong formalin does so. A final concentration of 1% in the suspension does not cause difficulties [102], and thorough washing on the filter, or permitting the paper to dry and let the formaldehyde evaporate, is useful. An alternative is to kill the organisms with gentle heating, [65] so that a fixative is unnecessary, or by a small amount of thimerosal. The organism must be dead for good ninhydrin penetration to occur, so staining the living eggs or cercariae is not to be recommended. There must then be time for ninhydrin in the aqueous phase to diffuse into the schistosome, and finally heating and drying produce the colour reaction. The writer finds that incubating filters with the ninhydrin in closed petri dishes for a few hours and then removing the lids ensures that both stages occur. The temperature of heating can be from 37° C to 100° C, depending on readily available facilities. The papers are re-damped for examination. If they are left exposed to light in a damp state the blue colour fades rapidly, but papers stored dry and in the dark retain it for several weeks. Eggs on papers varnished with a varnish dissolved in ethyl acetate (nail varnish, in fact) retained their colour for over 2 years with no sign of fading. It is essential to use freshly made up ninhydrin solution — dissolved under a week previously and stored in the dark. It is found in practice that a reliable routine for ninhydrin staining, with a standard procedure, and solution made up freshly each Monday, may be readily established. It is more suited to a laboratory with a continuous, if small, programme of counting than to the occasional count once a month or so.

Various alternative means of staining have been described. When the schistosomes are in relatively pure aqueous suspension practically any general stain is adequate. Methylene blue, carbol fuchsin, eosin and many others give good results. The organisms are best killed by heat or a fixative and stained before filtration by a very dilute solution of the stain. The writer (unpublished) has had good results in urine studies by adding merthiolate-formaldehyde solution [104] to urines in the field, using equal volumes of sample and preservative. Commercial "Merthiolate (thimerosal) tincture "contains a red dye. The urines were left for a week, then diluted with an equal volume of water, allowed to sediment, and filtered, the container being washed out with water and this also filtered. This is applicable to cercarial suspensions and other stages. BROWNE and THOMAS [22] used lactophenol cotton blue for staining eggs extracted from liver homogenates, and suggested its more general application. We have found that in urine the cellular debris stains so much more readily with this dye than eggs that counting is difficult.

In general, no method other than the ninhydrin reaction, has been shown to be adequate for all stages of the life cycle though one may yet be found. More specialised stains are considered under the appropriate section.

2. Sedimentation and sampling equipment

Apparatus needed for these methods is of a conventional laboratory type, and only a few comments are needed. Pipettes need to have a wide mouth and glassware used for concentrated suspensions of organisms is best silicone-treated before use to avoid wetting of surfaces and adhesion of the parasites. Census of *Schistosomatium douthitti* cercariae has been difficult due to their extreme tendency to adhere to surfaces [77]. The use of polytetrafluoroethylene ("Teflon") beakers and tubes might avoid this, but has not so far been reported upon.

Where many routine estimations of similar samples are to be studied the use of automatic devices is useful. Machines are now available (e.g. Griffin Diluspence) to pipette a known volume of a sample and later expel it, washing out the pipette with a predetermined volume of diluent which is added to the sample.

Where sedimentation procedures involve centrifugation, rotation speeds may be checked by a small meter placed on the hub through the lid of some types. Short periods at any setting of the rheostat rarely allow the centrifuge to attain its steady state speed for that setting.

Pipetting is usually quite accurate enough for census purposes, but where multiple volume measures are required to give a single count it must be remembered that this multiplies the error of any one stage by the square root of the number of stages. Thus, if pipetting has an error of $\pm 10\%$, four pipettings of that accuracy for one count will have a total error of $\pm 20\%$.

The mixing of viscous and heterogeneous suspensions may be achieved by a Waring blender or by air bubbling. The simplest and perhaps best of the latter methods is in a cylindrical jar having a perforated plunger and a lid; the plunger is rapidly moved up and down from the bottom of the vessel to above the liquid surface (e.g. a "Horlicks Mixer").

3. Sections

For the census of stages within the host the use of serial tissue sections is an extremely accurate method that has been rather little used, partly because it is tedious to eliminate the effects of an egg or other stage appearing in several sections.

Ordinary thin paraffin sections may be used, or thicker ones from blocks in celloidin or in nitrocellulose [28]. The use of alternating sections of two thicknesses, which may be cut on a simply modified rotary microtome [110], allows of a correction for overlap of organisms between sections or permits a thin section to be cut at regular intervals through the block. The combination of thick sections and selective staining techniques for specific stages to be discussed later will, in the writer's opinion, allow of more detailed population analyses within the host but without the histological destruction that characterises digestion procedures.

The methodology suitable for particular stages may now be considered in detail.

III. Sampling and counting particular stages

A. Excreted eggs

The occasional schistosome egg is expectorated [36] or even excoriated [5], but for practical purposes the eggs pass out in the urine or faeces. Although each

20*

species of worm has its preferred site of oviposition, *S. haematobium* eggs are not uncommon in faeces, and the occasional *S. mansoni* egg reaches the urine. For census purposes the main problems are sampling in the case of the urine, and egg extraction for the faeces.

The urine is considered first. Egg output from the host varies with the time of day chiefly, and also with activity, and in an apparently random manner. In addition, systematic variation for several days may follow unaccustomed activities [41].

This may be overcome by taking urine samples from people following their normal occupations. A marked diurnal cycle with maximal output in the early afternoon has now been demonstrated for *S. haematobium* in Egypt [113], Tanzania [16, 51] and Ghana [78]. The slight available evidence suggests that day to day variation is least at the time of peak excretion [17] and that 10 ml of urine then contain roughly 2.5% of the day's egg output. For census purposes, therefore, 24 hour urine collections are desirable; daytime 12 hour collections need a relatively small correction to give an estimate of the daily output; and if single samples are to be used they should be collected during the peak output period (noon to 2 p.m.). Even more important than choosing peak output is rigidly to standardise collection times and relate them to the total daily output in the locality under study. The actual specimen to be collected has been the subject of various opinions. Although some workers have considered that most of the eggs are in the terminal urine this has occasionally led to practical absurdities such as asking patients "to collect the last 200 mls of urine voided . . .". The only published data on variations within the urinary stream are due to GOVE [43] in Rhodesia. He collected urine samples in a series of test tubes. Although his own concern was with diagnostic accuracy, analysis of his results shows that at low egg excretion rates the distribution of eggs in the stream is neither even, nor random, nor exclusively terminal. For egg census studies, therefore, the whole specimen passed is collected and well mixed subsamples are used for egg counting. Under suitable circumstances subjects should void at 11 a.m. or 12 noon, discarding the specimen, and again at 2 p.m. when the whole bladder contents are collected.

Little data on day to day variation is available. Analysis of data from SCOTT [109], STIMMEL and SCOTT [113] and BRADLEY [17] gives a coefficient of variation around 60—70% for comparable samples from the same patients on different days. The lowest coefficients of variation, were for peak period urines from STIMMEL and SCOTT's [113] patient.

Schistosome eggs sediment rapidly in urine and adequate mixing by shaking or air bubbling is necessary just prior to subsampling.

Methods for the enumeration of eggs in urine have recently been reviewed in detail [20]. Three main techniques have been used. The first, devised by BARLOW [4] and used extensively by SCOTT [107], employed centrifugation to sediment the eggs and methylene blue, as a stain. They were transferred to a slide and subsequently counted. Quantitative transfer of sediment was the most difficult step. More recent workers have tended to resuspend the urinary sediment in a known volume and subsample this with a pipette. Variations of this procedure have been used by GERRITSEN [41] and by BENNIE [10], but the simplest and most widely used variant is that of JORDAN [51]. 10 ml of urine are centrifuged and the deposit resuspended after all but 0.2 ml of the urine has been drawn off. A subsample of

60 cu mm is transferred to a slide for counting. Uemura (unpublished) has shown from Jordan's data that if replicate counts are to be performed the whole procedure should be repeated, as second and third subsamples by pipette are subject to systematic bias. Advantages of the method are its straightforward character using standard laboratory apparatus. Defects are the need for three accurate volume measurements in each estimation and the difficult procedure of evenly resuspending the urine sediment in a small volume. The preparations are not permanent so that subsequent rechecking of counts is not feasible.

Methods of the third type depend on filtration to separate the eggs. Several devices for doing this have now been described. The well mixed urine is sucked through a filter membrane, the eggs stained and counted [16, 18, 20, 22]. All have particular advantages and are adequate. The mode of use is more important than the shape of the apparatus and any of the commercially available holders from membrane filter manufacturers described above, especially type A, is suitable. Since schistosome eggs are very large by usual filtration standards almost any of the membranes available will retain them; the only problem is to find one that does not also retain the cellular debris being passed. The discussion of methods in section II above is relevant to the detailed methodology. The urine container and filter are washed out with saline containing a little detergent to lyse red cells. The eggs should be dead before staining. This is best achieved by storing the urine with 2% formalin in saline for a day or so before filtering. If the ninhydrin stained papers are heated with and then without covers to prevent evaporation, penetration of the eggs by reagent and the ninhydrin reaction itself occur serially. A one-step heating and drying process has often been used successfully but I believe that several examples of failure to stain have occurred due to too rapid drying before penetration occurred.

For census work, therefore, there are various suitable techniques, of which filtration is probably preferable unless morphological observations of the eggs are required, when a subsampling procedure may be used. Large urine volumes may be filtered by proportionate increase of the filtering surface or without this provided the urine is not heavily infected.

Since diurnal variation in S. mansoni and S. japonicum egg output, even if present, is obscured by the pattern of faecal excretion, the best sampling procedure is a 24 hour sample beginning immediately after a stool has been passed. For practical purposes a single random stool is the best that can usually be obtained and the assumption is made that egg density is even between stools. Scott [108] found, in Egypt, that from day to day there was less variation between counts expressed as eggs per gram than between 24 hour output levels, but Bell [8] showed the reverse in Tanzania. There seems little to choose between the two for most purposes and an estimate of the 24 hour stool production is in any case necessary for expressing output per unit of time.

The largest sample practically obtainable is homogenised in formalin, or fixed with formalin and homogenised in water. 2% formol saline is a suitable preservative. Sturrock [119] has shown that at least eight times the stool volume of diluent is needed for adequate mixing. Low speed mixing in a Waring blender seems not to damage the eggs, and use of a beverage mixer with a perforated plunger also is very satisfactory (Sturrock, personal communication).

Where a large number of hosts (microhabitats) are under study smaller faecal samples may be inevitable. The author has found that a one ml metal scoop and a universal container with 9 ml merthiolate-formalin stock solution [12] is very convenient. The scoop also acts as an impacter to help break up the faeces.

Methods for counting the schistosome eggs in a sample of homogenised stool are very numerous, and they have never all been compared simultaneously. Most tests have been concerned also with diagnostic accuracy rather than quantitative assessment. Only two types of procedure are unlikely to miss any eggs: dilution counting and filtration.

The dilution egg count as described by Stoll and Hausheer [118] for hookworm studies was extensively used by Scott [106, 107], for studies of *S. mansoni* in Egypt and has been more recently employed in Brazil [54, 55]. Disadvantages are the small size of sample examined, between 0.005 G and 0.03 G depending on the number of replicates performed, and the need for three accurate volume measurements. Oliver-Gonzáles and Hernández-Morales [75], modified the procedure by sieving the suspension and then sedimenting for 30 minutes, removing the upper $3/4$ of the supernatant and resuspending before subsampling. They thus achieved a concentration of four times without the likelihood of losing any eggs. With three replicate counts on each sample a total of 0.06 G of stool are examined, 0.04% or less of the daily output. For *S. japonicum* with a high fecundity per worm this is reasonable but for *S. mansoni* with a fecundity of about 300 eggs per female per day [73], light infections would certainly be missed.

To avoid this, concentration procedures have been widely used. They have the general defect of losing a variable proportion of the eggs. The work of Maldonado and Acosta-Matienzo [69] shows how extensive this may be. Concentration methods recovered 2.4% to 70% of the *S. mansoni* eggs present in stool samples. Blagg and coworkers [12] achieved very high diagnostic yields of schistosome eggs by their MIFC concentration procedure, and if a concentration method is to be used at all, it seems to the present author the most suitable one as it is both quick and reasonably effective. It was used in quantitative studies by Pesigan and associates [84], but the basis for their choice there was not given. All the more elaborate concentrations take time which, if counts are needed, would be better spent on replicate Stoll-type counts or filtration.

A variety of methods has been used to reduce the débris and increase the concentration of eggs in suspension of faeces for counting. Kuntz [56] used hypertonic saline maceration, a 60 mesh sieve, and repeated sedimentation, and Newsome [74] followed a similar sequence followed by hatching of eggs. In general there are almost as many variants as authors and though few modifications greatly alter the method even fewer have been adequately tested (or at any rate the tests published).

Filtration of stools followed by ninhydrin staining of the schistosome eggs was used for stool egg counts by Bell [7], though the procedure was earlier used as the last stage of an extraction by Rowan and Gram [102]. The advantage of Bell's approach was that, except for sieving off really big particles from the stool, no concentration procedure was employed. A higher concentration of faeces per unit area scanned is possible with a filter paper than on a Stoll slide. A faecal concentration of $2.5-5$ mg/cm^2 is readily managed, as compared with 1 mg/cm^2 on a Stoll slide. The blue staining of eggs permits of rapid scanning.

Again, the precise apparatus used to hold the filters may be varied to suit particular needs. That of BELL [7] filters through 32 cm² of paper, and commercial holders can be obtained to cover 10 or 6 cm². Whatman 1 or 541 and S and S 404 are suitable papers for this purpose.

Large volumes of urine may be studied by the above methods suitably enlarged. Large volumes of sewage or stool, however, give unmanageably large amounts of débris and some type of concentration procedure is needed. The most carefully devised and tested one is that of ROWAN and GRAM [102]. In their apparatus homogenised sewage flows over saline of a higher specific gravity and schistosome eggs sediment through this layer. After repeating the procedure to clean the deposit, the eggs are deposited on a filter paper and stained with ninhydrin. They showed that over half of the eggs added to sewage were extracted by this means, and that the extraction fraction was reasonably constant for a particular sewage system. Any of the traditional concentration methods can also be used where it is necessary to examine large masses of stool or sewage. The one essential is to run a series of local standards by adding known numbers of schistosome eggs to a stool and determining the extraction efficiency of the chosen procedure.

B. Free miracidia

The detection of free-swimming schistosome miracidia by physical means does not appear to have been successfully accomplished in *natural waters*. This is not surprising as they are very fragile organisms. Attempts to filter them out of water by suction methods have left only smears on the filter paper and even with formalin fixation first they are difficult to separate from the many ciliates and other freshwater organisms. As under natural circumstances miracidia must be relatively scarce in water bodies these lines of attack are not promising. *S. mansoni* miracidia are photopositive in their responses and might be extractable by this means using the apparatus devised by KLOCK [53] for cercarial extraction. This would not apply to the miracidia of *S. haematobium* which are relatively unresponsive to light stimulation.

It appears, therefore, that bioassay is the only technique showing much promise for the future, and CHERNIN and DUNAVAN's [27] work suggests that miracidia show a considerable ability to find their hosts. The observations of MACCLELLAND [64] on recovery rates of marked snails in muddy ponds do not favour paint label techniques but his 3″ diameter snail cages with perspex ends and mosquito gauze sides were of value. The efficiency of such a sentinel snail system should ideally be calibrated in a similar habitat to that under study but to which known numbers of viable eggs have been added. If very heavy infection rates are encountered amongst sentinel molluscs, a closer estimate of the infecting miracidial densities is obtained by exposing experimental animals to the cercariae from individual snails, and calculating the proportion of bisexual infections. Since miracidia give rise to potentially unisexual cercariae, the total developing miracidial input may be estimated from this proportion. Alternative procedures for use when more than one miracidium is likely to have penetrated are considered in the next section.

The enumeration of miracidia liberated from a sample of infective urine, stool, or organ in the laboratory is more straightforward. Where the viable eggs are in a

pure state hatching may be observed in a Syracuse dish under a dissecting microscope. The number of miracidia hatching may be determined, as an alternative, by
performing egg counts on the sample by filtration, before and after exposure to
water for a period, and the hatch found by difference. Alternatively, miracidia
after fixation and staining with lactophenol cotton blue are readily seen on a
cellulose ester filter [22].

Photopositive and negatively geotropic species may be concentrated by placing
the viable eggs within a blackened side-arm flask, adding water, and illuminating

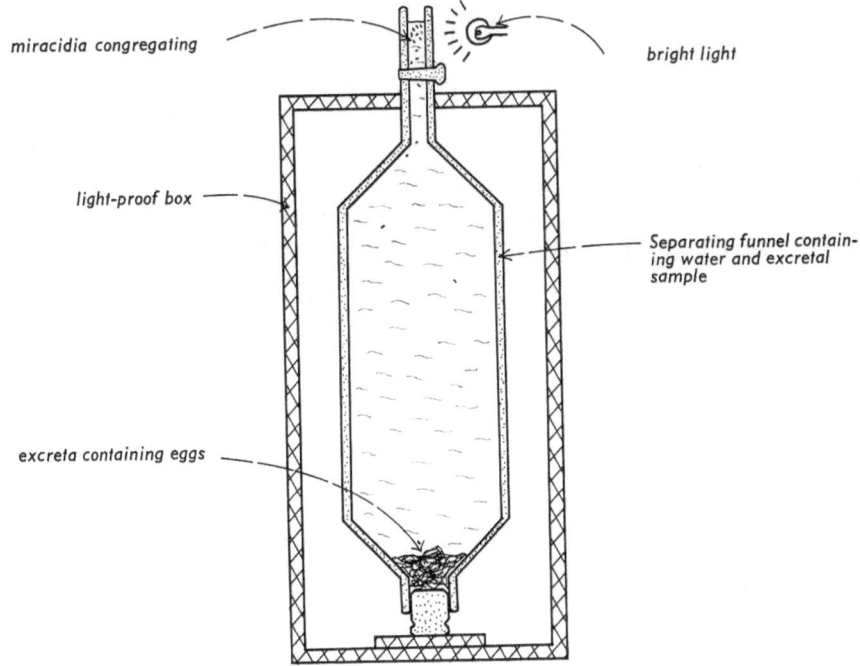

miracidia congregating   bright light

light-proof box   Separating funnel contain-
                                                             ing water and excretal
                                                             sample

excreta containing eggs

Fig. 3. Miracidial concentrating device; after Chaia [25]

the side-arm [67]. This is very widely used in transmission work. A rather more
elaborate version was developed by Chaia [25] who added the excreta to a separating funnel, stoppered and inverted it into a dark container, opened the now
upward-pointing exit stopcock and filled it with water to just above the stopcock.
A light was directed at this upper part and the hatching miracidia rose into it
(Fig. 3). Shutting the tap retained them in the stem from which they could be
poured off. This again depends on suitable taxic reactions to light or gravity. *S.
japonicum* is negatively geotactic [49] and the careful analysis of Chernin and
Dunavan [27] has shown that *S. mansoni* react to both gravity and light but the
former is more important. *S. haematobium* miracidia do not rise to the surface of
illuminated waters. Fortunately eggs of this species are most readily obtained in
fairly pure suspension. When hatching is to be undertaken in the laboratory a
variety of factors need control, or measurement: age of eggs, environment of
storage before experiment [70], aeration [68], pH for *S. japonicum* [49] but not
S. mansoni [71], and the reverse with light affecting *S. mansoni* and not *S.*

japonicum. Temperature has a smaller effect. Since in studies of dynamics of natural populations the prevailing natural conditions are relevant these should be simulated rather than the optimum sought. The use of plastic cylinders containing the excretal samples, closed with cellulose ester or other membranes, and immersed in natural waters has not been adequately explored.

The actual technique of counting rather concentrated miracidia requires fixation if large numbers are to be counted. 1% chlorobutanol has been used for immobilizing miracidia [123] but formalin is adequate for most purposes. Staining is with lactophenol cotton blue [22] or neutral red [50] before filtration, or by ninhydrin afterwards. The former is preferable.

At least for studies of *S. haematobium* miracidial densities in natural waters, two methods only seem feasible: animal exposure, or observations of human behaviour combined with measurements of egg output and means of detecting whether urine actually reaches the water, by feeding trace substances capable of subsequent detection by fluorimetry or by other sensitive chemical analyses.

C. Developing stages in molluscs

The use of sentinel snails to sample the miracidial content of natural waters has been mentioned. The methods used for their subsequent study are the same as those for examination of wild snails. Provided that snails put in a given habitat will only be exposed to schistosome miracidia, or that other trematode miracidia likely to be encountered are morphologically separable, the numbers of miracidia penetrating may be determined by sectioning the snails. Molluscan tissue, especially of the foot and head regions where most schistosomes penetrate, is very diffuse and thicker sections than are usually cut provide a manageable way of doing this. The miracidia are easily seen. Possibly the use of fluorescent antibody methods might speed this process if carried out on a large enough scale.

Serial sections are also a means for study of the sporocyst and immature cercariae. Alternative methods are dissection and squashes. Dissection is tedious and requires care. Sometimes it is possible to separate out the sporocyst and then count the contained cercariae. Squashes are rather crude, and give a preparation contaminated with snail tissues. They may be used in a precise manner at the mother sporocyst level if the date of infection is known [27].

Methods for intra-host census of trematodes in snails are, therefore, at a rather empirical level and have received little attention. One more complex method has been devised, by McCAULEY [62]. He ground the apex off from shells with a spire and by gently blowing into the aperture, protruded the hepatopancreas from the apex for examination. It was then sucked back and the hole sealed with paraffin or tacky wax. The snails *(Oxytrema silicula)* survived remarkably well, unless infection by Saprolegniales occurred. The method might have some application in schistosome work, but as the mother sporocyst is not in the hepatopancreas for this genus, its use for screening snails early in infection, yet allowing subsequent maturation, is not possible.

D. Free cercariae

Two lines of investigation have been followed in attempts to extract and count cercariae in natural waters: filtration with nets or membranes and attracting

cercariae to light. Both were attempted by BRACKETT [15] who immersed an
opaque frame without top or bottom into lake water, transferred the upper layers
to a pail and used light to concentrate the cercariae. He also tried netting but
found that the cercariae either poured through or were so damaged as to be un-
manageable. A continuous centrifuge was as bad. It is likely that many other
workers subsequently had similar experiences and failed to publish them, and only
in the last few years have reasonably effective methods been devised, chiefly
through the work of ROWAN, who has recently [101] summarised the various
methods he has devised. His techniques have so far mainly found application in
the Western hemisphere, due to the extreme turbidity of African waters in transmission foci. African workers have concentrated on biological assay of cercariae
by immersion of susceptible experimental animals [125].

ROWAN has developed three filtration devices using paper of 18.5 cm diameter.
His first model [98] employed pressure filtration; this has been replaced by suction
in later [101] models with less damage to the cercariae. These two later forms of
apparatus do not differ in major respects other than that one has a motor vacuum
pump and the other a hand pump as used for inflating tyres, with reversed valves.
An ordinary Buchner funnel is used without the top overlying the S and S 404
paper. Ninhydrin staining is used, and the paper heated till steaming but not
dried. Up to 20 litres of water may be filtered. RAYBOULD [91] has attempted to
use Rowan's cercariometer in East Africa but without success because of silt and
plankton clogging the paper, and other workers have had similar difficulties
(unpublished). In work with S. haematobium RAYBOULD [91] had some success
with a sand and water filter but [92] in later experiments using bolting silk and
metal screens he found that cercariae passed through even 25 micron holes and he
eventually abandoned work on this topic [93]. It would be interesting to know how
long this crossing of a 25 μ mesh takes, as it is clearly an active process with the
normal cercaria wider than this. If it is rather slow it might be possible to filter
water rather fast and then place the filter sieve on a petri dish of water to allow
cercariae to free themselves.

At the other extreme, PESIGAN and associates [85] used Millipore membranes
with extremely small pores and collected cercariae of S. japonicum from natural
waters. Their membrane appears unnecessarily fine for the purpose.

The morphological separation of related species of cercariae is notoriously
difficult, and animal exposure is the only reliable method of specific determination.
VERCAMMEN-GRANDJEAN [121] drew attention to the regular pattern of fine hairs
on the cercarial body of S. mansoni, but his suggestion that this could be applied
to taxonomy has not been followed up. Schistosome cercariae can be separated
from those of other families by their morphology on ninhydrin-stained filters.
ROWAN [100] has produced a more elaborate staining procedure using buffered
bromthymolblue which will separate S. mansoni from S. matthei fairly reliably
when mixed populations are on the same paper. The reagents are easy to prepare
but the steps of the procedure are somewhat numerous and should be followed very
carefully as given in the original paper.

RAYBOULD [91, 92] investigated the attractive power of electrodes for S.
haematobium cercariae with negative results, and also confirmed their well known
lack of positive phototaxis. S. mansoni does respond to light however and KLOCK

[53] has designed a complex maze, through which natural waters may be passed, with light to attract cercariae and concentrate them under a stereoscopic microscope. His limited trials showed that it could detect a single cercaria in 5 litres of water and may be of value in the field, though it is large, bulky and fragile. The cercariometer is preferable in clear waters. BOURNS [14] used a much simpler version of the illuminated container, in which cercariae are attracted into a side arm extension of cellophane. The technical innovations are slight, but BOURNS makes the important point that small changes of light intensity may produce positive phototaxis in some species which may be completely missed when more drastic changes are made.

Since *S. haematobium* lives in turbid waters and is non-phototaxic its estimation in natural waters is peculiarly difficult and not solved as yet.

By contrast, the enumeration of cercariae liberated by a snail in a rather small volume of water in the laboratory poses few problems, and has been reviewed recently MACCLELLAND [65]. Often an aliquot from a suspension of live cercariae is needed, and it is fortunate that automatic stirring with a teflon-coated magnet has been shown not to kill or reduce the infectivity of cercariae [96]. The sample for counting is removed with a pipette and the cercariae are killed, with acetic acid [37], Bouin's fluid [1], or heat [63]. GIOVANNOLA [42] added 0.2 parts of 5% alcoholic iodine to the cercariae to kill and stain them, and PELLEGRINO and coworkers [83] used 2% aqueous acetic acid and 5% formalin to which 1 G/litre of methylene blue had been added. MACCLELLAND [63, 65] filtered cercariae through Whatman No. 1 paper and stained with ninhydrin. I have found that staining with methylene blue or cotton blue before filtration is also reasonable.

All these variations are satisfactory. To reduce the number of procedures in use in a laboratory it is most convenient to filter the live or fixed cercariae and stain with ninhydrin (after thermal killing if necessary). LAGRANGE [57] found that very dilute aqueous lucanthone and nile blue sulphate were toxic to cercariae. If the process results in also staining them this might provide an effective pre-filtration procedure for dilute suspensions.

Certain cercariae, as of *Schistosomatium douthitti*, adhere to surfaces and the air-water interface so firmly [76] that a loop is better for sampling the population.

The problems of assessing cercarial production in natural habitats by snails could usefully be attempted, as for miracidia, by enclosing molluscs in lucite cylinders sealed with membrane filters and leaving them in the habitats for 24 hours or so. Cercarial shedding in the laboratory is influenced by pH, light and temperature though their relative importance is uncertain and certainly varies with the parasite species. A diurnal cycle of emergence is present, with forenoon maxima in *S. mansoni* and an evening rise in *S. japonicum* [65, 125]. By forced emergence using artificial light it is possible to obtain large numbers of cercariae on one day followed by a period of low emergence. BAUMAN and coworkers [6] have in fact observed a cycle of three days heavy shedding and three of low output for *S. japonicum* These various observations suggest that it is difficult to simulate reliably in the laboratory the natural rates of output in snails, and that for census purposes emergence over a period of at least several days should be assessed. The way in which cercariae are hoarded by the host and its possible importance in relation to weather changes from day to day in nature have not been investigated.

Census of cercariae awaiting release from albino snails [94] by simple transillumin-ation would elucidate this.

Sampling of cercarial populations has been carried out by exposure of sus-ceptible laboratory animals in East and South Africa [86, 124, 125] Puerto Rico [90], and many other areas. It is an excellent procedure for demonstrating varia-tions in transmission at different times, but has not been used to determine absolute cercarial densities. For this purpose the system would need calibrating with known numbers of cercariae. Since currents have an effect on infection rates, both by bringing more cercariae past the sentinel animals and by reducing cercarial in-fectivity at flow rates in excess of about one metre per second [90] there is not a constant relation in most waters between cercariometrical counts and animal infection results. Since the two procedures measure rather different things they are best used together where possible, to determine the infectivity of a site in terms both of cercariae per unit volume and infection per sampling unit. The develop-ment of a non-living sampling device with some "vertebrate characters" is greatly needed. BOLWIG's [13] work showed that S. haematobium cercariae respond to human sebum in narrow tubes and I have reproduced this effect in a two-dimen-sional system (unpublished work). If the attractant or settling factor [20] can be determined it should be possible to produce a membrane sampler which will allow census of penetrating cercariae separately from the losses occurring during subse-quent development in the host. An alternative approach is considered in the next section.

The actual process of mouse exposure is conveniently carried out in wire gauze cylinders supported upright in annuli of cork some 6″ across and 1″ deep. A group of these can be kept together in a floating wooden frame. Immersion procedures are impossible in rough weather on open water.

ROWAN's [101] suction cercariometer and animal exposure are therefore the methods of choice for cercarial population studies.

E. Attachment and penetration

The enumeration of penetrating cercariae follows naturally from the preceding section. Since attractive membrane systems have not yet been devised, live animals or their skins need to be exposed, in natural waters or laboratory containers. STIREWALT and HACKEY [116] showed that cadaver skin 18 hours post-mortem was penetrated in a similar manner to normal living human skin, but otherwise living vertebrates have been used. Two aspects need discussion: the mode of exposure and the means of assessing numbers of cercariae penetrating.

Numerous means of exposing experimental animals, especially mice, to schisto-some cercariae have been described. It should not be forgotten however that the aim is to estimate the number likely to penetrate human skin, which is far from a homogeneous substance and has not been compared with animal skin except by STIREWALT and HACKEY [116]. The best procedure seems to be to use as stand-ardised a method as possible in the hope that eventually it may be compared with penetration of man. If unphysiological methods, suitable for transmission studies rather than census, be omitted, the main means of exposure are simple partial immersion, tail exposure, and exposure of either the front or back. All have some advantages. WATSON and AZIM [122] maintained that partial immersion was most effective of a series of techniques which they compared. It has the advantage also of being the means used in floating cage exposures. An important demonstration was that clipping of the host fur seems not to affect susceptibility of animals to infection [117]. The tail immersion method of Olivier and STIREWALT [77] gives very reproducible results. Their original method for holding the mice has been followed by an elaborate and almost over-restricting device [115] and a rather more easily made holder [11]. Ether anaesthesia is used for exposing mice by some but not all workers. Exposure of the shaved abdomen [33] or back [79, 80] gives good recovery rates but for census work an easier procedure is preferable. It seems to the writer that for field work partial immersion and for laboratory work tail immersion provide fairly readily standardised census procedures, even though they may not give rise to maximal parasite loads. STIREWALT [114] found that baby mice were more susceptible to cercarial infection than adults and more extensive experiments [87] have confirmed these findings for *S. mansoni*. PURNELL [87] has also shown the importance of host rearing media and exposure water temperature on infection levels. Hardwood shavings used for rearing mice greatly reduced the recovery rate of worms after exposure. All these facts underline the large number of variables needing control if biological means of population census are used. Even if exposures are to be made to large numbers of cercariae in small water volumes, there is much to be said for carrying out this procedure in the natural habitat. The choice of host will depend on schistosome species and though statements such as "hamsters are better hosts of *S. haematobium* than are mice" can be made, comparison with man has not yet been made and in most circumstances he is the relevant standard.

If cercariae are to be identified to species the obvious way of examination is by perfusion of the host when they have matured or somewhat before. If we are interested in the changes in parasite population between penetration and subsequent development this is clearly not helpful. Animals can be exposed to known numbers of cercariae and the residual ones still in the water after exposure counted, to give the penetrating number by subtraction, but this lumps those settling but not penetrating with those actually passing through the epidermis. Another method is needed.

LEWERT and LEE [58] in studies of the mechanism of penetration, found that if mice were injected, intravenously, with 1 ml of 1% saline solution of Evans blue dye per 100 G of mouse, prior to exposure, intensely blue spots appeared at the sites of cercarial penetration. The method has been used in subsequent similar studies [72] and appears reliable. It has not been studied quantitatively but could be perhaps applied in field studies. There would then be no delay between exposure of animals and the results, instead of a gap of several months. The mice could be kept then for subsequent species identification of any penetrating schistosomes. In the experiments published, cercariae penetrated through a limited shaved area on the abdomen. Field exposure would be of a larger area and further work would be needed to define the best procedure. The Evans blue should be injected 15 minutes before exposure. COUTINHO-ABATH [30] has shown that the inflammatory response to penetrating cercariae is greatest in mice fed a high protein diet; mice for the Evans blue method should perhaps be given casein supplements.

F. Developing and Adult Worms

Schistosome worms in the tissues may be observed in squash preparations, dissected out of the mesenteric or other blood vessels, or left to emerge from manually minced tissues incubated in saline. All these procedures are time consuming and rather inefficient in small laboratory animals; in man and the primates they are exceedingly tedious. The alternative is to perfuse the vessels of the abdomen and pelvis in such a way as to wash out all the worms, which are then recovered from the perfusate by sedimentation, dilution-haemolysis or filtration, or any combination of these. Though FAUST and MELENEY [38] perfused some organs of animals to recover schistosomes the first fully described method for perfusion is that of YOLLES and coworkers [127] and subsequent procedures are mostly simplified variants of their methods. They displaced the perfusion medium (0.75% sodium citrate in 0.85% saline) from a large carboy by compressed air and perfused each organ separately after appropriate ligatures had been applied. Later [128] the procedure was extended to other organs. Two main modifications have been subsequently described. PAN and HUNTER [79, 80] simplified the fluid source to a large bottle connected through a tap to a T-piece, to a 100 ml syringe and to a needle hub. The syringe was filled from the reservoir and the tap closed. Perfusion pressure was provided by manually emptying the syringe. They used numerous ligatures and divided the backbone at two sites to leave only the trunk. Undoubtedly the procedure is excellent and extracts almost all worms. However, the authors themselves allow $1-1^{1}/_{2}$ hours per animal and this has limited its applicability. The method of RUIZ [103] is similar.

The other modification is the "Perf-0-Suction" procedure of RADKE and associates [88], fully described in 1961 [89]. The animal is held by plastic clothespins (5 cm size for mice, 7.5 cm for hamsters) arranged at the corners of a rectangle 8 cm by 14 cm on a plastic board. Perfusion is with 0.85% saline delivered via an automatic pipetting machine (Brewer) in 3 ml quantities 21 times each minute. Animals are killed with chloroform. The abdomen is opened and the diaphragm and part of the chest wall excised. The perfusing fluid is introduced into the thoracic aorta through a 23 gauge needle and the hepatic portal vein is cut. Ligatures are not applied to vessels. The perfusing needle passes through the rib cage and is thus held firm. Intermittent periods of perfusion are used at first and later these may be extended. The perfusate is removed through a rubber tube by suction. The tube passes to a receiving vessel consisting of a large separating funnel containing saline. The tube dips under the saline level so that worms pass directly into it and suction is applied through another hole in the stopper. After being allowed to settle, the worms are withdrawn through the separating funnel tap. The procedure was found [89] to extract 98% of S. mansoni from mice and 84.2% of those in hamsters. This method and minor modifications of it seems the most generally useful for census of adult schistosomes. Minor improvements concern anticoagulants, skinning, and alternative pressure sources. The use of 7.5 mg chlorobutanol intraperitoneally in 0.5 ml of water for mice combines host anaesthetic effects with relaxing the parasites [48]. Citrate and heparin may be added to the perfusing fluid to prevent blood clots forming. WILKS (personal communication) has incised the experimental animals' skin circumferentially at diaphragm level and by retracting the skin forwards and backwards over the animal avoids any exposed fur during perfusion, so reducing the chance of losing worms. A hand or motor driven roller pump provides a useful alternative to the Brewer automatic pipette.

The quantitative extraction of schistosome worms from human cadavers is an urgent problem, but has recently been achieved for *S. mansoni* in the portal-mesenteric system of man by CHEEVER (personal communication) who will shortly publish the method.

G. Eggs in tissues

There is an astonishing variety of procedures for extracting schistosome eggs from tissues, particularly the liver, but these have two defects for census work. Firstly, the methods were devised to give a *good yield* of live eggs, for infection and use as antigens, and their authors were not primarily concerned to preserve every egg. Secondly, even where the aim was to count eggs, remarkably few workers have tested their methods for egg destruction and none have compared their counts on digests with those from serial sections.

Three methods will be considered; mild or no digestion, caustic alkali digestion, and sectioning methods.

The mildest form of extraction, only applicable to the unfixed liver, involves practically no digestion at all and yields whole granulomata rather than eggs [81]. The fresh liver is cut into small pieces with removal of vessels, and is homogenized in 150 ml of saline in a Waring blender for 3 minutes, followed by repeated sedimentation in saline. The loss by this procedure has not been determined and must surely be very dependent on the rate of rotation of the homogenizer blades.

Almost every worker who extracts liver eggs from tissue publishes a new method. The main types of procedure are homogenization followed by sedimentation [29, 95] or sieving [44] or both. This may be combined with enzymic digestion using trypsin [9], trypsin and collagenase [105], pepsin [34], trypsin and pepsin [111], pepsin and sodium hydroxide [47, 73], or trypsin followed by filtration [21]. Since none of these methods has been shown to give quantitative extraction, and no one has compared them in detail with each other, it is impossible to recommend one above the others. If the procedure of RITCHIE and BERRIOS-DURAN [11] can be shown to be quantitative, which is doubtful, it has the great virtue of simplicity.

The alternative mode of digestion uses potassium or sodium hydroxide on unfixed tissue (no digestion method is much good for formalin-fixed material). This has been used in numerous autopsy studies on man in Rhodesia [3, 39, 40], summarised and extended by ALVES [2]. It is much to be regretted that these studies did not include attempts to enumerate the numbers of eggs in the various organs. ALVES [2] digested organs in over 10 times their volume of 10% potassium hydroxide at 40° C for at least 48 hours; GELFAND and ROSS [39, 40] incubated at 37% for 24 hours. In one of the few checks on these digestion procedures CHEEVER and WARREN [26], incubating liver in 5% potassium hydroxide at 37° C, after previously freezing the liver, found that egg counts fell by 10% after 24 hours and 60% after 48 hours, though at room temperature counts fell less than 10% in 48 hours. They therefore digested tissue for 4—8 hours only. These observations cast doubt upon the effects of earlier drastic digestions. If live eggs are not needed the method of Cheever and Warren [26] is that of choice for most tissues, though enzymic methods are presumably still more gentle. The eggs may be enumerated either by filtering, staining before or after, and counting, or by directly counting an aliquot in a Sedgewick-Rafter chamber or one of the variety of counting chambers available for agricultural nematology.

When small tissue samples are to be examined, squashes, if thin enough, give good results. It is essential to have plates compressible by wing-nuts, and acrylic resins ("Perspex" or "Lucite") are more readily worked than glass. I have found it convenient to use a perspex plate that screws in place of the mechanical stage slide holder of a microscope (Wild, M20). A grid is engraved on the upper plate.

The use of sections in enumeration of eggs in tissues has been little used, and could be applied more widely. It does not destroy the tissues and is compatible with orthodox histological procedures. Thick sections — 50 or 100 microns — are excellent if combined with selective stains. The sections are best cut after collodion embedding or else on a freezing microtome. General principles have already been discussed. The specific staining of schistosome eggs has become feasible since it was found that S. mansoni egg shells are Ziehl-Nielsen positive in the same manner as tubercle bacilli [60]. It had earlier [112] been shown that methyl green pyronin formed a rather specific trematode egg-shell stain due to reaction with hydroxyphenols. Since these are no longer free after a tanning process has occurred in the egg shells this method is not of great value once the eggs have been laid a while. The PAS — Schiff staining procedure applied to schistosome eggs has been a source of some confusion [52, 64] and is not of use for our purpose. Brygoo and his co-workers have placed the Ziehl-Nielsen procedure on a practical basis [23]. They showed that S. haematobium is Z-N negative [23] and extended this work [24] to use crystal violet and methyl green to colour the egg shell of S. haematobium. Rousset, Houin and Buttner [97] have subsequently recommended modifications of the technique and use saturated aqueous methyl blue as a counterstain. Brygoo and coworkers [24] use Bouin-fixed material sectioned and passed to 70% alcohol saturated with Lithium carbonate for five minutes. Both groups then wash the sections in water and immerse in tenth normal hydrochloric acid for one minute, wash, stain in strong cold carbol fuchsin for 30 minutes, and then wash in 1% acid alcohol to a pale pink colour. Brygoo and associates [24] then wash in water and stain for 10 minutes in methyl green 1% in acetic acid solution before dehydrating mounting. Rousset and coworkers [97] follow the acid alcohol differentiation by mordanting in 1% aqueous phosphomolybdic acid for 5 minutes, stain in saturated aqueous methyl (not methylene) blue for $^1/_2$—2 minutes, wash in water and then through 1% aqueous acetic acid for 5 minutes, 0.1% acetic in absolute alcohol, alcohol and toluene to mount in balsam. They found that the fuchsin remained in S. japonicum, S. mansoni, S. nasalis, and Bilharziella polonica; whilst S. haematobium, S. bovis, S. matthei, S. spindalis, S. indicum and Trichobilharzia ocellata all stained blue. This is at present the method of choice for showing up schistosomes in sections, though in suitably equipped laboratories small fragments of bilharzial material may be detected by the fluorescent antibody technique applied to sections, beautifully demonstrated by Lichtenberg [59].

Digestion and filtration or dilution counting, sections, and squash preparations are all good methods for performing egg counts on some tissues.

IV. Demographic methods

The age-grouping of schistosomes is in some ways far easier than for mammalian populations, because of the wide morphological variations between different stages of the life cycle: egg, miracidium, sporocysts, cercaria, schistosomule, adult worm. Some of these stages are so brief that further sub-division on an age basis is rarely needed, miracidia and cercariae for example, though we may wish to characterise them physiologically as able or unable to penetrate and develop in a host. In the study of intra-host dynamics, age-grouping of eggs and schistosomules is desirable and feasible. For adult worms it is much more needed yet at present impossible.

Eggs have been graded on their developmental state by various workers, most usefully by PELLEGRINO and his co-workers [82, 83] who divided them as follows, Table 2, and in their 1962 paper [83] provided very fine photomicrographs of these stages. They treated infected animals with chemotherapy affecting adult worms only and followed the relative proportions of different stages, the "oogram". Their data are adequate for a rough timescale of development of the egg to be drawn up [83].

The developing schistosomules in experimental animals have been grouped into numerous stages for *S. japonicum* [38] and *S. mansoni* though workers differ on detail. The timing of these stages was recorded in the animals studied, though it is variable with host and parasite species.

The best hope of working with eggs and worms at other stages of precisely known age seems to be dependent on labelling techniques. Various substances may be incorporated into living organisms when they are laid, or at some specific time

Table 2. *Classification of the stages of Schistosoma mansoni eggs; after* PELLEGRINO *et al. [83]*

(a) Eggs		
I. Infertile		
II. Fertile		
A. Viable		
i. Immature.	Stage 1	Embryo $1/_3$ of transverse diameter of egg
	Stage 2	Embryo $1/_2$ of transverse diameter of egg
	Stage 3	Embryo $2/_3$ of length of egg
	Stage 4	Embryo practically fills egg
ii. Mature		With flame cells and cilia active, contracting.
iii. With disturbed embryonic development		
B. Dead		
i. Immature:	semitransparent	Half clear; half dark
	granular	Fatty granules present
	darkened	Entirely black
	with retracted embryo	Clear irregular embryo outline
ii. Mature:	recently dead:	with distintegrating miracidium roughly granulated eggs with retracted miracidium
	calcified	Clear and glassy appearance
(b) Shells		
From hatching		
From miracidial destruction		
(c) Parasitic nodules where egg was.		

subsequently and form labels of greater or less permanence. Tetracycline has been used as a label for filariae [120] but has not been reported as a trematode label as yet. The work of DARKEN [31, 32] on incorporation of fluorescent markers into fungi and bacteria might find application to schistosomes. Radioisotopes have been used as labels [35] but mainly to follow migrations of parasites. However, the writer (in preparation) investigating the hypothesis that adult flukes might take up nucleic acid bases from the host circulation has labelled eggs with radioactive thymidine. The method is tedious but precise as a tool for intra-host dynamic studies. The persistence of labelling in the adult fluke has not yet been determined. Since all stages of schistosomes have no "hard parts" growing by regular secretion of materials, the search for inherent age measures – corresponding to fish scale rings, the annual rings of the Lofoten Island limpets, or otolith layers – is likely to prove disappointing and various forms of age-cohort labelling seem to offer the best hopes of an analytical method. Natural genetic marker chromosomes for adults have not yet been explored.

V. Conclusion

It is seen that very many potential census methods are available, though most have been developed with different aims in mind. Many have been intended to give a "good yield" for purposes of transmission maintenance or antigen preparation, rather than to give either a complete sample or reproducible fraction of the schistosome population. Extraction methods vary but their later steps tend to converge onto either resuspension and subsample counting or filtration. Since the manner of carrying out the technique is at least as important for reproducibility as the choice of method, one of these two should be chosen and used for all stages being counted, if possible. The first step of any study involving census work should be to determine the accuracy of the methods used in that particular situation. For this reason published coefficients of variation of various procedures in the hands of their inventors have been largely omitted from this account. Reasonable methods are now available for most stages, except cercariometry in turbid waters in Africa and the enumeration of miracidia in natural waters other than by snail exposure.

The need for precise census work in *transmission* studies has been made clear by the recent attempts at model systems [45, 66] and has been recognised for some time by workers in the field. There is an equal need for parasite numbers *in the hosts* to be studied rigorously in attempts to understand the pathogenetic and immunological mechanisms in bilharzial infections.

Acknowledgements

The preparation of this account was made possible by World Health Organisation assistance, for which I am most grateful. Dr. N. E. WILKS very kindly read the draft manuscript.

References

[1] ABDEL AZIM, M., and S. G. COWPER: On the maintenance of strains of Schistosoma mansoni, S. haematobium, and S. matthei in the laboratory in Egypt, with special reference to the use of gerbils. Brit. J. Exp. Path. 31, 577—589 (1950).

[2] ALVES, W.: The distribution of Schistosoma eggs in human tissues. Bull. Wld Hlth. Org. 18, 1092—1097 (1958).

[3] — R. W. WOODS, and M. GELFAND: The distribution of bilharzia ova in the male genital tract. Cent. Afr. J. Med. 1, 166—167 (1955).

[4] BARLOW, C. H.: A new method for examining urine for helminth eggs. Amer. J. Hyg. 14, 212—217 (1931).

[5] —, and H. E. MELENEY: A voluntary infection with Schistosoma haematobium. Amer. J. Trop. Med. Hyg. 29, 79—87 (1949).

[6] BAUMAN, P. M., H. J. BENNETT, and J. W. INGALLS: The molluscan intermediate host and schistosomiasis japonica II. Amer. J. Trop. Hyg. Med. 28, 567—575 (1948).

[7] BELL, D. R.: A new method for counting Schistosoma mansoni eggs in faeces. Bull. Wld. Hlth. Org. 29, 525—530 (1963).

[8] — Daily variation in egg output. Ann. Rep. East Afr. Inst. Med. Res. 1962—1963. p. 35, Nairobi, 1963

[9] BÉNEX, J.: Méthode pratique de récolte d'oeufs de schistosomes par digestion enzymatique. Bull. Soc. Path. Exot. 53, 309—314 (1960).

[10] BENNIE, I.: Urinary schistosomiasis. The best time to obtain specimens. The effect of specific therapy on egg output. S. Afr. Med. J. 23, 97—100 (1949).

[11] BERRIOS-DURAN, L. A.: An efficient device for exposing mice to schistosome cercariae and holding small animals for post mortem examination. J. Parasit. 41, 641—642 (1955).

[12] BLAGG, W., E. L. SCHLOEGEL, N. S. MANSOUR, and G. I. KHALAF: A new concentration technic for the demonstration of protozoa and helminth eggs in faeces. Amer. J. Trop. Med. Hyg. 4, 23—28 (1955).

[13] BOLWIG, N.: An experimental study of the behaviour and host-recognition in Schistosoma cercariae. S. Afr. J. Sci. 51, 338—344 (1955).

[14] BOURNS, T. K. R.: A method for collecting cercariae. J. Parasit. 49, 370 (1963).

[15] BRACKETT, S.: Studies on schistosome dermatitis VI. Notes on the behaviour of schistosome cercariae. Amer. J. Hyg. 31 D, 64—73 (1940).

[16] BRADLEY, D. J.: Standardization of egg counting techniques. Ann. Rep. East Afr. Inst. Med. Res. 1961—1962 p. 31—33, Nairobi 1962.

[17] — A quantitative approach to bilharzia. E. Afr. Med. J. 40, 240—249 (1963).

[18] — A simple and rapid method for counting schistosome eggs in urine. Trans. Roy. Soc. Trop. Med. Hyg. 58, 291 (1964).

[19] — The analysis of larval forms in the trematoda and marine bottom invertebrates. In: Science and Medicine in Central Africa, pp. 343—350. G. J. SNOWBALL. (Ed.) Oxford: Pergamon 1965.

[20] — The measurement of bilharzial prevalence and egg output — aims and techniques, with an account of a field method. Bull. Wld Hlth. Org. (in press).

[21] BROWNE, H. G., and J. I. THOMAS: A method for isolating pure, viable schistosome eggs from host tissues. J. Parasit. 49, 371—374 (1963).

[22] — — A filter counting technique for helminth eggs. Exp. Parasit. 15, 485—490 (1964).

[23] BRYGOO, E. R., A. CAPRON, and J. C. RANDRIAMALALA: Sur quelques méthodes de coloration sélective des coques d'oeufs d'helminthes parasites de l'homme. Bull. Soc. Path. Exot. 52, 655—664 (1959).

[24] — and J. C. RANDRIAMALALA: Difference de colorabilité au Ziehl entre les oeufs de Schistosoma mansoni et ceux de Schistosoma haematobium. Bull. Soc. Path. Exot. 52, 26 (1959).

[25] CHAIA, G.: Technica para concentracão de miracidios. Rev. Bras. Malar. 8, 355—357 (1956).

[26] CHEEVER, A. W., and K. S. WARREN: Hepatic blood flow in mice with acute hepatosplenic schistosomiasis mansoni. Trans. Roy. Soc. Trop. Med. Hyg. 58, 406—412 (1964).

[27] CHERNIN, E., and C. A. DUNAVAN: The influence of host-parasite dispersion upon the capacity of Schistosoma mansoni miracidia to infect Australorbis glabratus. Amer. J. Trop. Med. Hyg. 11, 455—471 (1962).

[28] CHESTERMAN, W., and E. H. LEACH: Low viscosity nitrocellulose for embedding tissues. Quart. J. Micr. Sci. 90, 431—434 (1949).

[29] COKER, C. M., and F. LICHTENBERG: A revised method for isolation of Schistosoma mansoni eggs for biological experimentation. Proc. Soc. Exp. Biol. 92, 780—782 (1956).

[30] COUTINHO-ABATH, E.: Influence of protein uptake on the penetration of cercariae of Schistosoma mansoni in the skin of normal and experimentally infected mice. Rev. Inst. Med. Trop. S. Paulo **4**, 230—241 (1962).

[31] DARKEN, M. A.: Natural and induced fluorescence in microscopic organisms. Appl. Microbiol. **9**, 354—360 (1961).

[32] — Absorption and transport of fluorescent brighteners by microorganisms. Appl. Microbiol. **10**, 387—393 (1962).

[33] DEWAARD, F., and N. E. H. VERMEULEN: Penetration of the mammalian skin by cercariae of Schistosoma mansoni. Trop. Geogr. Med. **13**, 82—88 (1961).

[34] DEWITT, W. B., and K. S. WARREN: Hepato-splenic schistosomiasis in mice. Amer. J. Trop. Med. Hyg. **8**, 440—446 (1959).

[35] DISSANAIKE, A. S.: The use of radioisotopes in the study of helminth life cycles. In Radioisotopes in Tropical Medicine. International Atomic Energy Agency, Vienna 1962.

[36] FARID, Z., J. W. GREER, K. G. ISHAK, A. M. EL NAGAH, P. C. LE GOLVAN, and A. H. MOUSA: Chronic pulmonary schistosomiasis. Amer. Rev. Tuberc. **79**, 119—133 (1959).

[37] FAUST, E. C., and W. A. HOFFMAN: Studies on schistosomiasis mansoni in Puerto Rico III. Biological studies. 1. The extra-mammalian phases of the life cycle. Puerto Rico J. Publ. Hlth. **10**, 1—47 (1934).

[38] —, and H. E. MELENY: Studies on schistosomiasis japonica. Amer. J. Hyg. Monogr. Ser. 3, 1—339 (1924).

[39] GELFAND, M., and W. F. ROSS: The distribution of schistosome ova in the alimentary tract in subjects of bilharziasis. Trans. Roy. Soc. Trop. Med. Hyg. **47**, 215—217 (1953).

[40] — — The distribution of schistosome ova in the genitourinary tract in subjects of bilharziasis. Trans. Roy. Soc. Trop. Med. Hyg. **47**, 218—220 (1953).

[41] GERRITSEN, T., A. R. P. WALKER, B. DE MEILLON, and R. M. YEO: Long term investigations of blood loss and egg load in urinary schistosomiasis in the adult African Bantu. Trans. Roy. Soc. Trop. Med. Hyg. **47**, 134—140 (1953).

[42] GIOVANNOLA, A.: Some observations on the emission of cercariae of Schistosoma mansoni (Trematoda; Schistosomatidae) from Australorbis glabratus. Proc. Helminth. Soc. Wash. **3**, 60—61 (1936).

[43] GOVE, R. B.: The distribution of the eggs of Schistosoma haematobium in the urinary system. Trans. Roy. Soc. Trop. Med. Hyg. **56**, 74—76 (1962).

[44] GRIFFITHS, R. B., and W. N. BEESLEY: A technique for the collection of large numbers of Schistosoma mansoni ova. Trans. Roy. Soc. Trop. Med. Hyg. **49**, 301 (1955).

[45] HAIRSTON, N. G.: Population ecology and epidemiological problems. In: CIBA Foundation Symposium, Bilharziasis, pp. 36—62. G. E. W. WOLSTENHOLME, and M. O'CONNOR. (Eds.) London: Churchill 1962.

[46] — B. HUBENDICK, J. M. WATSON, and L. J. OLIVIER: An evaluation of techniques used in estimating snail populations. Bull. Wld Hlth. Org. **19**, 661—672 (1958).

[47] HSU, H. F., and S. Y. L. HSU: Distribution of eggs of different geographic strains of Schistosoma japonicum. Amer. J. Trop. Med. Hyg. **9**, 240—247 (1960).

[48] HUNTER, G. W.: The use of anticoagulants and chlorobutanol for the recovery of adult schistosomes from mice. J. Parasit. **46**, 206 (1960).

[49] INGALLS, J. W., G. W. HUNTER, D. B. McMULLEN, and P. M. BAUMAN: Molluscan intermediate host and schistosomiasis japonica 1. Observations on the conditions governing hatching of eggs of Schistosoma japonicum. J. Parasit. **35**, 147—151 (1949).

[50] ITO, J.: Studies on hatchability of Schistosoma japonicum eggs in several external environmental conditions. Jap. J. Med. Sci. Biol. **8**, 175—184 (1955).

[51] JORDAN, P.: Periodicity of ova output and intensity of infection (S. haematobium). Ann. Rep. East Afr. Inst. Med. Res. 1959—1960: p. 25. Nairobi 1960.

[52] KATZ, F. F., and G. M. CARRERA: The reaction of Schistosoma mansoni egg shells to periodic acid-Schiff staining procedure. J. Parasit. **43**, 24 (1957).

[53] KLOCK, J. W.: A method for the direct quantitative recovery of Schistosoma mansoni cercariae from natural waters of Puerto Rico. Bull. Wld Hlth. Org. **25**, 738—740 (1961).

[54] KLOTZEL, K.: Splenomegaly in schistosomiasis mansoni. Amer. J. Trop. Med. Hyg. **11**, 472—476 (1962).

[55] — Some quantitative aspects of diagnosis and epidemiology in schistosomiasis mansoni. Amer. J. Trop. Med. Hyg. **12**, 334—337 (1963).

[56] KUNTZ, R. E.: Passage of eggs by hosts infected with Schistosoma mansoni, with emphasis on rodents. J. Parasit. **47**, 905—909 (1961).
[57] LAGRANGE, E.: Une méthode simple d'essai des anti-bilharziens in vitro. C. R. Soc. Biol. **154**, 1498—1499 (1960).
[58] LEWERT, R. M., and C. L. LEE: Studies on the passage of helminth larvae through host tissues. J. Infect. Dis. **95**, 13—51 (1954).
[59] LICHTENBERG, F. v.: Studies in granuloma formation. III. Antigen sequestration and destruction in the schistosome pseudotubercle. Amer. J. Path. **45**, 75—93 (1964).
[60] LICHTENBERG, F., and M. LINDENBERG: An alcohol-acid-fast substance in eggs of Schistosoma mansoni. Amer. J. Trop. Med. Hyg. **3**, 1066—1076 (1954).
[61] LILLIE, R. D.: Reactions of various parasitic organisms in tissues to the Baur, Feulgen, Gram, and Gram-Weigert methods. J. Lab. Clin. Med. **32**, 76—88 (1947).
[62] McCAULEY, J. E.: A new method for examining snails for trematode parasites. J. Parasit. **44**, 243—244 (1958).
[63] McCLELLAND, W. F. J.: Production of cercariae. Ann. Rep. East Afr. Inst. Med. Res. 1960—1961: p. 12, Nairobi 1961.
[64] — Intermediate host-parasite relationships. Ann. Rep. East Afr. Inst. Med. Res. 1962 to 1963: p. 17—18, Nairobi 1963.
[65] — The production of cercariae by Schistosoma mansoni and S. haematobium and methods for estimating the numbers of cercariae in suspension. Bull. Wld Hlth. Org. **33**, 270—276 (1965).
[66] MACDONALD, G.: The dynamics of helminth infections with special reference to schistosomes. Trans. Roy. Soc. Trop. Med. Hyg. **59**, 489—506 (1965).
[67] McMULLEN, D. B., and P. C. BEAVER: Studies on schistosome dermatitis IX. Amer. J. Hyg. **42**, 128—154 (1945).
[68] MAGATH, T. B., and D. R. MATHIESON: Factors affecting the hatching of ova of Schistosoma japonicum. J. Parasit. **32**, 64—68 (1946).
[69] MALDONADO, J. F., and J. ACOSTA-MATIENZO: A comparison of fecal examination procedures in the diagnosis of schistosomiasis mansoni. Exp. Parasit. **2**, 294—310 (1953).
[70] — —, and J. THILLIET: Biological studies on the miracidium of Schistosoma mansoni. Part 2. Behaviour of unhatched miracidium in undiluted stools under diverse environmental conditions. Puerto Rico J. Publ. Hlth. **25**, 153—174 (1949).
[71] — —, and F. VELEZ-HERRERA: Ibid. Part 4. The role of pH in hatching and longevity. Puerto Rico J. Publ. Hlth. **26**, 85—91 (1950).
[72] MILLEMANN, R. E., and S. E. MERGENHAGEN: Studies on the penetration of schistosome cercariae. I. Action of the antihistamine promethazine hydrochloride. J. Parasit. **46**, 155—163 (1960).
[73] MOORE, D. V., and J. H. SANDGROUND: The relative egg producing capacity of Schistosoma mansoni and Schistosoma japonicum. Amer. J. Trop. Med. Hyg. **5**, 831—840 (1956).
[74] NEWSOME, J.: Investigation of anti-schistosome opsonins in vivo. Trans. Roy. Soc. Trop. Med. Hyg. **58**, 58—62 (1964).
[75] OLIVER-GONZALEZ, J., and F. HERNANDEZ-MORALES: Quantitative determination of Schistosoma mansoni ova in feces from patients under treatment with antimonial drugs. Puerto Rico J. Publ. Hlth. **22**, 210—216 (1946).
[76] OLIVER, L.: A comparison of infections in mice with three species of schistosomes, Schistosoma mansoni, Schistosoma japonicum and Schistosomatium douthitti. Amer. J. Hyg. **55**, 22—35 (1952).
[77] —, and M. A. STIREWALT: An efficient method for exposure of mice to cercariae of Schistosoma mansoni. J. Parasit. **38**, 19—23 (1952).
[78] ONORI, E.: Observations on variations in Schistosoma haematobium egg output, and on the relationship between the average egg output of infected persons and the prevalence of infection in a community. Ann. Trop. Med. Parasit. **56**, 292—296 (1962).
[79] PAN, C. T., and G. W. HUNTER III.: A modified perfusion technique for the recovery of schistosomes. J. Lab. Clin. Med. **37**, 815—816 (1951).
[80] PAN, C. T., E. H. KAUFMAN, and G. W. HUNTER III.: A technique for infecting small mammals with Schistosoma japonicum. J. Lab. Clin. Med. **37**, 817—819 (1951).

[81] Pellegrino, J., and Z. Brener: Method for isolating schistosome granulomas from mouse liver. J. Parasit. **42**, 564 (1956).

[82] — C. A. Oliviera, and J. Faria: The oögram in the study of relapse in experimental chemotherapy of schistosomiasis mansoni. J. Parasit. **49**, 365—370 (1963).

[83] — — —, and A. S. Cunha: New approach to the screening of drugs in experimental Schistosoma mansoni in mice. Amer. J. Trop. Med. Hyg. **11**, 201—215 (1962).

[84] Pesigan, T. P., M. Farooq, N. G. Hairston, J. J. Jauregui, E. G. Garcia, A. T. Santos, B. C. Santos, and A. A. Besa: Studies on Schistosoma japonicum infection in the Philippines. I. General considerations and epidemiology. Bull. Wld Hlth. Org. **18**, 345—455 (1958).

[85] — N. G. Hairston, J. J. Jauregui, E. G. Garcia, A. T. Santos, B. C. Santos, and A. A. Besa: Ibid. 2. The molluscan host. Bull. Wld Hlth. Org. **18**, 481—578 (1958).

[86] Pitchford, R. J., and P. S. Visser: Results of exposing mice to schistosomiasis by immersion in natural water. Trans. Roy. Soc. Trop. Med. Hyg. **56**, 294—301 (1962).

[87] Purnell, R.: Vertebrate host-parasite relationships. Ann. Rep. East Afr. Inst. Med. Res. 1963—1964: p. 20—23, Nairobi 1965.

[88] Radke, M. G., L. A. Berrios-Duran, and K. Moran: A perfusion procedure (Perf-0-Suction) for recovery of schistosome worms. J. Parasit. **43**, Suppl. 26—27 (1957).

[89] — — — A perfusion procedure (Perf-0-Suction) for recovery of schistosome worms. J. Parasit. **47**, 366—368 (1961).

[90] — L. S. Ritchie, and W. B. Rowan: Effects of water velocities on worm burdens of animals exposed to Schistosoma mansoni cercariae released under field and laboratory conditions. Exper. Parasit. **11**, 323—331 (1961).

[91] Raybould, J. N.: A method for the detection of schistosome cercariae in natural waters. Ann. Rep. East Afr. Inst. Malaria and Vector-borne Diseases 1960—1961: 23—24, 1961.

[92] — A method for the detection of schistosome cercariae in natural waters. Ann. Rep. East Afr. Inst. Malaria and Vector-borne Diseases 1961—1962: 23, 1962.

[93] — Difficulties in the detection of Schistosoma haematobium cercariae in natural waters. Ann. Rep. East Afr. Inst. Malaria and Vector-borne Diseases 1962—1963: 20, 1963.

[94] Richards, C. S.: Emergence of cercariae of Schistosoma mansoni from Australorbis glabratus. J. Parasit. **47**, 428 (1961).

[95] Ritchie, L. W., and L. A. Berrios-Duran: A simple procedure for recovering schistosome eggs in mass from tissues. J. Parasit. **47**, 363—365 (1961).

[96] Ritchie, L. S., S. Garson., and W. B. Knight: The biology of Schistosoma mansoni in laboratory rats. J. Parasit. **49**, 571—577 (1963).

[97] Rousset, J. J., R. Houin, and A. Buttner: Acido-alcoolo-resistance de divers oeufs de schistosomes. Modification de la technique de Brygoo, Capron et Randriamalala. Ann. Parasit. Hum. Comp. **37**, 866—869 (1962).

[98] Rowan, W. B.: A simple device for determining population density of Schistosoma mansoni cercariae in infected waters. J. Parasit. **43**, 696—697 (1957).

[99] — Daily periodicity of Schistosoma mansoni cercariae in Puerto Rican waters. Amer. J. Trop. Med. Hyg. **7**, 374—381 (1958).

[100] — A quantitative field technique for differentiating South African Schistosoma matthei cercariae from those of S. mansoni. J. Parasit. **47**, 406 (1961).

[101] — The ecology of schistosome transmission foci. Bull. Wld Hlth. Org. **33**, 63—71 (1965).

[102] —, and A. L. Gram: Quantitative recovery of helminth eggs from relatively large samples of feces and sewage. J. Parasit. **45**, 615—621 (1959).

[103] Ruiz, J. M.: Processo rapido de perfusão do sistema porta de mamiferos para coleta de equistossomatideos, aplicavel aos trabalhos de campo. Mem. Inst. Butantan **25**, 29—33 (1953).

[104] Sapero, J. J., and D. K. Lawless: The "M.I.F." stain preservation technique for the identification of intestinal protozoa. Amer. J. Trop. Med. Hyg. **2**, 613—619 (1953).

[105] Scorza, J. V.: Eine neue Methode zur Isolierung von Schistosoma japonicum Eiern durch Enzyme. Z. Tropenmed. Parasit. **12**, 196—207 (1961).

[106] Scott, J. A.: Dilution egg counting in comparison with other methods for determining the incidence of Schistosoma mansoni. Amer. J. Hyg. **25**, 546—565 (1937).

[107] Scott J. A.: The incidence and distribution of the human schistosomes in Egypt. Amer. J. Hyg. 25, 566—614 (1937).

[108] — The regularity of egg output of helminth infestation with special reference to Schistosoma mansoni. Amer. J. Hyg. 27, 155—175 (1938).

[109] — Egg counts as estimates of intensity of infection with Schistosoma haematobium. Tex. Rep. Biol. Med. 15, 425—430 (1957).

[110] Sloane, J. F., and J. E. Harris: A twin-knife microtome attachment. Quart. J. Micr. Sci. Ser. 3, 92, 347—350 (1951).

[111] Smithers, S. R.: The isolation of viable schistosome eggs by a digeston technique. Trans. Roy. Soc. Trop. Med. Hyg. 54, 68—70 (1960).

[112] Smyth, J. D.: Specific staining of egg shell material in trematodes and cestodes. Stain Technol. 26, 255—256 (1951).

[113] Stimmel, C. M., and J. A. Scott: The regularity of egg output of Schistosoma haematobium. Tex. Rep. Biol. Med. 14, 440—458 (1956).

[114] Stirewalt, M. A.: Effects of age of the host on mouse infections with Schistosoma mansoni with especial reference to cercarial penetration. J. Parasit. 38, Suppl. 34 (1952).

[115] —, and J. F. Bronson: Description of a plastic mouse restraining cage. J. Parasit. 41, 328 (1955).

[116] —, and J. R. Hackey: Penetration of hosts kin by cercariae of Schistosoma mansoni. 1. Observed entry into skin of mouse, hamster, monkey and man. J. Parasit. 42, 565—580 (1956).

[117] — R. E. Kuntz, and A. S. Evans: The relative susceptibilities of the commonly used laboratory animals to infection by Schistosoma mansoni. Amer. J. Trop. Med. 31, 57—82 (1951).

[118] Stoll, N. R., and W. C. Hausheer: Concerning two options in dilution egg counting: small drop and displacement. Amer. J. Hyg. 6. March. Suppl. 134—145. (1926).

[119] Sturrock, R. F.: Hookworm studies. Ann. Rep. East Afr. Inst. Med. Res. 1961—1962: 36, Nairobi 1962.

[120] Tobie, J. E., and H. K. Beye: Fluorescence of tetracyclines in filarial worms. Proc. Soc. Exp. Biol. Med. 104, 137—140 (1960).

[121] Vercammen-Grandjean, P. H.: Sur la chaetotaxie de la larve infestante de Schistosoma mansoni. Ann. Parasit. Hum. Comp. 26, 412—414 (1951).

[122] Watson, J. M., and M. A. Azim: Comparative efficiency of various methods of infecting mice with Schistosoma mansoni. Ann. Trop. Med. Parasit. 43, 41—46 (1949).

[123] Watts, N. P., and G. A. Boyd: Schistosoma mansoni miracidium under phase contrast microscopy. Stain Technol. 25, 157—160 (1950).

[124] Webbe, G.: Population studies of intermediate hosts in relation to transmission of bilharziasis in East Africa. In: CIBA Foundation Symposium Bilharziasis, pp. 7—22. G. E. W. Wolstenholme and M. O'Connor. (Eds.) London: Churchill 1962.

[125] — Transmission of bilharziasis. 2. Production of cercariae. Bull. Wld Hlth. Org. 33, 155—162 (1965).

[126] World Health Organization. Snail control in the prevention of bilharziasis. Geneva 1965.

[127] Yolles, T. K., D. V. Moore, D. L. DeGiusti, C. A. Ripsom, and H. E. Meleney: A technique for the perfusion of laboratory animals for the recovery of schistosomes. J. Parasit. 33, 419—426 (1947).

[128] — —, and H. E. Meleney: Post-cercarial development of Schistosoma mansoni in the rabbit and hamster after intraperitoneal and percutaneous infection. J. Parasit. 35, 276—294 (1949).

The addresses of firms referred to in the text, are:

Millipore Filter Corporation, Bedford, Mass. 07130, USA
Griffin and George, Ealing Road, Alpenton, Wembley Middlesex, England
Henry Simon Ltd., Cheadle Heath, Stockport, England
A & S Thomas, West Washington Square, Philadelphia, Pennsylvania 19105, USA
Fisons Scientific Apparatus Ltd., Loughborough, Leicestershire, England
Whatman Filters, H. Reeve Angel and Company Ltd., 9 Bridewell Place, London, EC 4, England
S & S Filters, Carl Schleicher and Schull, Dassel-Kreis, Einbeck, West Germany

A Comparison of Techniques for the Recovery of Schistosome Eggs in Autopsy Material

S. Brumdutt Bhagwandeen* and R. Elsdon-Dew**

During an assessment of the incidence of Bilharziasis in the Durban area, the material from 900 autopsies was examined for ova by three different techniques. This note gives a comparison of the results.

Materials and methods

The bladder and rectum were removed from Indian and African cadavers of the age group 2–65 years. Of these 700 were routine hospital examinations and the remainder medico legal autopsies.

1. Direct Snip method

Fresh snips of material from bladder and rectal mucosa were crushed between two microscope slides.

2. Histology

The same cases were examined by the paraffin techniques sections being cut at 6 μ and stained by H and E.

3. Digestion

Twenty grams each of the remainder of the bladder and of the rectum were digested overnight in 10% caustic potash at 60° C and the centrifuged deposit examined.

Results

Though digestion gave the highest proportion (Table 1), this was not significantly greater than that obtained by the simpler "snip" method. Digestion however permits quantitative estimation. Either method permits identification of the species of ovum, which is not always possible on histology. Table 2 gives the species incidence encountered by the two methods.

Thus, except possibly for S. *mattheei* there is, despite the difference in size of sample, but little to choose between the two methods. The size of the sample

Table 1. *Incidence of bilharziasis as determined by three different methods in 900 autopsies*

Method	No.	Bladder % + ve.	No.	Rectum % + ve.	No.	Composite % + ve.
Snip	217	24	165	18	268	30
Histology	185	21	98	11	211	23
Digestion	237	26	178	20	277	31

* Department of Pathology, University of Natal. Durban, South Africa
** Amoebiasis Research Unit, Institute for Parasitology, Durban, South Africa. The Institute for Parasitology is sponsored by the following bodies: The South African Council for Scientific and Industrial Research. The University of Natal. The Natal Provincial Administration. The United States Public Health Service (Grant Al 01592).

Table 2. *Incidence of various schistosome species as determined by two methods in 900 autopsies*

Species	No.	Snip % + ve.	No.	Digestion % + ve.
S. *haematobium* only	231	26	249	28
S. *mansoni* only	37	4	28	3
S. *haematobium* and S. *mansoni*	21	2	30	3
S. *mattheei* [always associated)	7	1	20	2
All positives	248	30	277	31

Table 3. *Egg load on tissue digestion in 900 autopsies*

Eggs per gm	Bladder S. *haematobium*	Rectum S. *haematobium*	S. *mansoni*	*Mixed*
10^6	1	—	—	—
10^5—10^6	10	—	—	—
10^4—10^5	87	5	2	5
10^3—10^4	86	19	1	7
10^2—10^3	48	65	20	8
10—10^2	19	17	8	4
1—10	14	15	3	1
Total	235 +	121	34	25

examined at histology (of the order of 5 mgm.) probably accounts for the relatively poor return given by histology, which does however reveal the nature of the lesion.

As a matter of interest the quantitative results are shown in Table 3.

An additional case with pure S. *mansoni* infection of the bladder was seen. S. *mattheei* was encountered in eleven cases in the bladder and in 9 in the rectum always in association with other species.

The comparatively low loads of S. *mansoni* encountered in Durban will be noted.

Summary and conclusions

Though all three techniques have their place in the survey of autopsy material for bilharziasis the relative simplicity of "snip" makes it the method of choice where quantitative methods are not required.

Acknowledgements. The authors have to thank, Dr. T. M. ADNAMS, Superintendent and Dr. R. M. A. NUPEN acting medical superintendent of King Edward VIII Hospital for facilities and Prof. J. WAINWRIGHT, Head of the Department of Pathology, University of Natal for advice and criticism.

This work was partly financed by a generous grant to one of us (S.B.B.) by Roshe Products.

Summary and Conclusions
The need for research in Bilharziasis

F. K. Mostofi*

In the opening chapter I have discussed the problems of evaluating the disability resulting from bilharzial infection. In the ensuing chapters my distinguished colleagues have reviewed the life cycle, the diagnosis, the clinical, pathological, radiological, immunological and experimental aspects of bilharziasis. I would like now to summarize the clinicopathological aspects and to emphasize the need for research.

A. Stage of cercarial invasion

In the stage of cercarial invasion when penetration and migration occur, the natives in an endemic area may manifest no symptoms but the new visitor may show dermatitis which may be quite severe after reinfection. The type, the severity, the time of onset of clinical symptoms, and the pathological changes are thus dependent on the experience of the host. If this is an initial infection, little local reaction may be encountered. If it is a reinfection or if the patient has been previously sensitized, in addition to the local reaction, there may be serious systemic manifestations.

It is of interest to note that if the host and the parasite are not compatible, as occurs in accidental penetration of the skin by nonpathogenic species, a local reaction is produced with congestion, cellular infiltration with polymorphonuclear leukocytes, eosinophils, lymphocytes, and plasma cells resulting in local destruction of the cercariae.

Respiratory symptoms — cough, bloody sputum, and even asthmatic attacks — are occasionally observed at this stage, attributed to the passage of cercariae through the pulmonary capillaries. Toxic manifestations, rarely observed in people living in endemic areas, may be encountered in 15 to 25 days. These consist of fever, abdominal pain, and diarrhea. The migration of cercariae may also result in reaction in other organs with little or no clinical symptoms. If the schistosomulae become impacted, there is thrombosis and its sequelae, otherwise little is known of the reaction of tissue to the living organism.

Study of the clinical and pathological findings at this stage, especially among children, is extremely important, for as Bogliolo [v. s.][1] has said, the host response is already qualitatively and quantitatively established in this phase.

B. Stage of maturation

Wright [v. s.] has discussed the life cycle in detail. The period of maturation and oviposition varies depending on the species of the parasite. The exact period

---

* Armed Forces Institute of Pathology, Washington, D. C. 20305 U.S.A.
[1] The references in this chapter are, for the most part, to the other chapters in the monograph. In such cases, v. s. (vide supra) is used to denote the reference.

is unknown for S. hematobium but it is suspected to be 8 to 12 weeks after invasion. For S. Mansoni it is 30 to 35 days and for S. Japonicum, 25 to 28 days. The completion of maturation and early oviposition is difficult to recognize clinically. There may be no symptoms, the symptoms may be mild, or they may be severe and toxic, depending on the intensity of the infection and the severity of immunological response. Anorexia, nausea, vomiting, diarrhea, abdominal colic, headache, backache, generalized malaise, marked eosinophilia, and alterations in plasma proteins with increase in the alpha 2 globulins and in the gamma globulin have been observed.

ANDRADE and CHEEVER [v. s.] have reported granulomas with central areas of necrosis and eosinophilic infiltration scattered over the intestinal serosa, liver, and lungs and small superficial ulcers in the intestines (small and large). Both of these authors and BOGLIOLO [v. s.], who has examined liver biopsies in 2 or 3 patients, have observed intense hepatitis without any apparent relationship to schistosomulae. The spleen may be enlarged, probably secondary to reticuloendothelial hyperplasia on an immunological basis. The complement fixation reaction, the fluorescent antibody and the intradermal reactions become positive about the third, sixth, and ninth weeks, respectively. The pathology and the pathogenesis of the lesions produced at this stage in man remain to be studied.

C. Stage of established infection

The majority of investigators consider massive oviposition, accompanied by a corresponding egg excretion as the basic cause of the symptoms, signs, and the pathological processes. Oviposition and the appearance of clinical manifestations occur earliest in S. Japonicum and latest in S. hematobium. The severity of symptoms varies considerably with the species, the race, and sex of the schistosome; the number, frequency, and severity of exposures; the load of infection, the nutritional state, race, immunity and resistance of the patient. There may be no signs or symptoms. Headache, backache, generalized aches, pains, anorexia, nausea, vomiting, diarrhea, hematuria, burning on urination, cough, bloody sputum, and hepatosplenomegaly may be mild or severe.

Despite the variable manifestations, the stage is heralded by the excretion of eggs in the urine (S. hematobium) and feces (S. hematobium, S. Mansoni and S. Japonicum).

The diagnosis of bilharziasis, in its acute or chronic stage, is dependent on clinical and laboratory findings. Since the clinical picture is not clearly defined, we must depend on laboratory diagnosis. SADUN [v. s.] has summarized the efforts in developing cutaneous and serological tests (complement fixation, serum flocculation, plasma card test, fluorescent antibody reaction and others) for rapid and reliable diagnosis. He has emphasized that as yet no suitable tests exist for the detection of early infection and of chemotherapeutic cures. JORDAN and BRADLEY [v. s.] have emphasized the importance of demonstration of ova in urine and feces and its variable reliability in providing accurate data on the presence, prevalence, and intensity of infection.

In the stage of established infection, bilharziasis may be mild and/or asymptomatic, manifested only by the excretion of ova in urine or stools, by a strong skin reaction to the injected schistosome antigens, or by the finding of histological evidence of infection especially in the urinary tract, the intestine or the liver. The economic significance of such subclinical infection is unkown.

In the symptomatic phase, bilharziasis may involve any organ with serious consequences to the individual patient. However, there are four organ systems which are most frequently involved and in which the disability may assume epidemic proportions.

1. *Urogenital manifestations.* Although urinary bilharziasis has been known from time immemorial, FAIRLEY [2] first recorded the symptoms: in 60% the earliest symptom was urethral pain on micturition; in the other 40% the pain was deep seated or perineal, associated with aching in the loins and frequency. About 4 weeks after the commencement of pain a terminal hematuria is noted.

MAKAR, GELFAND, FORSYTH, ELWI, ISHAK, GAZAYERLI, EDINGTON, and PAYET and CAMAIN [v. s.] have described the clinical and pathological findings in the urogenital tract. Of the three species, S. hematobium is the only one that is involved, and in man the urogenital system constitutes the principal site of involvement with S. hematobium. The chief clinical symptoms are proteinuria and occasionally dysuria and terminal hematuria. In the earliest stages the bladder mucosa shows congestion and edema and there may be superficial thin-walled ulcers. The migration of the eggs in the vesical wall results in a foreign body granulomatous reaction with eosinophils, macrophages, multinucleated giant cells, lymphocytes, and plasma cells. Cystoscopically, these appear as pinpoint shiny tubercles surrounded by a fine network of capillaries. These are most commonly encountered at the base, the trigone at the ureteral orifices, the lateral walls, and the dome. Conglomerations of these tubercles form bilharzial nodules. The older granulomas are replaced by fibrosis.

As MAKAR, ELWI, GELFAND, and MIDDLEMISS [v. s.] have discussed, the specific lesion of the bilharzial bladder is the calcifications of the bladder wall. Visible through the thin atrophic vesical mucosa as sandy patches and readily demonstrable by x-ray, the process represents calcification of the large numbers of eggs deposited in the wall. Secondary infection and extensive ulceration are further manifestations of the vesical response.

The early reversible changes of inflammatory reaction, tiny ulcers, and granulomas lead to the irreversible changes of fibrosis, calcification, and extensive ulceration. However, the mechanism which determines the extent and magnitude of fibrosis and calcification and the role of infection or ova in the development of calcification are not clearly understood.

It is of interest to note, as GELFAND, MAKAR, and FORSYTH [v. s.] have pointed out, that in many cases the bladder capacity is not reduced or, in fact, altered in any way. In spite of the gross fibrosis and calcification, no changes in function are detectable and there are no signs or symptoms. MAKAR and ELWI [v. s.] have called attention to the involvement of the bladder neck, prostate, and seminal vesicles resulting in obstruction and later hydronephrosis. On the other hand, neither in Egypt nor in Rhodesia is there universal agreement on the existence and significance of vesical neck involvement.

In addition to these reactions the vesical mucosa may respond by hyperplasia, proliferation, and "metaplasia".

Overgrowth of the granulation and the fibroadipose tissue of the lamina propria results in "vesical bilharziomata" or "bilharzial polyp," and proliferation of the epithelium leads to the formation of Brunn's nests, and cystitis cystica and glandularis. In addition, the mucosa frequently shows squamous change. Glandular and mucous "metaplasia" may also be seen, but rarely.

MAKAR, GELFAND, GAZAYERLI, ELWI, and ISHAK [v. s.] have discussed the relationship of bilharziasis to cancer of the bladder. Suffice it to say that in Egypt, Rhodesia, and Lourenco Marques there is a high incidence of cancer of bladder and since there is also an associated high incidence of vesical bilharziasis, the two are believed by many to be related to each other. Indeed, these investigators consider the relationship as highly probable. Yet, as GELFAND, ELSDON-DEW, EDINGTON, and PAYET and CAMAIN [v. s.] have pointed out, in certain parts of the Middle East, in South and in West Africa, the incidence of cancer of the bladder is quite low and appears to be unrelated to bilharziasis. Even in Egypt, Rhodesia, and Lourenco Marques there have been no systematic epidemiological studies to determine if in fact it is infection with bilharziasis or some other factor that is responsible for the development of bladder cancer.

The majority of severe lesions of the ureter occur in the intramural and lower segments of the ureter with resultant stricture and stenosis. Dilatation of the ureter and ureterovesical incompetence are frequently observed in Egypt, East Africa, and Rhodesia but the pathological basis for the change is unknown, and it is not known whether these lesions also occur in other geographie areas.

According to GELFAND [v. s.] over 30% of patients in Rhodesia affected with vesical bilharziasis showed dilatation of the ureters, but stenosis was found only occasionally. MAKAR (v. s.) found 30% of children examined in Egypt and FORSYTH [v. s.] observed 20% of those in Tanzania to show roentgenological changes in the urinary tract with varying degrees and incidences of hydronephrosis.

Bladder neck fibrosis, fibrosis of the bladder wall, and stenosis of the ureter could easily explain hydronephrosis seen in many of the patients; however, GELFAND [v. s.] has observed hydronephrosis without these basic lesions, and hydronephrosis has not been related to the intensity of infection. The nature of the pathological changes in these organs, the correlation of pathological findings with incidence and egg load both in the biopsy and autopsy material, and the specific clinical course of these patients remain to be determined.

In addition to hydronephrosis the kidney may show two other lesions. Renal oviposition, known to have occurred in man as early as 1200 to 1040 B. C., produces the usual granulomata. Another renal lesion reported by GELFAND and PAYET and CAMAIN [v. s.] is interstitial nephritis but the genesis of this lesion, its etiology, and the specific pathology have not yet been determined. Involvement of genital organs, the prostate, testes, fallopian tubes, cervix, and vagina have also been reported, but the pathological changes have not been adequately defined.

These observations would seem to indicate that the involvement of urogenital tract secondary to S. hematobium is a serious and disabling disease in many parts of Africa. However, ELSDON-DEW [v. s.] has been impressed that although over 60% of children showed eggs in their urine, in only a very small fraction of autopsies in King Edward VIII Hospital in Durban could deaths be attributed to urinary bilharziasis. This is in sharp contrast to the findings of PRATES [4] who, a few hundred miles away, observed urinary tract lesions in over 80 % of his autopsies.

EDINGTON's [v. s.] experience may throw some light on the discrepancy. In his own autopsy material in Ibadan, Edington found four deaths due to bilharziasis (only one involving the urinary tract) in over 3000 autopsies, whereas in an adjacent holoendemic area 50 % of those examined showed x-ray evidence of urinary tract involvement.

Obviously, we need comprehensive long range longitudinal studies on human patients with vesical bilharziasis and we need application of modern technics of experimental medicine and pathology to evaluate the role of bilharziasis in urinary tract pathology.

2. *Hepatic changes.* MOUSA, ELWI, GELFAND, PAYET and CAMAIN, MIYAKE, BOGLIOLO, DE PAOLA and WINSLOW, RODRIGUEZ and his associates, and ANDRADE and CHEEVER [v. s.] have described liver involvement in bilharziasis. All three species affect the liver, but S. Mansoni and S. Japonicum are the two chief pathogens. Although MOUSA [v. s.] has seen hepatic involvement in 15 % of S. hematobium infections, GELFAND [v. s.] is not convinced that S. hematobium causes hepatic cirrhosis even though ova are deposited in this organ.

The liver appears to be involved quite early in the course of infection. Within 15 to 25 days after exposure and before maturation and oviposition, an intense hepatitis has been reported with focal cloudy swelling, fatty degeneration, parenchymal necrosis, and hyperplasia of Kupffer's cells. Occasional granulomas are reported with central necrosis and eosinophilic infiltration. The inflammatory reaction usually subsides, and with oviposition the nature of hepatic involvement changes.

It is in the chronic form that involvement of the liver results in serious clinical and pathological sequelae.

The clinical symptoms consist of general weakness, gradual weight loss, epigastric discomfort, pain, and heaviness, abdominal distention, and diarrhea. Later, the manifestations are those of portal hypertension with splenomegaly, and edema of the lower extremities, but preservation of liver function. In the early stages, there may be hepatomegaly, usually of the left lobe; later, the liver may be smaller, and there may be dilatation of abdominal and esophageal veins and gastrointestinal bleeding. The external surface may be smooth or it may show tubercle-like nodules, it may be coarsely granular (Symmers' pipe stem cirrhosis), or it may be finely nodular (Hashim's fine nodular cirrhosis). Cut surfaces show dense periportal fibrosis with maintenance of lobular architecture. Microscopically, few or many granulomas may be seen, and there may be large areas of necrosis with eosinophilic infiltration around the ova but these may be rare or absent. There is hyperplasia of Kupffer's cells, deposition of brown pigment, occlusion of small veins, thrombophlebitis with recanalization of large portal branches, narrowing of portal vein by phlebosclerosis, intimal thickening of arteries, and formation of new blood vessels (angiomatoids). The portal obstruction is presinusoidal as shown by RODRIGUES and his associates [v. s.].

ANDRADE and CHEEVER [v. s.] have called attention to the fact that the vascular lesions may result in parenchymatous changes especially during episodes of gastrointestinal hemorrhage and shock when extensive areas of necrosis are seen.

Superimposed on the pre-existing basic fibrosis these necrotic areas may mislead into the diagnosis of post necrotic cirrhosis.

MIYAKE [v. s.] recognized three gross types of severe liver involvement in S. Japonicum: the lobular type resembling hepar lobatum with coarsely indented liver; the granular type with nodular or granular surface resembling atrophic cirrhosis; and the mixed type. ANDRADE and CHEEVER [v. s.] have described a white granuloma with central necrosis and peripheral eosinophilia in association with ova of S. Mansoni and a diffuse non-specific portal inflammation or slight portal fibrosis, usually observed in either asymptomatic or symptomatic intestinal bilharziasis. ANDRADE and CHEEVER [v. s.] distinguish the bilharzial lesion from other types of cirrhosis by its dense periportal fibrosis, while the lobular structure of the liver is maintained albeit with subcapsular foci of regeneration and occasional foci of fibrosis. ANDRADE and CHEEVER have not seen HASHIM's fine diffuse fibrosis.

DE PAOLA and WINSLOW [v. s.], in comparing the livers of patients infected with schistosomes from Africa and Latin America, observed the full spectrum of changes ranging from minor alterations with rare granuloma, with or without eggs, and minimal fibrosis to typical Symmers fibrosis, inluding advanced forms, with angiomatoids, focal necrosis, and active hepatitis. No geographical differences were recognized.

GELFAND [v. s.] found many cases of Mansonal infestation in adult patients but could not relate it to cirrhosis. Secondly, he found cirrhosis in other parts of East Africa where bilharziasis is rarely encountered. In infected juveniles, however, needle biopsy of the liver showed bilharzial eggs and inflammatory reaction in a significant number of cases, suggesting that the irreparable damage done at this stage may result in death of a substantial number of these children with few surviving to adulthood; a situation comparable to that suspected in S. hematobium infection of the urinary tract in East African children.

The presence of ova or dead parasites in a hepatic granuloma would seem to establish a definite cause — and — effect relationship between the parasite and the lesion. GEAR [v. s.] has contributed materially to the pathology and pathogenesis of hepatic changes through experimental induction of infection in several rodents. S. hematobium and S. Mansoni both caused a subacute and chronic progressive, often fatal, disease. The characteristic lesions consisted of multinucleated giant cells formed around an egg or the remnants of an egg, surrounded by a zone of polymorphonuclear and eosinophilic leukocytes and a peripheral zone of monocytes, lymphocytes, plasma cells, and eventually fibroblasts which form a capsule of fibrous tissue.

Portal hypertension, as seen in many of these patients, is certainly disabling. However, the complete absence of eggs or adult parasites, the presence of only insignificant numbers of eggs in human livers, and the existence of other possible factors in the pathogenesis of the hepatic lesions have raised many questions on the true etiology of the hepatic changes. Is it the migrating schistosomulae that cause the hepatitis of the early stage? Are the changes always present? In the chronic form is it the worm, the viable or the dead eggs, the toxins, the antigen-antibody reaction, or the effects of therapy that cause the hepatic fibrosis? Until these questions are adequately answered, the role of bilharziasis in the genesis of the hepatic lesions remains to be determined, as does its public health significance.

Splenomegaly is encountered early (15 to 25th day) before oviposition but is more severe thereafter. Except rarely, Symmers' fibrosis is associated with splenomegaly. The spleen shows hyperplasia of reticuloendothelial cells, dilatation of venous channels and infiltration with eosinophils. However, the specific pathology and the pathogenesis have not been clearly defined.

3. *Cardiopulmonary bilharziasis*. All three species affect the cardiopulmonary system and the manifestations seem to be identical. ZAKY, ELWI, GAZAYERLI, GELFAND, ANRADE, MENEZES, and MIDDLEMISS [v. s.] have described the cardiopulmonary manifestations of bilharziasis. ZAKY [v. s]. believes it always develops in conjunction with hepatosplenomegaly. Clinically, the patients gradually develop evidence of cor pulmonale and congestive heart failure. Thirty-three per cent of patients suffering from bilharziasis show pulmonary lesions.

Grossly, the most frequently observed pulmonary lesions is the tubercle or nodule in relation to vessel walls. The lungs may be congested. Focal or confluent lesions may be seen around the bronchioles, there may be focal hemorrhages, or the lungs may show extensive fibrosis. Microscopically, there may be nothing but tubercle formation or there may be congestion, focal or confluent pneumonia, focal hemorrhages, or pulmonary fibrosis of varying degrees.

The most important and interesting lesions are those involving the pulmonary arterial system and designated by some as bilharzial Ayerza's disease. The arterioles may show thrombosis, necrosis of the wall, and infiltration with eosinophils, monocytes, macrophages and multinucleated giant cells with varying degrees of necrotizing pneumonic process at the periphery.

With healing there may be recanalization. The newly formed vessels may hypertrophy to produce angiomatoids. The involved arterioles may be partly or completely replaced by fibrous tissue, and eventually fibrosis of the surrounding tissue may ensue.

The changes may be focal and of little clinical significance or they may be diffuse and generalized resulting in atherosclerosis of pulmonary arteries, arteriolar and arterial medial hypertrophy, and fibrous or fibroblastic intimal thickening with resultant pulmonary fibrosis. Pulmonary hypertension may lead to right-sided heart failure and as such may cause severe disability. The exact mechanism and the specific etiological factors responsible for the lesion have not been established.

Cyanosis and clubbing of the fingers are rare, but ANDRADE and CHEEVER [v. s.] have called attention to a new syndrome in hepatosplenic schistosomiasis consisting of marked cyanosis in patients who show no evidence of pulmonary hypertension. These authors believe that cyanosis is probably related to multiple minute pulmonary arteriovenous fistulae.

Both ova and worms may be found in the lungs. Since S. hematobium is already in the systemic circulation, it is easy for it to gain access to the lungs. In S. Mansoni and S. Japonicum, the mechanism of pulmonary invasion is not clear. Where hepatosplenic bilharziasis has resulted in establishing porto-systemic collateral circulation, adult schistosomes and eggs may pass from the portal to the pulmonary circulation. Although the living worm is believed to be harmless, the low oxygen saturation and the venous blood conditions in the pulmonary arteries militate against the survival of the worm, and the death of the parasite may be responsible for at least some of the events.

There are, however, several disturbing features. In the more advanced cases it is often difficult, if not impossible, to find ova or worms. This led ANDRADE and CHEEVER [v. s.] to consider the reaction as allergic or hyperimmune in nature or due to repeated migration of schistosomulae through the lungs. All three species invade the lungs and S. hematobium is the most frequent invader, but pulmonary lesions are more frequently associated with S. Mansoni. The number of advanced cases is relatively small and, similar diffuse pulmonary lesions have been reported in areas where bilharziasis is rare or absent.

Thus to establish the relationship between bilharziasis and cor pulmonale we need to study the progression of the disease not only clinically but pathologically by means of lung biopsies of living patients and of autopsies of those who die of other causes. Experimental studies are also indicated to correlate the pulmonary findings with egg and worm counts and to determine the role of immune reaction.

4. *Intestinal bilharziasis.* Intestinal bilharziasis has been reported in Asia, Africa, and Latin America. ELWI, GELFAND, ELSDON-DEW, BHAGWANDEEN, AN-DRADE and CHEEVER, BOGLIOLO and others [v. s.] have described the clinical and pathological findings.

Intestinal symptoms begin during the stage of maturation before oviposition and are characterized by nausea, vomiting, abdominal colic, and diarrhea, which is not bloody until the initiation of oviposition when the symptoms become severe. At this stage the intestinal lesions are said to consist of numerous small superficial necrotic and hemorrhagic mucosal ulcers mostly in the jejunum and ileum and completely unrelated to the number of ova in the mucosa. Although the reaction is generally regarded as analogous to the Schwartzman phenomenon, the basic mechanism for the development of the symptoms and the nature of the precise pathological changes have not been established.

Intestinal bilharziasis may also be disabling during the stage of established infection, but as in other manifestations of bilharziasis, there is considerable variation in the severity of clinical symptoms and the extent of the pathological findings.

In Africa, where both S. hematobium and S. Mansoni occur, the former has a greater tendency to settle in the colon, but it is the latter which is held chiefly responsible for the symptoms; in the Far East, the principal agent is S. Japonicum and in Latin America, S. Mansoni.

Pathologically confirmed intestinal bilharziasis may be asymptomatic or symptomatic, the distinction being based on whether the patient has abdominal complaints. The asymptomatic form comprises by far the larger group. The disease involves chiefly the rectosigmoid and appears to be of greater severity in Egypt. The symptoms range from tenesmus, cramping, and small amounts of mucus to extensive bleeding, diarrhea, painful defecation, prolapse, and obstruction.

ELWI, GELFAND, BHAGWANDEEN, ANDRADE and CHEEVER and BOGLIOLO [v.s.] have reported ulceration, sandy patches, fibrosis, granulomata, and polyps of the rectosigmoid. Polyps vary from 2 mm to 24 mm in length, average 8 mm in diameter, and are usually multiple. An occasional polyp has a mulberry-like

338 F. K. Mostofi:

appearance. Obstruction and hemorrhage are the two chief manifestations of the polyp and these may necessitate surgical intervention. Intestinal bleeding may also result as a complication of portal hypertension.

BOGLIOLO (v. s.) has called attention to the fact that in the chronic intestinal forms, bouts of hemorrhagic necrosis of intestinal mucosa similar to those seen in the toxemic stage may accompany the acute exacerbation of the symptoms.

It is of interest to note that outside Egypt, intestinal symptoms due to bilharziasis are infrequent even though eggs may be found in the feces or in the rectal biopsy. Secondly, intestinal polyps, reported in more than 40 % of Egyptian patients and considered characteristic of the third stage of bilharzial infection in Egypt, are not observed with this frequency elsewhere in or outside of Africa. Thirdly, oviposition (principally S. hematobium, but S. Mansoni as well) and calcification in the intestinal wall without any tissue response appear to be the most common pathological findings. Fourthly, although carcinoma of rectosigmoid has been described secondary to S. Japonicum, no relationship between intestinal bilharziasis and carcinoma of the colon has been reported elsewhere.

There is need to determine whether the intestinal symptoms, signs, and pathology are in fact due to bilharziasis. Is S. hematobium actually as harmless in the intestinal tract as it seems? What causes the gastrointestinal symptoms of early stages? What are the factors which result in the lack of clinical manifestations and pathology despite the presence of ova in the intestinal wall? What are the factors which bring about the severe intestinal manifestations in Egypt in contrast to other areas?

FAUST and MELENEY [3] have contributed materially to the study of the intestinal pathology in experimental infection with S. Japonicum, but similar studies for S. Mansoni and S. hematobium, both in man and in experimental animals are desired to elucidate the spectrum of pathological changes from early infection, to the late stages.

In this brief summary attention has been focused on the clinical and pathological manifestations of bilharziasis in four organ systems, because these are the areas which are involved most frequently and resultant the disability may assume epidemic proportions. Bilharziasis also affects a number of other sites with serious results for the individual patient, but with little or no public health significance since such involvement is of sporadic nature.

The need for research

The main controversy in pathophysiology of bilharziasis has centered on the basic mechanism of tissue reaction. Failure to demonstrate the eggs or the parasite in tissue sections, inability to clearly correlate the clinical or the pathological changes to the number of parasites or the egg, lack of a satisfactory method of assaying the total egg or parasite load in an organ, absence of clearly defined host response to the egg or the parasite, failure to separate reactions which are allergic from those which are due to physical presence of the cercaria, schistosomula, the adult parasite or the egg, the existence of other possible factors in the clinico-pathological changes observed in these patients, and sparsity of controlled uniformly collected, clinical and pathological observations from various endemic areas, are responsible factors in this controversy.

ANDRADE [1] has made a major contribution to the clarification of the problem by calling attention to the three categories of lesions: the hypoergic, the normergic and the hyperergic; however, further confirmation of ANDRADE's observations and support from experimental and clinicopathological studies are necessary.

VON LICHTENBERG's [v .s.] classic study of the tissue responses in highly susceptible, susceptible and resistant animals, and the study of histopathological and immunological changes resulting from single and multiple initial and subsequent infections provide the tools with which the pathology of the disease can be clearly defined. ANDRADE [1], MOORE, and VON LICHTENBERG [v. s.] have demonstrated that the cuticle, the apical glands, the intestinal lining and the intestinal contents of adult worms, and the cephalic penetration glands of miracidia are the major sources of antigen and that this is a metabolic antigen. Although these studies have shown that the immunological response in bilharzial infection is similar to that seen in bacterial infection and in transplantation field, all efforts to correlate antiboyd titers, intensity of infection, and acquisition of immunity have failed. What is greatly needed, as SADUN [v. s.] has pointed out, is the application of the more imaginative and sophisticated technics for the isolation and definition of the specific antigenic components – detection of the specific antigen in the parasite and the protective antibody in the host – basic biochemical studies that have been long overdue!

Another equal, if not greater, need is for information on the nature, pattern, and frequency of various manifestations – clinical and pathological – in different endemic areas. Clinical history, physical, and laboratory examinations must be carried out and the results recorded in a uniform manner to provide comparable reliable information. However, such studies, conducted alone, will give us a superficial picture of bilharzial morbidity. We must also assess the pathological lesions observed in various stages of infection. Such an assessment, however, must be conducted and recorded in a uniform manner to provide comparable data. Full utilization of biopsy and autopsy methods and the application of modern histopathological technics are essential.

Such clinicopathological studies must be correlated simultaneously with comparable biological, epidemiological, and environmental observations. The physiological and the structural responses of human tissue must be clearly correlated with the developmental stages of the specific species of the parasite and the incidence and the severity of the infection. Environmental factors which may modify the response must be carefully evaluated.

We must study not only the pathophysiology of bilharziasis in man, but that of the parasite and the snail, to understand the basic nature of the tissue response. The need for a truly holistic approach to the problem is obvious.

It is self evident also that while some of the studies, especially the experimental, can be carried out in institutes and universities in Europe and the United States, truly comprehensive clinicopathological investigations must be conducted in the field – in Africa, in Latin America, and in Asia. While in certain regions good facilities exist for such studies, in many instances the trained personnel, the equipment or the financial means are presently not available. These must be provided. But even with these, unless a cooperative research program is organized on an international level the results would not be comparable.

22*

What is needed then is an internationally organized, staffed, and financed cooperative program for clinical, pathological, and experimental research in bilharziasis. In no other field is there a greater challenge than in the understanding, control and conquest of bilharziasis. In addition to humanitarian and scientific merits, such an approach is essential to determine the public health significance of bilharziasis.

References*

[1] ANDRADE, Z. A., e G. RODRIGUEZ: Manifestacoes pseudo-neoplasticas da esquistossomose intestinale. Arch. Bra. Med. **44**, 437—444 (1954).
[2] FAIRLEY, N. H.: Observations on the clinical appearance of bilharziasis in Australian troops and the significance of symptoms noted. Quart. J. Med. **12**, 391—403 (1919).
[3] FAUST, E. C., and H. E. MELENEY: Studies on schistosomiasis japonica. Amer. J. Hyg. Monograph series no. 3 (1924).
[4] PRATES, M. D.: The rates of cancer of bladder in the Portuguese East Africans. Acta Un. Int. Cancr. **18**, 643—647 (1962).

* [v. s.] has been used to denote reference to the preceeding chapters in this monograph.

Subject index

The terms schistosomiasis and bilharziasis, though synonymous, are listed separately according to the usage of the authors of the various chapters. Each entry has the note *see also* bilharziasis/schistosomiasis; thus if the reader desires to find references to the history of schistosomiasis, he should look under "schistosomiasis, history of" and also under "bilharziasis, history of".

The common schistosomal species names (*S. mansoni*, *S. hematobium*, and *S. japonicum*) are used to indicate both the organism and the pathologic changes they cause. For example, the entry "*Schistosoma mansoni*, symptoms, incidence of" would mean the incidence of various symptoms in patients infested with *S. mansoni*.

The page numbers in *italics* refer to tables.

Brühlsche Universitätsdruckerei Gießen